Handbook of Parathyroid Diseases

Aliya A. Khan • Orlo H. Clark
Editors

Handbook of Parathyroid Diseases

A Case-Based Practical Guide

Foreword by John T. Potts, Jr., MD

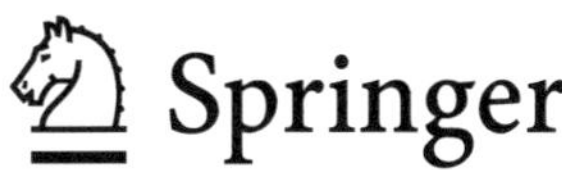 Springer

Editors
Aliya A. Khan, MD, FRCPC, FACP, FACE
Professor of Clinical Medicine
Department of Endocrinology
and Metabolism
McMaster University
Hamilton, ON, Canada
aliya@mcmaster.ca

Orlo H. Clark, M.D, FACS
Professor of Surgery
Department of Surgery
University of California
San Francisco
San Francisco, CA, USA
orlo.clark@ucsfmedctr.org

ISBN 978-1-4614-2163-4   e-ISBN 978-1-4614-2164-1
DOI 10.1007/978-1-4614-2164-1
Springer New York Dordrecht Heidelberg London

Library of Congress Control Number: 2011945773

Springer is part of Springer Science+Business Media (www.springer.com)

*I dedicate this book to my parents
Mohammed Abdul Aziz Khan and Zahida
Siddiqi Khan*

Aliya A. Khan, MD

*I dedicate this book to my parents Orlo Holly
Clark MD and Elizabeth Herrick Clark*

Orlo H. Clark, MD

Foreword

Hyperparathyroidism has undergone a dramatic shift in clinical presentation from the cases typically seen in the first two thirds of the previous century, following recognition of the disease in the late 1920s and its successful treatment by surgical removal of the overactive parathyroid gland. The disease, as then identified, was characterized by overt signs and symptoms of bone, renal, and other organ dysfunction, such as severe osteitis fibrosa and kidney stones. Hyperparathyroidism, as recognized today, has largely transformed into a milder but more frequently recognized disorder, often termed asymptomatic hyperparathyroidism to reflect the virtual absence of symptoms typically associated with the disease.

Despite much progress in definition of the physiology of calcium homeostasis, as well as the genetic pathogenesis of hyperparathyroidism, its diagnosis, and surgical management, uncertainty persists about optimum management of asymptomatic hyperparathyroidism. The disease may remain clinically stable for many years and bone mineral density, although often reduced from that of euparathyroid subjects of the same age, may remain remarkably constant for many years. These findings led in recent years to the view that medical monitoring may be sufficient in these patients, rather than recommending surgery. For several reasons, however, the pendulum seems to be swinging back toward the view that surgical correction rather than medical monitoring may be appropriate in many of these patients because of concern about subtle organ deterioration, even in the absence of overt symptoms.

This volume presents 17 chapters dealing with fundamental and clinical issues pertinent to disease recognition, pathogenesis and pathophysiology, and surgical and medical management. Chapters 5, 6, and 9 focus particularly on the disease features that are central to the key management decision, surgery versus medical monitoring. Guidelines felt useful have been developed through several consensus meetings of experts in the field. These deal with (1) criteria for formally recommending surgery and (2) criteria to be followed if medical observation is elected. Also reviewed is the current status of medical therapies, should disease manifestations require efforts of intervention rather than mere medical monitoring in patients who are medically unsuitable or unwilling to undergo surgical correction.

Concerns about eventual skeletal deterioration as well as subtle neuropsychiatric and cardiovascular features of even mild hyperparathyroidism, coupled with clear evidence of improved bone density with surgery and suggestive but still somewhat inconclusive evidence regarding the presence and reversibility with surgery of neuropsychiatric and cardiovascular features is leading most endocrinologists and surgeons to now favor surgery. The possibility of medical monitoring, however, is still regarded as an option awaiting further study of the presence and reversibility of subtle disease features.

One chapter deals with hypoparathyroidism, a deficiency rather than excess of parathyroid action. Hypoparathyroidism has long been unusual among endocrine deficiency disorders, in that replacement therapy with the missing hormone is not offered because of the need for parenteral therapy and the short half life of hormone after administration. Effective current therapies are reviewed. There is however, renewed interest in exploring treatment with recently available, longer acting form of parathyroid hormone.

John T. Potts, Jr., MD
Jackson Distinguished Professor of Clinical Medicine
Harvard Medical School
Director of Research and Physician-in-Chief Emeritus
Massachusetts General Hospital

Preface

The purpose of the Handbook of Parathyroid Diseases is to present a concise yet comprehensive overview of our current knowledge in the area of parathyroid function, hormone regulation, and medical and surgical management of disease states. Many advances have been made in particular over the past decade in our understanding of molecular biology, physiology, genetics, cell signaling, hormone regulation, imaging, surgical, and pharmacologic intervention. These advances are conveyed to the practitioner in an easy-to-read format which is both practical and user friendly. This book will be of great value to students, residents, and physicians in endocrinology, surgery, radiology, nuclear medicine, pediatrics, primary care, internal medicine, biochemistry, and pathology. The handbook will educate the reader using a case-based approach presenting current evidence in the field. The material is presented in easy-to-read and understandable language with liberal use of tables and textboxes whenever possible. Complex concepts are conveyed in simple and clear language. Leading national and international experts have contributed to this state-of-the-art book which is unique in its depth of knowledge and practicality.

Hamilton, ON, Canada   Aliya A. Khan, MD
San Francisco, CA, USA   Orlo H. Clark, MD

Contents

Contributors

Andrew Arnold, MD Center for Molecular Medicine, University of Connecticut, School of Medicine, Farmington, CT, USA

Maria Luisa Brandi, MD Department of Internal Medicine, University of Florence, Centro di Riferimento Regionale sui Tumori Endocrini Ereditari, Azienda Ospedaliero-Universitaria Careggi, Florence, Italy

Jean-Hugues Brossard, MD Department of Medicine, Centre de recherche, Centre hospitalier de l'Université de Montréal (CHUM)-Hôpital Saint-Luc, Université de Montréal, Montreal, QC, Canada

Edward M. Brown, MD Division of Endocrinology, Diabetes and Hypertension, Department of Medicine, Harvard Medical School, Brigham and Women's Hospital, Boston, MA, USA

Naifa Lamki Busaidy, MD, FACP Department of Endocrine Neoplasia & Hormonal Disorders, University of Texas M. D. Anderson Cancer Center, Houston, TX, USA

Loredana Cavalli, MD Department of Internal Medicine, University of Florence, Florence, Italy

Tiziana Cavalli, MD Department of Internal Medicine, University of Florence, Florence, Italy

Orlo H. Clark, MD, FACS Department of Surgery, University of California, San Francisco, San Francisco, CA, USA

Pierre D'Amour, MD, FRCPC Department of Medicine, University of Montreal, Montreal, QC, Canada

Beth S. Edeiken, MD Department of Diagnostic Radiology, The University of Texas M. D. Anderson Cancer Center, Houston, TX, USA

Pieter Evenepoel, MD Department of Medicine, Division of Nephrology, University of Leuven, Leuven, Belgium

Alberto Falchetti, MD Department of Internal Medicine, University of Florence, Florence, Italy

Rachel Farkas, MD Department of Surgery, University of Rochester Medical Center, Rochester, NY, USA

Ghada El-Hajj Fuleihan, MD, MPH Calcium Metabolism and Osteoporosis Program, WHO Collaborating Center for Metabolic Bone Disorders, Department of Medicine, American University of Beirut-Medical Center, Riad El Solh, Beirut, Lebanon

Swaroop Gantela, MD Human Neuroimaging Laboratory, Baylor College of Medicine, Houston, TX, USA

Francesca Giusti, MD Department of Internal Medicine, University of Florence, Florence, Italy

Elizabeth G. Grubbs, MD Department of Surgical Oncology, Unit 1484, The University of Texas M. D. Anderson Cancer Cente, Houston, TX, USA

Maria K. Gule, MD Department of Surgical Oncology, Unit 1484, The University of Texas M. D. Anderson Cancer Cente, Houston, TX, USA

David A. Hanley, MD, FRCPC Department of Medicine, University of Calgary, Calgary, AB, Canada

Aliya A. Khan, MD, FRCPC, FACP, FACE Department of Endocrinology and Metabolism, McMaster University, Hamilton, ON, Canada

Edmund Kim, MD Department of Nuclear Medicine, The University of Texas M. D. Anderson Cancer Center, Houston, TX, USA

Amit Lahoti, MD Section of Nephrology, Department of General Internal Medicine, University of Texas M. D. Anderson Cancer Center, Houston, TX, USA

Kelly Lauter, BA, MD Center for Molecular Medicine, University of Connecticut, School of Medicine, Farmington, CT, USA

E. Michael Lewiecki, MD, FACP, FACE Department of Medicine, New Mexico Clinical Research and Osteoporosis Center, Albuquerque, NM, USA

Laura Masi, MD Department of Medicine, University of Florence, Centro di Riferimento Regionale sui Tumori Endocrini Ereditari, Azienda Ospedaliero-Universitaria Careggi, Florence, Italy

Paul D. Miller, MD Colorado Center for Bone Research, Lakewood, CO, USA

Jacob Moalem, MD Department of Surgery, University of Rochester Medical Center, Rochester, NY, USA

Brett J. Monroe, MD Department of Diagnostic Radiology, The University of Texas M. D. Anderson Cancer Center, Houston, TX, USA

Janice L. Pasieka, MD, FRCSC, FACS Department of Surgery and Oncology, Divisions of General Surgery and Surgical Oncology, University of Calgary, North Tower, Foothills Medical Center, Calgary, AB, Canada

Nancy D. Perrier, MD, FACS Department of Surgical Oncology, Unit 1484, The University of Texas M. D. Anderson Cancer Cente, Houston, TX, USA

D. Sudhaker Rao, M.B.B.S., FACP, FACE Bone & Mineral Metabolism, Bone & Mineral Research Laboratory, Henry Ford Medical Center, New Center One, Henry Ford Hospital, Detroit, MI, USA

Dolores Shoback, MD Endocrine Research Unit, San Francisco Department of Veterans Affairs Medical Center, University of California, San Francisco, CA, USA

Cord Sturgeon, MD Section of Endocrine Surgery, Department of Surgery, Northwestern University Feinberg School of Medicine, Chicago, IL, USA

Frederic Triponez, MD Thoracic and endocrine surgery, University Hospital of Geneva, Geneva, Switzerland

Thinh Vu, MD Department of Diagnostic Radiology, The University of Texas M. D. Anderson Cancer Center, Houston, TX, USA

Storm Weaver, MD Department of Surgical Oncology, The University of Texas M. D. Anderson Cancer Center, Houston, TX, USA

Meei J. Yeung, MD, FRACS Department of Surgery, Monash University Endocrine Surgery Unit, Melbourne, Australia

John Yoo, MD, FRCS(C), FACS Department of Otolaryngology-Head and Neck Surgery, University of Western Ontario, London, ON, Canada

J.E.M. Young, BSc, MD, FRCS, FACS Department of Surgery, McMaster University, Hamilton, ON, Canada

Kyle Zanocco, MD Section of Endocrine Surgery, Department of Surgery, Northwestern University Feinberg School of Medicine, Chicago, IL, USA

Chapter 1
Mechanisms Underlying Extracellular Calcium Homeostasis

Edward M. Brown

Keywords Calcium • PTH • Calcitonin • Vitamin D • 1,25(OH)$_2$D$_3$ • Calcium-sensing receptor • Calcium regulation by kidney • Bone • Intestine • Parathyroid chief cells • Fibroblast growth factor-23 • Phosphate • Calcium-binding protein • Calbindin • Magnesium • RANKL • Osteoprotegrin • Phosphatonins • Osteocyte • Osteoblast • Osteoclast • Alpha klotho

Calcium (Ca^{2+}) is indispensable for all living things. In complex, multicellular organisms, calcium serves key roles in both the intra- and extracellular spaces [1]. In humans and other mammals, for example, notable extracellular roles of calcium ions include promoting plasma membrane integrity and serving as an important cofactor in proteins, such as adhesion molecules, clotting factors, and secreted enzymes (i.e., trypsin) [1]. It is also an essential component, along with phosphate ions, of the mineral phase of bone [2, 3]. The combination of a collagenous matrix and its associated insoluble mineral phase confers upon bone both hardness and strength, thereby enabling the skeleton to protect vital internal structures (i.e., the brain and heart) and to facilitate ambulation and other directed movements [2]. Intracellular Ca^{2+} likewise serves numerous critical roles [4], including activating exocytosis (the so-called stimulus-secretion coupling) and muscle contraction ("stimulus-contraction coupling") and participating in the propagation of action potentials in some nerve cells. Ca^{2+} serves more generally as a key intracellular second messenger [3, 5], regulating a host of cellular processes (mitosis, energy metabolism, gene expression, cell death, etc.) through its interaction with intracellular Ca^{2+} sensors, such as calmodulin [6].

E.M. Brown, M.D. (✉)
Division of Endocrinology, Diabetes and Hypertension, Department of Medicine,
Harvard Medical School, Brigham and Women's Hospital, EBRC 223A,
221 Longwood Ave., Boston, MA 02115, USA
e-mail: embrown@partners.org

A.A. Khan and O.H. Clark (eds.), *Handbook of Parathyroid Diseases:
A Case-Based Practical Guide*, DOI 10.1007/978-1-4614-2164-1_1,
© Springer Science+Business Media, LLC 2012

The numerous roles of Ca^{2+} in living organisms highlight the importance of ensuring adequate and stable Ca^{2+} concentrations in bodily fluids in order to provide a sufficient source of Ca^{2+} for both its extracellular and intracellular functions (extracellular Ca^{2+} is the ultimate source of all intracellular Ca^{2+}) [7]. Tetrapods (animals with four extremities, e.g., birds, mammals, amphibians, and reptiles) have evolved a finely tuned homeostatic system designed to maintain near constancy of the extracellular ionized calcium concentration (Ca_o^{2+}) [2, 7, 8]. The purpose of this chapter is to provide an overview of how this system functions under normal circumstances. This provides a backdrop for subsequent chapters detailing various aspects of primary hyperparathyroidism (PHPT), a hypercalcemic disorder caused by hyperfunction of one or more parathyroid glands [9]. Indeed, a key aspect of PHPT is abnormal Ca_o^{2+} sensing by pathological parathyroid tissue, which "resets" the Ca_o^{2+} homeostatic system to maintain varying degrees of hypercalcemia [10–12]. While not a major focus of this chapter, recent important advances have taken place in our understanding of phosphate homeostasis [13, 14]. Since several of the key regulators of phosphate metabolism, e.g., fibroblast growth factor-23 (FGF-23) and alphaklotho (α-klotho), also modulate Ca_o^{2+} homeostasis, these interactions are covered briefly, stressing the essential and intimate links that have been emerging between these two homeostatic systems.

Key Elements of Ca_o^{2+} Homeostasis

The Ca_o^{2+} homeostatic system has three essential elements. Figure 1.1 shows how these elements function in a coordinated manner to maintain near constancy of Ca_o^{2+}. The first component is one or more Ca_o^{2+} sensors that detect perturbations in Ca_o^{2+} from its normal level [7, 8]. The best characterized Ca_o^{2+}-sensing mechanism is the extracellular calcium-sensing receptor (CaSR), a G protein-coupled receptor that is expressed in many, if not all, of the tissues participating in Ca_o^{2+} homeostasis [15, 16]. These include the parathyroid hormone (PTH)-secreting parathyroid chief cells [15], calcitonin (CT)-secreting thyroidal C cells [17], and various cell types in kidney [18], intestine [19, 20], and bone [21]. The CaSR's functions in these tissues are described in more detail subsequently.

The second key element of the Ca_o^{2+} homeostatic mechanism are hormones that are directly or indirectly regulated by Ca_o^{2+} sensors and modulate Ca^{2+} transport into or out of the extracellular fluid (ECF). The first of these is PTH, which acts on the kidney to increase distal tubular reabsorption of Ca^{2+} and proximal tubular synthesis of $1,25(OH)_2D_3$ as well as on bone to stimulate net release of skeletal Ca^{2+} (accompanied in an obligatory manner by phosphate) [2]. Vitamin D_3 is synthesized in the skin and also absorbed from the diet in the small intestine; it then undergoes largely unregulated 25-hydroxylation in the liver prior to its precisely regulated 1-hydroxylation in the kidney [22]. The synthesis of $1,25(OH)_2D_3$ is stimulated by PTH, hypocalcemia, and hypophosphatemia and inhibited by hypercalcemia, hyperphosphatemia, and $1,25(OH)_2D_3$ itself [2, 22]. The latter, therefore, feeds back

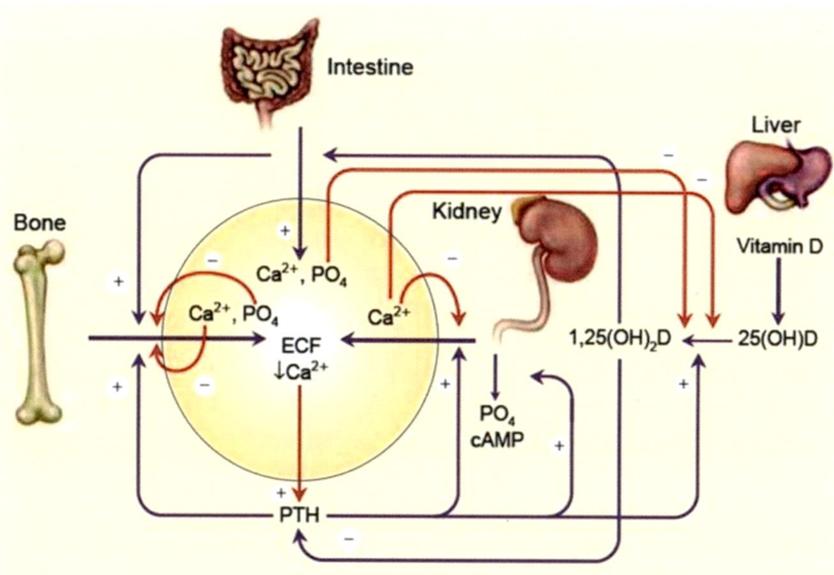

Fig. 1.1 Schematic representation of the system maintaining Ca_o^{2+} homeostasis. In response to hypocalcemia, PTH is released into the circulation (*plus* indicates stimulation). It acts on the kidney to promote increased distal tubular reabsorption of Ca^{2+}, enhanced synthesis of $1,25(OH)_2D_3$ from the $25(OH)D_3$ that is produced in the liver, and phosphaturia. The $1,25(OH)_2D_3$ formed in the kidney stimulates intestinal absorption of Ca^{2+} and phosphate and acts with PTH to increase net release of Ca^{2+} from bone. Increased influx of Ca^{2+} into the ECF from bone and intestine, coupled with reduced loss of Ca^{2+} via the kidney, restores Ca_o^{2+} to normal. In addition to the actions of the Ca_o^{2+}-regulating hormones just described (i.e., PTH and $1,25(OH)_2D_3$), Ca^{2+} and phosphate themselves exert direct actions on the tissues and organs involved in Ca_o^{2+} homeostasis, as indicated by the *arrows* from these ions to the respective target tissue. Many of the actions of Ca_o^{2+} are mediated by the CaSR. In addition to the actions of PTH and $1,25(OH)_2D_3$ that are illustrated, FGF-23 (not shown) is stimulated by hyperphosphatemia and $1,25(OH)_2D_3$ and, in turn, promotes phosphaturia, inhibits the 1-hydroxylation of 25-hydroxyvitamin D, and reduces the secretion of PTH (see text for additional details). Reproduced in modified form with permission from Brown EM. Mechanisms underlying the regulation of parathyroid hormone secretion in vivo and in vitro. Curr Opin Nephrol Hypertens. 1993; 2: 541–51

on its own synthesis in a negative manner. $1,25(OH)_2D_3$ is the most biologically active form of vitamin D_3 in the body. Its sequential, regulated synthesis enables it to act as the second major Ca_o^{2+}-elevating hormone (along with PTH) by increasing intestinal Ca^{2+} (and phosphate) absorption and activating bone resorption [2, 22]. CT is a potent hypocalcemic hormone in some species, such as rodents, primarily owing to its capacity to inhibit bone resorption [23]. Its importance in Ca_o^{2+} homeostasis in humans is probably marginal [24], although in pharmacological doses it has found some utility in treating hypercalcemia, Paget disease of bone, and osteoporosis prior to the advent of the much more efficacious bisphosphonates [25, 26].

The third component of the Ca_o^{2+} homeostatic system is the cells within kidney, bone, and intestine that effect vectorial transport of Ca^{2+} into or out of the ECF.

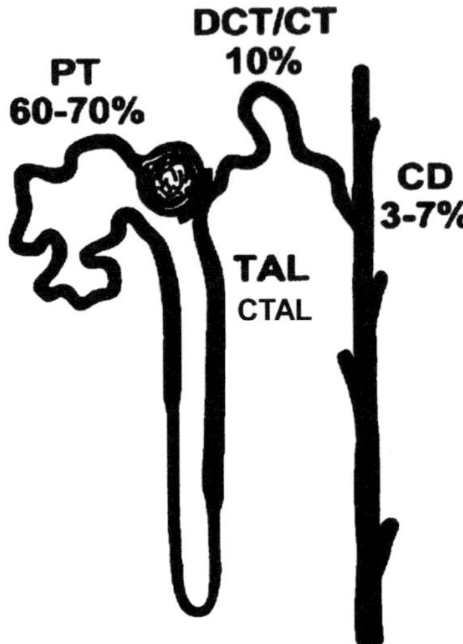

Fig. 1.2 Segments of the nephron relevant to Ca_o^{2+} homeostasis and their contribution to Ca^{2+} reabsorption along the entire length of the renal tubule (see text for details). Passive reabsorption of Ca^{2+} in the proximal tubule (PT), which is largely unregulated, accounts for 60–70% of Ca^{2+} reabsorption while regulated reabsorption in CTAL and DCT (as well as the connecting tubule (CT) just distal to the DCT) comprises 20 and 10%, respectively. At most, ~5% of Ca^{2+} is reabsorbed in the collecting duct (CD). Courtesy of S.C. Hebert, M.D.

The major sites of hormonally regulated Ca^{2+} transport in the kidney are the cortical thick ascending limb (CTAL) of Henle's loop and the distal convoluted tubule (DCT) (Fig. 1.2) [27, 28], where PTH and/or $1,25(OH)_2D_3$ increase tubular reabsorption of Ca^{2+}, thereby conserving bodily Ca^{2+} stores. In the proximal small intestine and, to some extent, in the colon, $1,25(OH)_2D_3$ increases transepithelial absorption of Ca^{2+} [29]. This capacity to assimilate Ca^{2+} from the environment is a critical component of the Ca_o^{2+} homeostatic system because the kidney cannot completely reabsorb all Ca^{2+} filtered at the glomerulus, and there is some obligate loss of Ca^{2+} into intestinal secretions. Adequate dietary Ca^{2+} is particularly key during somatic growth because of the accompanying increase in requirements for Ca^{2+} in the growing skeleton and soft tissues. The ability to regulate the fluxes of Ca^{2+} into and out of the skeleton is also essential for maintaining Ca^{2+} homeostasis. When dietary Ca^{2+} is limited, for example, skeletal Ca^{2+}, mobilized in response to increased circulating levels of PTH and $1,25(OH)_2D_3$, becomes a critical internal reservoir of Ca^{2+} to sustain normocalcemia [2].

Integrated Control of Ca_o^{2+} Homeostasis

The information presented to this point can be summarized by delineating the manner in which the Ca_o^{2+} homeostatic system responds to hypo- or hypercalcemia. A decrease in Ca_o^{2+} is detected by the CaSR in the parathyroid chief cells leading

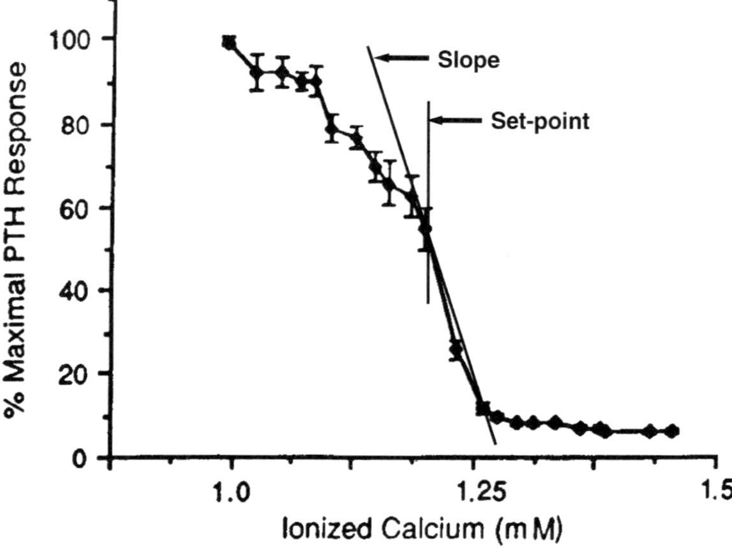

Fig. 1.3 Sigmoidal relationship between serum-ionized calcium concentration and circulating intact PTH (iPTH) levels in normal human subjects. Hypocalcemia was first induced by intravenous administration of ethylenediaminetetraacetic acid (EDTA) and then hypercalcemia by infusion of calcium gluconate; serum levels of calcium and iPTH were determined at frequent intervals. Note the steepness of the slope at the midpoint of the curve. This midpoint is defined as the set point, which is closely related to the level at which Ca_o^{2+} is set in vivo. The serum-ionized Ca^{2+} in mM should be multiplied by 8 to yield mg/dl total Ca^{2+}. See text for details. Reproduced with permission from Brown EM [34]. Extracellular Ca^{2+} sensing, regulation of parathyroid cell function, and role of Ca^{2+} and other ions as extracellular (first) messengers. Physiol Rev 1991; 71: 371–411

to an acute increase in PTH secretion. The steepness of the inverse sigmoidal relationship between Ca_o^{2+} and PTH (Fig. 1.3) [11] ensures large changes in PTH for small changes in Ca_o^{2+}, thereby contributing to the narrow range over which serum Ca^{2+} is maintained. The midpoint or set point of the Ca_o^{2+}–PTH relationship, in turn, is closely related to the level at which Ca_o^{2+} is "set" in vivo.

The increase in the circulating PTH level elicited by hypocalcemia stimulates release of Ca^{2+} from bone and has at least three actions on the kidney: (1) promoting phosphaturia in the proximal tubule, (2) increasing distal tubular reabsorption of filtered Ca^{2+}, and (3) enhancing renal synthesis of $1,25(OH)_2D_3$ from $25(OH)D_3$ [2]. The first two of these are rapid, occurring within minutes, while the last requires several hours of exposure to an elevated PTH level [30]. There is also PTH-independent "buffering" of changes in extracellular calcium by bone through poorly understood mechanisms, possibly involving the CaSR [31], that restore Ca_o^{2+} to its baseline level following induced reductions or increases in the serum calcium concentration by administration of EGTA or calcium, respectively [32]. Thus, a brief episode of hypocalcemia may be corrected solely through increased renal Ca^{2+} conservation and mobilization of Ca^{2+} from bone. More prolonged hypocalcemia, in contrast, may necessitate a $1,25(OH)_2D_3$-mediated increase in intestinal absorption of Ca^{2+} [as well as phosphate, whose intestinal absorption is also stimulated by $1,25(OH)_2D_3$] [2]. Furthermore, $1,25(OH)_2D_3$, like PTH, stimulates net release of Ca^{2+} and phosphate from bone, further increasing the availability of Ca^{2+} for restoring normocalcemia. Increased influx of Ca^{2+} into the ECF from intestine and bone, coupled with renal Ca^{2+} conservation, normalizes Ca_o^{2+} and closes this negative feedback loop. The phosphaturic action of PTH can be conceptualized as a mechanism to rid the body of any excess phosphate released from bone or absorbed from the intestine as part of the homeostatic response just noted that is directed at normalizing Ca_o^{2+}. Clearly, however, there are additional potent mechanisms that contribute to maintaining the circulating level of phosphate within its desired homeostatic range (see below). In contrast to the catabolic effects of sustained elevations in PTH on the skeleton, intermittent administration of PTH or its N-terminal fragment, PTH [1–34], produces an anabolic effect, thereby serving as the basis for treating osteoporosis with daily injections of PTH [33].

In most cases, an increase in circulating PTH in response to hypocalcemia is sufficient to restore normocalcemia within minutes to a few hours. There are a variety of clinical situations, however, such as markedly low Ca^{2+} intake or vitamin D deficiency, in which more prolonged and quantitatively larger increases in PTH levels are needed to restore and maintain normocalcemia. This can be accomplished through a temporal hierarchy of responses of the parathyroid glands to low Ca_o^{2+} and/or associated $1,25(OH)_2D_3$ deficiency [34]. Following the initial release of stored PTH from the parathyroid chief cells in response to hypocalcemia, which occurs within seconds and lasts for 60–90 min, there is reduced intracellular degradation of PTH after 20–30 min [35], increased expression of the PTH gene over hours to a day or so, and, finally, enhanced parathyroid cellular proliferation over weeks to months or more [34, 36]. Increases in circulating PTH and in parathyroid cellular mass of 100-fold or more occur not infrequently in the setting of severe hyperparathyroidism, as in patients with chronic kidney disease.

The response of the Ca_o^{2+} homeostatic system to hypercalcemia is in many ways the mirror image of its response to hypocalcemia, but likely places a different emphasis on the various components of the homeostatic mechanism. A high Ca^{2+}-induced decrease in circulating PTH promotes increased renal Ca^{2+} excretion, reduced intestinal Ca^{2+} absorption as $1,25(OH)_2D_3$ levels fall, and decreased net skeletal Ca^{2+} release. Additional homeostatic mechanisms that come into play in this setting include a direct calciuric action of hypercalcemia on the kidney mediated by the CaSR in the distal tubule (as opposed to that resulting solely from lower PTH levels—see below) [28, 37] and, in species in which CT is biologically important, CaSR-induced stimulation of CT secretion, which then inhibits bone resorption. Of note, mice with knockout (KO) of the PTH gene defend against hypercalcemia induced by a Ca^{2+} load (e.g., increased dietary Ca^{2+} intake) as well as normal mice, emphasizing that a robust defense against hypercalcemia, including a marked increase in renal Ca^{2+} excretion, does not absolutely require the capacity to inhibit PTH secretion [38]. The two major mechanisms in this defense against hypercalcemia are calcium-evoked renal calcium excretion and CT secretion.

Cellular and Molecular Mechanisms Underlying the Direct Regulation of the Secretion/Production of Ca_o^{2+}-Regulating Hormones by the CaSR

Regulation of PTH and CT secretion by the CaSR. The CaSR regulates several aspects of parathyroid function, all of which are relevant to the control of Ca_o^{2+} homeostasis. Proof of the CaSR's role in these processes, as well as in the others described below, has come from studies in CaSR knockout mice [39] and/or in humans heterozygous or homozygous for inactivating mutations in the CaSR [40] as well as from the use of specific CaSR activators ("calcimimetics") or blockers ("calcilytics") [41]. The CaSR mediates the regulation by Ca_o^{2+} of the following processes: the acute PTH secretory response, expression of the PTH gene, and para-thyroid cellular proliferation—all of which are inhibited by hypercalcemia and stimulated by hypocalcemia, as just noted. The CaSR regulates expression of the PTH gene by a posttranscriptional mechanism [42]. However, the intracellular mechanism(s) by which the CaSR regulates PTH secretion and parathyroid cellular proliferation remains murky, although the former involves G proteins of the $G_{q/11}$ pathway and products of the PLA_2 and lipoxygenase pathways [43, 44] and the latter likely involves the cell cycle regulator, cyclin D1 [45]. Activation of the CaSR also upregulates the expression of both the CaSR and the vitamin D receptor (VDR) genes [46]. Since $1,25(OH)_2D_3$, acting via the VDR, inhibits PTH gene expression and parathyroid cellular proliferation, there is a potential feed-forward mechanism, whereby activation of either receptor enhances the activation of the other.

The CaSR also mediates the increase in intracellular degradation of PTH that takes place during hypercalcemia. This control of hormonal degradation by the ambient level of Ca_o^{2+} increases the ratio of inactive fragments of PTH to biologi-cally active PTH(1–84) that is secreted as Ca_o^{2+} increases [35]. With the availability of "second-generation," two-site immunoradiometric assays for PTH in the late 1980s, the so-called intact PTH assays [47], it was originally thought that only PTH(1–84) was recognized. However, it subsequently turned out that large frag-ments of the hormone, such as PTH(7–84), are also immunoreactive in these assays, comprising ~30% of the circulating PTH recognized by the initial "intact" assays in normal individuals and a higher percentage in patients with renal insufficiency, in whom clearance of the fragments is slowed [48]. The more recently developed, "third-generation," the so-called whole PTH assays do not recognize PTH(7–84) [49], but these latter assays have not been proven to be clearly superior to the sec-ond-generation "intact" PTH assays for diagnosing disorders of Ca_o^{2+} homeostasis, such as primary hyperparathyroidism.

The CaSR is also expressed by the thyroidal C cells [17] and has been shown to mediate the stimulatory effect of Ca_o^{2+} on CT secretion [50]. It remains puzzling how hypercalcemia, acting via the CaSR, has diametrically opposed actions on hormonal secretion by parathyroid and C cells, inhibiting PTH secretion and stim-ulating CT secretion, respectively, with both actions being homeostatically appro-priate. The precise sequence of steps by which the CaSR exerts these divergent effects of Ca_o^{2+} on PTH and CT secretion remains to be fully elucidated, but likely involves the receptor's capacity to couple to a wide range of intracellular signaling systems [51].

Direct regulation of 1,25(OH)$_2$D$_3$ production by Ca^{2+}$_o$. The CaSR is expressed along most, if not all, of the kidney tubule ("nephron") [18]. The sites most relevant to this discussion are the proximal tubule, the CTAL, and the DCT (Fig. 1.2). In the proximal tubule, elevation of Ca_o^{2+} directly inhibits the 1-hydroxylation of 25(OH)D$_3$, in addition to indirectly inhibiting it by lowering PTH [52]. Since 1,25(OH)$_2$D$_3$, acting via the VDR in the proximal tubule, reduces expression of the 25(OH)D$_3$ 1-hydroxylase enzyme, CaSR-mediated upregulation of the VDR [53] may explain, at least in part, the high Ca_o^{2+}-induced inhibition of 1,25(OH)$_2$D$_3$ production. That is, even without a change in the circulating level of 1,25(OH)$_2$D$_3$, increased signaling through the VDR, owing to its upregulation, could inhibit 1-hydroxylation. The 1-hydroxylase enzyme is also present in the parathyroid cell as well as in a variety of others, i.e., skin, placenta, kidney, osteoblasts, and colon [54, 55]. The function and regulation of the local production of 1,25(OH)$_2$D$_3$ by the parathyroid and these other tissues is a subject of active investigation.

Cellular and Molecular Mechanisms Underlying the Homeostatically Regulated Transport of Ca^{2+} in Kidney, Intestine, and Bone

In response to the CaSR-mediated alterations in PTH and CT secretion and in synthesis of 1,25(OH)$_2$D$_3$ that are elicited by perturbations in Ca_o^{2+} from its normal level, there are resultant changes in the handling of Ca^{2+} by kidney, bone, and intestine that normalize Ca_o^{2+}, as described earlier. PTH and 1,25(OH)$_2$D$_3$ are the body's principal Ca_o^{2+}-elevating hormones. While CT has traditionally been designated as the principal Ca_o^{2+}-lowering hormone, it should be pointed out that Ca_o^{2+} itself can act in a hormone-like manner to regulate ion transport in a homeostatically appropriate manner by binding to its cognate receptor, the G protein-coupled CaSR. Viewed in this way, Ca_o^{2+} is a potent Ca_o^{2+}-lowering "hormone-like" factor, and it does so by inhibiting PTH secretion and 1,25(OH)$_2$D$_3$ formation, stimulating CT secretion and directly enhancing renal Ca^{2+} excretion. This section details the rapid progress that has taken place in our understanding of the cellular and molecular mechanisms by which PTH, 1,25(OH)$_2$D$_3$, and Ca_o^{2+}, acting via their respective receptors, regulate Ca^{2+} transport in kidney, intestine, and bone.

Mechanisms underlying the hormonal regulation of intestinal Ca^{2+} absorption. As noted above, hypocalcemia evokes a PTH-mediated increase in the circulating level of 1,25(OH)$_2$D$_3$. The latter is the sole hormonal mediator of the accompanying augmentation of intestinal Ca^{2+} absorption. PTH per se has no direct effect on intestinal absorption of mineral ions. Active transcellular absorption of Ca^{2+} in the intestine occurs by a three-step process (Fig. 1.4) [56]: (1) Transfer of Ca^{2+} from the intestinal

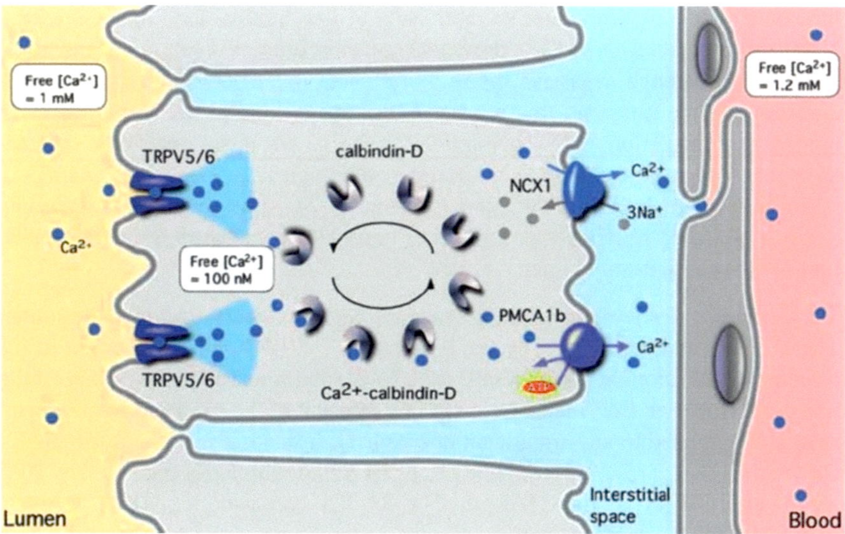

Fig. 1.4 Schematic model of the mechanisms for transcellular absorption of Ca^{2+} in the intestine and DCT. Ca^{2+} is absorbed across the apical/luminal membrane of the intestine utilizing TRPV6 and of the DCT using primarily TRPV5. Ca^{2+} then translocates to the basolateral membrane largely bound to the shuttle/buffer calbindin D_{9K} in intestine and calbindin D_{28K} in DCT, where it is pumped out of the cell by NCX1 and PMCA1b (see text for details). Reproduced with permission from Nijenhuis T, Hoenderup J, and Bindels R. TRPV5 and TRPV6 in Ca^{2+} (re)absorption: regulating Ca^{2+} entry at the gate. Pflugers Arch Eur J Physiol 2005; 451: 181–192

lumen across the apical membrane into the cytosol of the enterocyte, which is favored by the electronegativity of the cytosol relative to the intestinal lumen and by the ~10,000 lower level of the cytosolic Ca^{2+} concentration (Ca_i^{2+}) relative to Ca_o^{2+} in the lumen. Transcellular Ca^{2+} transport takes place principally in the proximal small intestine, especially the duodenum, but also, to some extent, in the colon. Apical Ca^{2+} uptake occurs via a Ca^{2+}-permeable channel, called TRPV6 [56, 57]. (2) Diffusion of Ca^{2+} ions to the basolateral cell membrane, likely bound to the Ca^{2+}-binding protein, calbindin D_{9K}, which may serve both as a "shuttle" for Ca^{2+} and as a buffer against excessively large, potentially toxic increases in Ca_i^{2+} occurring during the transcellular transfer of large amounts of Ca^{2+}. (3) Ejection of Ca^{2+} across the basolateral cell membrane via a Ca^{2+}-ATPase (PMCA1b) and Na^+-Ca^{2+}-exchanger (NCX1). In general, knockout mouse models have supported this model, although mice with KO of calbindin D_{9K} can still absorb Ca^{2+} nearly normally [58], either because calbindin D_{9K} is not absolutely required for transcellular intestinal Ca^{2+} absorption or because other mechanisms can compensate for the lack of calbindin D_{9K}.

$1,25(OH)_2D_3$ enhances active transport of Ca^{2+} in the intestine by upregulating all three of the steps just enumerated owing to increases in expression of their respective genes [59]. $1,25(OH)_2D_3$ can also stimulate rapid (within minutes) increases in intestinal Ca^{2+} transport through an incompletely understood mechanism [60]. Active transcellular Ca^{2+} transport is a relatively high-affinity, saturable process that is most important quantitatively at low luminal Ca^{2+} concentrations. At higher luminal levels of Ca^{2+}, the active transport process is saturated, and transport of Ca^{2+} through a passive, paracellular route (e.g., between cells) becomes dominant. In the intestine, this process is not susceptible to the same degree of homeostatic regulation as the transcellular pathway, but it can contribute substantially to intestinal absorption of Ca^{2+} in some pathological states, such as milk-alkali syndrome, in which there is excessive Ca^{2+} intake [2]. At present, the CaSR has no firmly established role in regulating either transcellular or paracellular Ca^{2+} transport in the gastrointestinal tract.

Mechanisms underlying the hormonal regulation of Ca^{2+} reabsorption in the kidney. The bulk of the Ca^{2+} filtered by the glomerulus (~60–70%) is reabsorbed in the proximal tubule along with other salts (i.e., NaCl) and water by passive paracellular transport. However, Ca^{2+} reabsorption in this segment of the nephron is not homeostatically regulated to any significant degree [61]. Instead, it is the reabsorption of Ca^{2+} in the CTAL (15–20%) [62] and DCT (10–15%) [63] that is regulated by PTH and/or $1,25(OH)_2D_3$. In the CTAL, the Na^+-K^+-$2Cl^-$ cotransporter, NKCC, actively transports Na^+, K^+, and Cl^- across the apical membrane of the tubular epithelium (Fig. 1.5). Some of the K^+ is recycled back across the apical membrane by the K^+ channel, *rat outer medullary potassium (K^+)* (ROMK) channel. This recycling of positive charge into the lumen combined with the net transfer of two Cl^- and one Na^+ across the basolateral membrane (e.g., excess negative charge) generates a net-positive potential across the tubular epithelium (i.e., positive on the inside relative to the outside of the tubule) [28]. This potential difference drives the reabsorption of Na^+, Ca^{2+}, and Mg^{2+} through a passive paracellular pathway [62]. Some investigators ascribe a significant component of transcellular Ca^{2+} transport to the CTAL [37], but most investigators believe that the paracellular pathway is the dominant route for tubular reabsorption of Ca^{2+} and Mg^{2+} in this nephron segment. A key component of this pathway is the protein, paracellin-1 or claudin-16 [64], through which Ca^{2+} and Mg^{2+} permeate the paracellular route. The validity of this model is strongly supported by experiments in nature affecting essentially all of the molecular components just enumerated (e.g., NKCC, ROMK, a basolateral Cl^- channel, and claudin-16) in which there are inactivating mutations of the respective genes [65]. The wasting of Na^+, Ca^{2+}, and Mg^{2+} that results from genetically impaired transport of these ions manifests as various forms of Bartter's syndrome.

The CTAL is a key site, where PTH exerts its Ca^{2+}-conserving action, and the CaSR, which is located on the basolateral cell surface, has just the opposite effect, i.e., enhancing Ca^{2+} excretion [28]. These actions can be understood in terms of the model just described. PTH, by raising intracellular cAMP levels, activates the mechanism generating the lumen-positive potential, thereby stimulating paracellular reabsorption of Ca^{2+} and Mg^{2+} [66]. The CaSR, in contrast, reduces cAMP production and likely stimulates the formation of metabolites of arachidonic acid formed by the P450 pathway. Through these and possibly other signaling pathways, the CaSR inhibits the activity of the apical K^+ channel and, perhaps, NKCC, resulting in a decrease in the lumen-positive potential and, pari passu, in Ca^{2+} and Mg^{2+}

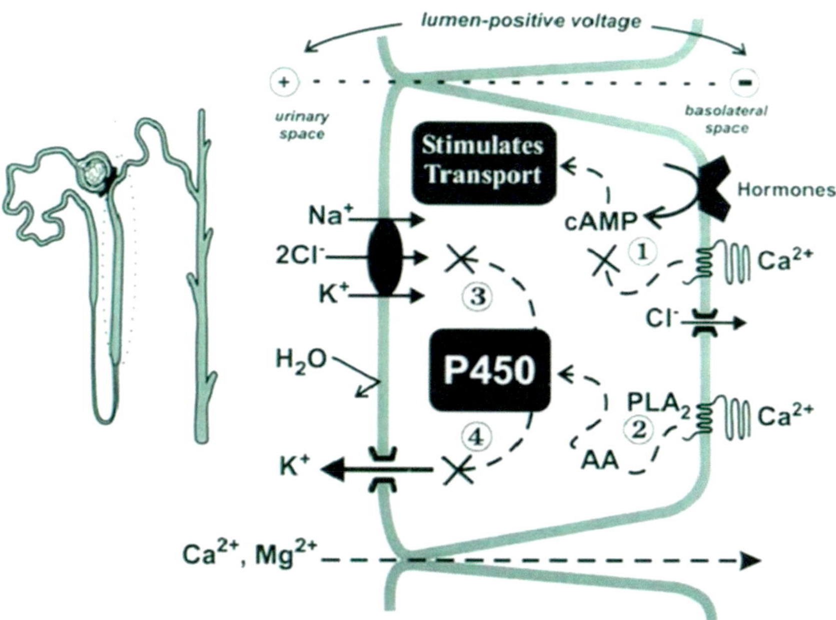

Fig. 1.5 Mechanisms underlying paracellular reabsorption of Ca^{2+} in CTAL and its inhibition by the CaSR. See text for details. The activity of the NKCC, combined with recycling of K^+ into the lumen through the apical K^+ channel and efflux of Cl^- at the basolateral aspect of the cell, generates a lumen-positive potential that drives the transport of Ca^{2+} and Mg^{2+} through the paracellular pathway via paracellin-1. The CaSR inhibits PTH-stimulated as well as basal reabsorption of Ca^{2+} by decreasing cAMP accumulation, generating metabolites of arachidonic acid (AA) via the P450 pathway and, perhaps, other mechanisms. The CaSR may also regulate the permeability of the paracellular pathway to calcium (and magnesium). Reproduced with permission from Brown EM, Hebert SC. Calcium receptor-regulated parathyroid and renal function. Bone 1997; 20: 303–309

reabsorption [28]. The CaSR's role in regulating divalent cation reabsorption in CTAL by this mechanism is supported by the identification of a form of Bartter's syndrome resulting from activating CaSR mutations [67] and, conversely, the demonstration of excessive reabsorption of Ca^{2+} and Mg^{2+} in CTAL in patients with inactivating CaSR mutations [7]. Thus, even though most reabsorption of divalent cations in the CTAL is via the "passive" paracellular route, there is nevertheless important physiological regulation of Ca^{2+} and Mg^{2+} reabsorption by this route that is highly pertinent to overall Ca^{2+} homeostasis. Furthermore, stimulation of this reabsorptive mechanism does not require changes in gene expression and can occur, therefore, within a matter of minutes.

Reabsorption of Ca^{2+} in the DCT takes place by active transcellular transport utilizing a mechanism very similar to that in the intestine (viz., Fig. 1.4) [68]. Luminal uptake of Ca^{2+} occurs through a Ca^{2+}-permeable channel, TRPV5, which is highly homologous to TRPV6 in the intestine. The Ca^{2+}-binding protein, calbindin D_{28K}, serves as the principal renal transcellular Ca^{2+} buffer/shuttle, rather than calbindin

D_{9K} [68]. Extrusion of Ca^{2+} again takes place via PMCA1b and NCX1. PTH increases the expression of all of these transporters [69] while $1,25(OH)_2D_3$ enhances the expression of TRPV5, calbindin D_{28K}, and NCX1 [59], thereby stimulating Ca^{2+} reabsorption in this nephron segment.

Mechanisms underlying the regulation of Ca^{2+} release from the skeleton. Rather than acting directly on osteoclasts to stimulate bone resorption and mobilize skeletal Ca^{2+} as part of the defense against hypocalcemia, PTH and $1,25(OH)_2D_3$ act indirectly, through the osteoblast [70]. Both hormones increase the expression by osteoblasts of the so-called RANKL (ligand for the receptor activator of NFκB) [71, 72]. Osteoblast-bound RANKL interacts with its receptor (RANK) on preexisting osteoclasts or their precursors, which are mononuclear cells of the monocyte/macrophage lineage [73]. In this way, RANKL not only enhances the resorptive activity of preexisting osteoclasts, but also promotes maturation and fusion of osteoclast precursors to form mature osteoclasts, if a more prolonged increase in bone resorption is homeostatically necessary. Another key participant in the RANKL–RANK system is a protein, called osteoprotegerin, which is likewise a product of osteoblasts [74]. It is soluble and binds to RANKL, forming an inactive complex, thereby acting as a "decoy" receptor for RANKL that prevents it from binding to RANK. As a consequence of their competition for RANKL, the ratio between the available amounts of OPG and RANK is an important determinant of the prevailing rate of bone resorption, with a high ratio of OPG/RANK suppressing and a low ratio stimulating it [71, 74]. Administration of OPG has been proposed as a treatment for conditions with excessive bone resorption, including osteoporosis [75]. Other factors produced by osteoblasts, such as monocyte/macrophage colony-stimulating factor (M-CSF) [76], as well as immunoglobulin-like receptors on osteoclasts and their precursors whose ligands are not yet fully elucidated, also contribute to osteoblast-mediated activation of osteoclasts [77]. Most investigators opine that osteoclast-mediated bone resorption is the predominant, if not sole, source of the Ca^{2+} mobilized acutely and chronically from bone in response to PTH. Others, however, argue that PTH can acutely mobilize mineral at the bone surface by modifying its solubility, without the requirement for bone resorption [78]. Perhaps, it is movements of calcium into and out of this compartment that is modulated by the CaSR through a PTH-independent mechanism that participates in the rapid uptake or efflux of calcium from bone [31]. The CaSR has been found in some, but not all, studies in both osteoblasts and osteoclasts (for review, see ref. 1), and may serve a homeostatically relevant role in stimulating bone formation [79] and inhibiting resorption [80], but additional work is needed to achieve a consensus regarding its role in Ca_o^{2+} homeostasis per se.

Bone resorption is not allowed to proceed indefinitely, however, without eliciting a compensatory increase in bone formation. Either one or more substances released from the bone matrix during bone resorption, e.g., TGF-β or bone morphogenetic proteins (BMPs) [81], or from osteoclasts themselves [82], promote chemotaxis and proliferation of osteoblast precursors, followed by their maturation, synthesis of collagen and other bone matrix proteins, and eventual mineralization of the newly formed bone matrix [2]. This process represents the "coupling" of bone resorption to subsequent bone formation to replace the missing bone. In some states, however, there can be insufficient coupling, with a resultant net loss of bone. The latter can occur with chronic elevations in PTH as in various forms of hyperparathyroidism, malignant osteolysis caused by overproduction of PTHrP by cancer cells, or multiple myeloma.

Recent Advances in Understanding the Mechanisms Regulating the Interactions Between Ca_o^{2+} and Phosphate Homeostasis

Progress in elucidating the mechanisms underlying phosphate homeostasis lagged for many years behind the corresponding advances in understanding Ca^{2+} homeostasis. Prior to 10–15 years ago, the only well-characterized phosphate-regulating hormone was PTH, which provided an inextricable linkage between Ca^{2+} and phosphate metabolism, as noted above. Studies of inherited [83] and acquired [84] human disorders resulting from unknown humoral factors that caused phosphate wasting lead to the identification of FGF-23 as an important new phosphate-regulating hormone. FGF-23 is the best characterized of a family of the so-called phosphatonins, which also includes secreted frizzle-related protein (sFRP-4), matrix extracellular phosphoglycoprotein (MEPE), and fibroblast growth factor-7 (FGF-7) [13, 85]. The dominant biological action of these factors is to regulate phosphate metabolism, principally by promoting renal phosphate wasting. For instance, FGF-23 production by osteocytes [85], its principal cell of origin, increases in response to hyperphosphatemia, at least in animals [86], permitting it to limit the rise of serum phosphate owing to its phosphaturic action.

It has also become clear, however, that the phosphatonins also modulate Ca_o^{2+} homeostasis. For instance, there is a feedback loop between $1,25(OH)_2D_3$ and FGF23, whereby $1,25(OH)_2D_3$ increases circulating FGF23 levels [87]; FGF23, in turn, feeds back to inhibit the 1-hydroxylation of $25(OH)D_3$ [88]. This loop can be understood in terms of its impact on phosphate homeostasis: in situations, where more $1,25(OH)_2D_3$ is needed to raise Ca_o^{2+}, for instance, it also increases the availability of phosphate from both intestine and bone, which might produce an excessive rise in serum phosphate concentration. An increase in FGF-23, therefore, would be homeostatically appropriate to limit the increase in serum phosphate. The FGF-23-induced inhibition of $1,25(OH)_2D_3$, in turn, would further serve to limit $1,25(OH)_2D_3$-mediated release of phosphate into the ECF from bone and intestine. However, the resulting decrease in $1,25(OH)_2D_3$ could potentially impact Ca_o^{2+} homeostasis by reducing availability of Ca^{2+} from bone and intestine. Indeed, patients with tumors overproducing FGF-23 can have, in addition to hypophosphatemia, frankly low levels of $1,25(OH)_2D_3$ [85]. Another way in which FGF-23 impacts Ca_o^{2+} homeostasis is by inhibiting PTH secretion [89], although the physiological relevance of this action and the extent to which it impacts parathyroid function acutely and chronically remain to be fully elucidated.

FGF-23 acts on its target tissues through one or more FGF receptors (subtypes 1c, 3c, and 4) [85]. α-Klotho is a recently described coreceptor for FGF-23 [90], which was originally described as an antiaging factor that was mutated in mice with a premature aging phenotype [91]. It has been recently suggested to have several actions relevant to Ca_o^{2+} homeostasis [92], including (1) promoting PTH secretion, (2) acting with FGF-23 via its coreceptor function to inhibit $1,25(OH)_2D_3$ formation, and (3) deglycosylating TRPV5 and, as a consequence, activating it by stabilizing the deglycosylated channel in the apical membrane of the epithelial cells of the DCT [93]. Of interest, the secretion of α-klotho by both parathyroid and kidney tissue was inhibited by raising Ca_o^{2+}, consistent with regulation of secretion of α-klotho by the CaSR or some other Ca_o^{2+}-sensing mechanism [92]. Increasingly, therefore, available data suggest the presence of a finely tuned mechanism, whereby the systems governing Ca_o^{2+} and phosphate homeostasis do not act in isolation. Instead, they act in an interrelated and integrated fashion designed to respond to a stress(es) on one or both systems with responses aimed at maximizing the chance of restoring and maintaining homeostasis of both systems [94]. No doubt our understanding of this highly coordinated system will increase greatly over the next several years.

References

1. Brown EM, MacLeod RJ. Extracellular calcium sensing and extracellular calcium signaling. Physiol Rev. 2001;81:239–97.
2. Bringhurst FR, Demay MB, Kronenberg HM. Hormones and disorders of mineral metabolism. In: Wilson JD, Foster DW, Kronenberg HM, Larsen PR, editors. Williams textbook of endocrinology. 9th ed. Philadelphia: W.B. Saunders; 1998. p. 1155–209.
3. Pietrobon D, Di Virgilio F, Pozzan T. Structural and functional aspects of calcium homeostasis in eukaryotic cells. Eur J Biochem. 1990;120:599–622.
4. Hofer AM, Brown EM. Extracellular calcium sensing and signalling. Nat Rev Mol Cell Biol. 2003;4:530–8.
5. Berridge MJ, Bootman MD, Roderick HL. Calcium signalling: dynamics, homeostasis and remodelling. Nat Rev Mol Cell Biol. 2003;4:517–29.
6. Klee CB, Means AR. Keeping up with calcium: conference on calcium-binding proteins and calcium function in health and disease. EMBO Rep. 2002;3:823–7.
7. Brown EM. Clinical lessons from the calcium-sensing receptor. Nat Clin Pract Endocrinol Metab. 2007;3:122–33.
8. Houillier P, Nicolet-Barousse L, Maruani G, Paillard M. What keeps serum calcium levels stable? Joint Bone Spine. 2003;70:407–13.
9. Bilezikian JP, Khan AA, Potts Jr JT. Guidelines for the management of asymptomatic primary hyperparathyroidism: summary statement from the third international workshop. J Clin Endocrinol Metab. 2009;94:335–9.
10. Cetani F, Picone A, Cerrai P, Vignali E, Borsari S, Pardi E, Viacava P, Naccarato AG, Miccoli P, Kifor O, Brown EM, Pinchera A, Marcocci C. Parathyroid expression of calcium-sensing receptor protein and in vivo parathyroid hormone-Ca(2+) set-point in patients with primary hyperparathyroidism. J Clin Endocrinol Metab. 2000;85:4789–94.
11. Brown EM. Four parameter model of the sigmoidal relationship between parathyroid hormone release and extracellular calcium concentration in normal and abnormal parathyroid tissue. J Clin Endocrinol Metab. 1983;56:572–81.
12. Hellman P, Carling T, Rask L, Akerstrom G. Pathophysiology of primary hyperparathyroidism. Histol Histopathol. 2000;15:619–27.

13. Berndt T, Kumar R. Novel mechanisms in the regulation of phosphorus homeostasis. Physiology (Bethesda). 2009;24:17–25.
14. Juppner H. Novel regulators of phosphate homeostasis and bone metabolism. Ther Apher Dial. 2007;11 Suppl 1:S3–22.
15. Brown EM, Gamba G, Riccardi D, Lombardi M, Butters R, Kifor O, Sun A, Hediger MA, Lytton J, Hebert SC. Cloning and characterization of an extracellular Ca(2+)-sensing receptor from bovine parathyroid. Nature. 1993;366:575–80.
16. Hu J, Spiegel AM. Structure and function of the human calcium-sensing receptor: insights from natural and engineered mutations and allosteric modulators. J Cell Mol Med. 2007;11:908–22.
17. Freichel M, Zink-Lorenz A, Holloschi A, Hafner M, Flockerzi V, Raue F. Expression of a calcium-sensing receptor in a human medullary thyroid carcinoma cell line and its contribution to calcitonin secretion. Endocrinology. 1996;137:3842–8.
18. Riccardi D, Hall AE, Chattopadhyay N, Xu JZ, Brown EM, Hebert SC. Localization of the extracellular Ca^{2+}/polyvalent cation-sensing protein in rat kidney. Am J Physiol. 1998;274:F611–22.
19. Chattopadhyay N, Cheng I, Rogers K, Riccardi D, Hall A, Diaz R, Hebert SC, Soybel DI, Brown EM. Identification and localization of extracellular Ca(2+)-sensing receptor in rat intestine. Am J Physiol. 1998;274:G122–30.
20. Gama L, Baxendale-Cox LM, Breitwieser GE. Ca^{2+}-sensing receptors in intestinal epithelium. Am J Physiol. 1997;273:C1168–75.
21. Chang W, Tu C, Chen T-H, Komuves L, Oda Y, Pratt S, Miller S, Shoback D. Expression and signal transduction of calcium-sensing receptors in cartilage and bone. Endocrinology. 1999;140:5883–93.
22. DeLuca HF. Overview of general physiologic features and functions of vitamin D. Am J Clin Nutr. 2004;80:1689S–96.
23. Woodrow JP, Sharpe CJ, Fudge NJ, Hoff AO, Gagel RF, Kovacs CS. Calcitonin plays a critical role in regulating skeletal mineral metabolism during lactation. Endocrinology. 2006;147:4010–21.
24. Hirsch PF, Baruch H. Is calcitonin an important physiological substance? Endocrine. 2003;21:201–8.
25. Kenny AM, Prestwood KM. Osteoporosis. Pathogenesis, diagnosis, and treatment in older adults. Rheum Dis Clin North Am. 2000;26:569–91.
26. Mosekilde L, Eriksen EF, Charles P. Hypercalcemia of malignancy: pathophysiology, diagnosis and treatment. Crit Rev Oncol Hematol. 1991;11:1–27.
27. Friedman PA. Calcium transport in the kidney. Curr Opin Nephrol Hypertens. 1999;8:589–95.
28. Hebert SC, Brown EM, Harris HW. Role of the Ca(2+)-sensing receptor in divalent mineral ion homeostasis. J Exp Biol. 1997;200:295–302.
29. Favus MJ. Intestinal absorption of calcium, magnesium and phosphorus. In: Coe FL, Favus MJ, editors. Disorders of bone and mineral metabolism. New York: Raven; 1992. p. 57–81.
30. Bilezikian JP, Canfield RE, Jacobs TP, Polay JS, D'Adamo AP, Eisman JA, DeLuca HF. Response of 1alpha,25-dihydroxyvitamin D3 to hypocalcemia in human subjects. N Engl J Med. 1978;299:437–41.
31. Huan J, Martuseviciene G, Olgaard K, Lewin E. Calcium-sensing receptor and recovery from hypocalcaemia in thyroparathyroidectomized rats. Eur J Clin Invest. 2007;37:214–21.
32. Lewin E, Wang W, Olgaard K. Rapid recovery of plasma ionized calcium after acute induction of hypocalcaemia in parathyroidectomized and nephrectomized rats. Nephrol Dial Transplant. 1999;14:604–9.
33. Neer RM, Arnaud CD, Zanchetta JR, Prince R, Gaich GA, Reginster JY, Hodsman AB, Eriksen EF, Ish-Shalom S, Genant HK, Wang O, Mitlak BH. Effect of parathyroid hormone (1–34) on fractures and bone mineral density in postmenopausal women with osteoporosis. N Engl J Med. 2001;344:1434–41.
34. Brown EM. Extracellular Ca^{2+} sensing, regulation of parathyroid cell function, and role of Ca^{2+} and other ions as extracellular (first) messengers. Physiol Rev. 1991;71:371–411.

35. Morrissey JJ, Hamilton JW, MacGregor RR, Cohn DV. The secretion of parathormone fragments 34–84 and 37–84 by dispersed porcine parathyroid cells. Endocrinology. 1980;107: 164–71.
36. Naveh-Many T, Rahamimov R, Livni N, Silver J. Parathyroid cell proliferation in normal and chronic renal failure rats. The effects of calcium, phosphate, and vitamin D. J Clin Invest. 1995;96:1786–93.
37. Ba J, Friedman PA. Calcium-sensing receptor regulation of renal mineral ion transport. Cell Calcium. 2004;35:229–37.
38. Kantham L, Quinn SJ, Egbuna OI, Baxi K, Butters R, Pang JL, Pollak MR, Goltzman D, Brown EM. The calcium-sensing receptor (CaSR) defends against hypercalcemia independently of its regulation of parathyroid hormone secretion. Am J Physiol Endocrinol Metab. 2009;297:E915–23.
39. Ho C, Conner DA, Pollak MR, Ladd DJ, Kifor O, Warren HB, Brown EM, Seidman JG, Seidman CE. A mouse model of human familial hypocalciuric hypercalcemia and neonatal severe hyperparathyroidism. Nat Genet. 1995;11:389–94. see comments.
40. Hauache OM. Extracellular calcium-sensing receptor: structural and functional features and association with diseases. Braz J Med Biol Res. 2001;34:577–84.
41. Nemeth EF. Calcimimetic and calcilytic drugs: just for parathyroid cells? Cell Calcium. 2004;35:283–9.
42. Levi R, Ben-Dov IZ, Lavi-Moshayoff V, Dinur M, Martin D, Naveh-Many T, Silver J. Increased parathyroid hormone gene expression in secondary hyperparathyroidism of experimental uremia is reversed by calcimimetics: correlation with posttranslational modification of the trans acting factor AUF1. J Am Soc Nephrol. 2006;17:107–12.
43. Bourdeau A, Moutahir M, Souberbielle J, Bonnet P, Herviaux P, Sachs C, Lieberherr M. Effects of lipoxygenase products of arachidonate metabolism on parathyroid hormone secretion. Endocrinology. 1994;135:1109–12.
44. Wettschureck N, Lee E, Libutti SK, Offermanns S, Robey PG, Spiegel AM. Parathyroid-specific double knockout of Gq and G11 alpha-subunits leads to a phenotype resembling germline knockout of the extracellular Ca^{2+}-sensing receptor. Mol Endocrinol. 2007;21:274–80.
45. Mallya SM, Arnold A. Cyclin D1 in parathyroid disease. Front Biosci. 2000;5:D367–71.
46. Rodriguez ME, Almaden Y, Canadillas S, Canalejo A, Siendones E, Lopez I, Aguilera-Tejero E, Martin D, Rodriguez M. The calcimimetic R-568 increases vitamin D receptor expression in rat parathyroid glands. Am J Physiol Renal Physiol. 2007;292:F1390–5.
47. Nussbaum SR, Potts Jr J, Wang CA, Zahradnik R, Lavigne JR, Kim L, Segre GV. A highly sensitive two-site immunoradiometric assay for parathyroid hormone (PTH) and its clinical utility in the evaluation of patients with hypercalcemia. Clin Chem. 1987;33:1364–7.
48. D'Amour P. Circulating PTH molecular forms: what we know and what we don't. Kidney Int. 2006;70(Suppl):S29–33.
49. Gao P, Scheibel S, D'Amour P, John MR, Rao SD, Schmidt-Gayk H, Cantor TL. Development of a novel immunoradiometric assay exclusively for biologically active whole parathyroid hormone (1–84): implications for improvement of accurate measurement of parathyroid function. J Bone Miner Res. 2001;16(4):605–14.
50. Fudge NJ, Kovacs CS. Physiological studies in heterozygous calcium sensing receptor (CaSR) gene-ablated mice confirm that the CaSR regulates calcitonin release in vivo. BMC Physiol. 2004;4:5.
51. Ward DT. Calcium receptor-mediated intracellular signalling. Cell Calcium. 2004;35:217–28.
52. Weisinger JR, Favus MJ, Langman CB, Bushinsky DA. Regulation of 1,25-dihydroxyvitamin D3 by calcium in the parathyroidectomized, parathyroid hormone-replete rat. J Bone Miner Res. 1989;4:929–35.
53. Maiti A, Beckman MJ. Extracellular calcium is a direct effecter of VDR levels in proximal tubule epithelial cells that counter-balances effects of PTH on renal Vitamin D metabolism. J Steroid Biochem Mol Biol. 2007;103:504–8.
54. Ritter CS, Armbrecht HJ, Slatopolsky E, Brown AJ. 25-Hydroxyvitamin D(3) suppresses PTH synthesis and secretion by bovine parathyroid cells. Kidney Int. 2006;70:654–9.

55. Zehnder D, Bland R, Williams MC, McNinch RW, Howie AJ, Stewart PM, Hewison M. Extrarenal expression of 25-hydroxyvitamin d(3)-1 alpha-hydroxylase. J Clin Endocrinol Metab. 2001;86:888–94.
56. Hoenderop JG, Bindels RJ. Epithelial Ca^{2+} and Mg^{2+} channels in health and disease. J Am Soc Nephrol. 2005;16:15–26.
57. Peng J-B, Chen XZ, Berger UV, Vassilev PM, Tsukaguchi H, Brown EM, Hediger MA. Molecular cloning and characterization of a channel-like transporter mediating intestinal calcium absorption. J Biol Chem. 1999;274:22739–46.
58. Lee GS, Lee KY, Choi KC, Ryu YH, Paik SG, Oh GT, Jeung EB. Phenotype of a calbindin-D9k gene knockout is compensated for by the induction of other calcium transporter genes in a mouse model. J Bone Miner Res. 2007;22:1968–78.
59. Hoenderop JG, Dardenne O, Van Abel M, Van Der Kemp AW, Van Os CH, St Arnaud R, Bindels RJ. Modulation of renal Ca^{2+} transport protein genes by dietary Ca^{2+} and 1,25-dihydroxyvitamin D3 in 25-hydroxyvitamin D3-1alpha-hydroxylase knockout mice. FASEB J. 2002;16:1398–406.
60. Norman AW, Bishop JE, Bula CM, Olivera CJ, Mizwicki MT, Zanello LP, Ishida H, Okamura WH. Molecular tools for study of genomic and rapid signal transduction responses initiated by 1 alpha,25(OH)(2)-vitamin D(3). Steroids. 2002;67:457–66.
61. Costanzo L, Windhager E. Renal tubular transport of calcium. In: Windhager E, editor. Handbook of physiology. New York: Oxford University Press; 1992. p. 1759–83.
62. Di Stefano A, Wittner M, Nitschke R, Braitsch R, Greger R, Bailly C, Amiel C, Roiel N, De Rouffignac C. Transepithelial Ca^{2+} and Mg^{2+} transport in the cortical thick ascending limb of Henle's loop of the mouse is a voltage-dependent process. Ren Physiol Biochem. 1993;16:157–66.
63. Hoenderop JG, Nilius B, Bindels RJ. Molecular mechanism of active Ca^{2+} reabsorption in the distal nephron. Annu Rev Physiol. 2002;64:529–49.
64. Landau D. Epithelial paracellular proteins in health and disease. Curr Opin Nephrol Hypertens. 2006;15:425–9.
65. Kamel KS, Oh MS, Halperin ML. Bartter's, Gitelman's, and Gordon's syndromes. From physiology to molecular biology and back, yet still some unanswered questions. Nephron. 2002;92 Suppl 1:18–27.
66. Di Stefano A, Wittner M, Nitschke R, Braitsch R, Greger R, Bailly C, Amiel C, Roinel N, de Rouffignac C. Effects of parathyroid hormone and calcitonin on Na^{+}, Cl^{-}, K^{+}, Mg^{2+} and Ca^{2+} transport in cortical and medullary thick ascending limbs of mouse kidney. Pflugers Arch. 1990;417:161–7.
67. Vargas-Poussou R, Huang C, Hulin P, Houillier P, Jeunemaitre X, Paillard M, Planelles G, Dechaux M, Miller RT, Antignac C. Functional characterization of a calcium-sensing receptor mutation in severe autosomal dominant hypocalcemia with a Bartter-like syndrome. J Am Soc Nephrol. 2002;13:2259–66.
68. Mensenkamp AR, Hoenderop JG, Bindels RJ. Recent advances in renal tubular calcium reabsorption. Curr Opin Nephrol Hypertens. 2006;15:524–9.
69. van Abel M, Hoenderop JG, van der Kemp AW, Friedlaender MM, van Leeuwen JP, Bindels RJ. Coordinated control of renal Ca(2+) transport proteins by parathyroid hormone. Kidney Int. 2005;68:1708–21.
70. Takahashi N, Akatsu T, Sasaki T, Nicholson GC, Moseley JM, Martin TJ, Suda T. Induction of calcitonin receptors by 1 alpha, 25-dihydroxyvitamin D3 in osteoclast-like multinucleated cells formed from mouse bone marrow cells. Endocrinology. 1988;123:1504–10.
71. Huang JC, Sakata T, Pfleger LL, Bencsik M, Halloran BP, Bikle DD, Nissenson RA. PTH differentially regulates expression of RANKL and OPG. J Bone Miner Res. 2004;19:235–44.
72. Kim S, Yamazaki M, Shevde NK, Pike JW. Transcriptional control of receptor activator of nuclear factor-kappaB ligand by the protein kinase A activator forskolin and the transmembrane glycoprotein 130-activating cytokine, oncostatin M, is exerted through multiple distal enhancers. Mol Endocrinol. 2007;21:197–214.
73. Bar-Shavit Z. The osteoclast: a multinucleated, hematopoietic-origin, bone-resorbing osteoimmune cell. J Cell Biochem. 2007;102:1130–9.

74. Boyce BF, Xing L. Functions of RANKL/RANK/OPG in bone modeling and remodeling. Arch Biochem Biophys. 2008;473:139–46.
75. McClung MR. Inhibition of RANKL as a treatment for osteoporosis: preclinical and early clinical studies. Curr Osteoporos Rep. 2006;4:28–33.
76. Yoshida H, Hayashi S, Kunisada T, Ogawa M, Nishikawa S, Okamura H, Sudo T, Shultz LD. The murine mutation osteoporosis is in the coding region of the macrophage colony stimulating factor gene. Nature. 1990;345:442–4.
77. Kim N, Takami M, Rho J, Josien R, Choi Y. A novel member of the leukocyte receptor complex regulates osteoclast differentiation. J Exp Med. 2002;195:201–9.
78. Talmage DW, Talmage RV. Calcium homeostasis: how bone solubility relates to all aspects of bone physiology. J Musculoskelet Neuronal Interact. 2007;7:108–12.
79. Chang W, Tu C, Chen TH, Bikle D, Shoback D. The extracellular calcium-sensing receptor (CaSR) is a critical modulator of skeletal development. Sci Signal. 2008;1:ra 1.
80. Mentaverri R, Yano S, Chattopadhyay N, Petit L, Kifor O, Kamel S, Terwilliger EF, Brazier M, Brown EM. The calcium sensing receptor is directly involved in both osteoclast differentiation and apoptosis. FASEB J. 2006;20:2562–4.
81. Wozney JM. Overview of bone morphogenetic proteins. Spine. 2002;27:S2–8.
82. Yano S, Mentaverri R, Kanuparthi D, Bandyopadhyay S, Rivera A, Brown EM, Chattopadhyay N. Functional expression of beta-chemokine receptors in osteoblasts: role of regulated upon activation, normal T cell expressed and secreted (RANTES) in osteoblasts and regulation of its secretion by osteoblasts and osteoclasts. Endocrinology. 2005;146:2324–35.
83. ADHR Consortium. Autosomal dominant hypophosphataemic rickets is associated with mutations in FGF23. Nat Genet. 2000;26:345–8.
84. Shimada T, Mizutani S, Muto T, Yoneya T, Hino R, Takeda S, Takeuchi Y, Fujita T, Fukumoto S, Yamashita T. Cloning and characterization of FGF23 as a causative factor of tumor-induced osteomalacia. Proc Natl Acad Sci U S A. 2001;98:6500–5.
85. Shaikh A, Berndt T, Kumar R. Regulation of phosphate homeostasis by the phosphatonins and other novel mediators. Pediatr Nephrol. 2008;23:1203–10.
86. Perwad F, Azam N, Zhang MY, Yamashita T, Tenenhouse HS, Portale AA. Dietary and serum phosphorus regulate fibroblast growth factor 23 expression and 1,25-dihydroxyvitamin D metabolism in mice. Endocrinology. 2005;146:5358–64.
87. Saito H, Maeda A, Ohtomo S, Hirata M, Kusano K, Kato S, Ogata E, Segawa H, Miyamoto K, Fukushima N. Circulating FGF-23 is regulated by 1alpha,25-dihydroxyvitamin D3 and phosphorus in vivo. J Biol Chem. 2005;280:2543–9.
88. Shimada T, Hasegawa H, Yamazaki Y, Muto T, Hino R, Takeuchi Y, Fujita T, Nakahara K, Fukumoto S, Yamashita T. FGF-23 is a potent regulator of vitamin D metabolism and phosphate homeostasis. J Bone Miner Res. 2004;19:429–35.
89. Ben-Dov IZ, Galitzer H, Lavi-Moshayoff V, Goetz R, Kuro-o M, Mohammadi M, Sirkis R, Naveh-Many T, Silver J. The parathyroid is a target organ for FGF23 in rats. J Clin Invest. 2007;117:4003–8.
90. Kuro-o M. Klotho as a regulator of fibroblast growth factor signaling and phosphate/calcium metabolism. Curr Opin Nephrol Hypertens. 2006;15:437–41.
91. Nabeshima Y. Klotho: a fundamental regulator of aging. Ageing Res Rev. 2002;1:627–38.
92. Imura A, Tsuji Y, Murata M, et al. alpha-Klotho as a regulator of calcium homeostasis. Science. 2007;316:1615–8.
93. Chang Q, Hoefs S, van der Kemp AW, Topala CN, Bindels RJ, Hoenderop JG. The beta-glucuronidase klotho hydrolyzes and activates the TRPV5 channel. Science. 2005;310:490–3.
94. Renkema KY, Alexander RT, Bindels RJ, Hoenderop JG. Calcium and phosphate homeostasis: concerted interplay of new regulators. Ann Med. 2008;40:82–91.

Chapter 2
Preoperative Parathyroid Imaging
for the Endocrine Surgeon

Elizabeth G. Grubbs, Beth S. Edeiken, Maria K. Gule, Brett J. Monroe,
Edmund Kim, Thinh Vu, and Nancy D. Perrier

Keywords Parathyroid classification system • Gland types • Pre-op imaging • US and Tc-99 MIBI imaging modalities • 4DCT. ultrasound-guided fine-needle aspiration biopsy • Tc-99 m MIBI half-life • SPECT/CT • Nuclear isotopes • Sensitivity • Preoperative localization

Introduction

Over the past decade, minimally invasive directed parathyroidectomy (DP) has become the operation of choice for most patients with sporadic primary hyperparathyroidism (PHPT). Using preoperative imaging as a tool to guide the operation, DP has many advantages over the traditional four-gland exploration. This minimally invasive approach may be performed under local anesthesia, requires less operative time, results in decreased postoperative pain, and offers improved aesthetics [1, 2].

E.G. Grubbs, MD • M.K. Gule, MD • N.D. Perrier, MD (✉)
Department of Surgical Oncology, Unit 1484, The University of Texas M. D. Anderson Cancer
Center, 1400 Pressler Street Boulevard, Houston, TX 77030, USA
e-mail: nperrier@mdanderson.org

B.S. Edeiken, MD • B.J. Monroe, MD • T. Vu, MD
Department of Diagnostic Radiology, The University of Texas M. D. Anderson Cancer Center,
Houston, TX 77030, USA

The University of Texas Medical School, 6431 Fannin, Houston, TX 77030, USA

E. Kim, MD
Department of Nuclear Medicine, The University of Texas M. D. Anderson Cancer Center,
Houston, TX 77030, USA

The University of Texas Medical School, 6431 Fannin, Houston, TX 77030, USA

A.A. Khan and O.H. Clark (eds.), *Handbook of Parathyroid Diseases:*
A Case-Based Practical Guide, DOI 10.1007/978-1-4614-2164-1_2,
© Springer Science+Business Media, LLC 2012

The DP approach has the added advantage of earlier hospital discharge and a decrease in the overall associated costs for the procedure.

Following biochemical confirmation of PHPT, a high-quality preoperative imaging evaluation for localization of one or more abnormal parathyroid glands is essential if a DP approach is considered. Ideally, the patient is referred to the surgeon prior to imaging so that the localization evaluation may be tailored to provide a roadmap that allows efficient and effective surgical intervention. It is important to remember that the diagnosis of PHPT is made by satisfying biochemical parameters, not by findings on a radiographic study. Positive imaging modalities help guide a surgeon where to begin a parathyroid exploration. Rapid intraoperative assay for intact parathyroid hormone (PTH) along with surgical expertise used to suggest when to cease the operation.

Candidates for DP

Success of DP is dependent on several key elements: (1) the patient must have biochemically proven primary hyperparathyroidism; (2) the PHPT should not be associated with multigland disease, such as that seen with multiple endocrine neoplasia (MEN or familial PHPT); and (3) there should be a lack of coexisting thyroid disease that would require concomitant surgical management.

Anatomic Considerations

The focused approach of DP requires a thorough knowledge of cervical anatomy and embryology. The DP technique is based on previous observations that the recurrent laryngeal nerve (RLN) is seldom anomalous and further that the inferior parathyroid gland is consistently anterior (ventral) to the RLN and the superior parathyroid gland posterior (dorsal) to the RLN [3]. Anatomic sites of the superior parathyroid gland are, in order of frequency, the cricothyroid junction, the dorsum of the upper pole of the thyroid, and the retropharyngeal space. The inferior parathyroid gland most commonly rests at the lower pole of the thyroid or in the cervical thymic tongue or descendent into the anterior mediastinum. Rarely, the inferior parathyroid gland resides in the upper neck (an undescended gland) or in the posterior or middle mediastinum.

Locations of enlarged parathyroid glands adhere to a definite pattern. Because the embryologic origin of the superior gland shares a common primordium in the fourth branchial pouch with the lateral thyroid, nondiseased superior parathyroid glands are invariably found in proximity to the posterior surface of the upper thyroid parenchyma. The relationship of a normal parathyroid gland to the thyroid capsule is critical to the potential position of a diseased gland. When located within the thyroid capsule, the diseased parathyroid gland remains in place and expands locally within the confines of the surgical capsule of the thyroid. When located outside of the capsule, enlarged parathyroid glands tend to displace into a dependent area (both posteriorly and caudally), especially in the tracheoesophageal groove, and their migration is met with little resistance.

The inferior parathyroid gland shares an embryologic origin with the thymus and both arise from the third branchial complex. An enlarged inferior parathyroid gland is located in the lateral-posterior aspect of the lower thyroid pole or descends with the thymus into the anterior mediastinum.

A common misconception is that a parathyroid gland located high in the neck is always a superior gland and that one low in the neck is an inferior gland. In fact, a superior enlarged parathyroid gland may descend caudally in the tracheoesophageal groove and be located near the lower pole of the thyroid or in the posterior mediastinum. In this situation, the gland frequently is suspended by a long, vascular pedicle from the inferior or superior thyroid artery rendering it to a posterior position in the neck near the esophagus or cervical spine.

Parathyroid Nomenclature

Parathyroid Classification System

As a means of improving communication between the various radiologic teams and the surgical team, a system of classification was created based on the most frequently encountered positions of enlarged parathyroid glands (Fig. 2.1) [3]. In this classification scheme, a type A gland is a "normal" superior gland in proximity to the posterior surface of the thyroid parenchyma. It may be compressed within the capsule of the thyroid. A type B gland is a superior parathyroid gland that has fallen posteriorly into the tracheoesophageal groove. There is minimal or no contact between the gland and the posterior surface of the thyroid tissue. On anterior views, the type B parathyroid gland is in the plane of the superior pole of the thyroid. An undescended gland high in the neck near the carotid bifurcation or mandible may also be classified as a type B gland. Because these glands are cephalad to the superior pole of the thyroid, they are referred to as B+ glands. A type C gland is a superior gland that has fallen posteriorly into the tracheoesophageal groove and lies at the level of or below the inferior pole of the thyroid. This places the type C gland posterior to the RLN. The type D gland ("difficult" or "dangerous") lies in the mid region of the posterior surface of the thyroid parenchyma, near the junction of the RLN and the inferior thyroid artery. The type D gland may be either a superior or inferior gland, depending on its exact relationship to the nerve. Whether this gland is an upper or lower parathyroid gland generally cannot be determined on imaging. These glands are in direct proximity to the nerve, as a result the dissection may be dangerous. The type E gland is an inferior gland in close proximity to the inferior pole of the thyroid parenchyma anterior to the trachea. Because these glands are relatively anterior in the neck and anterior and medial to the RLN, they are often

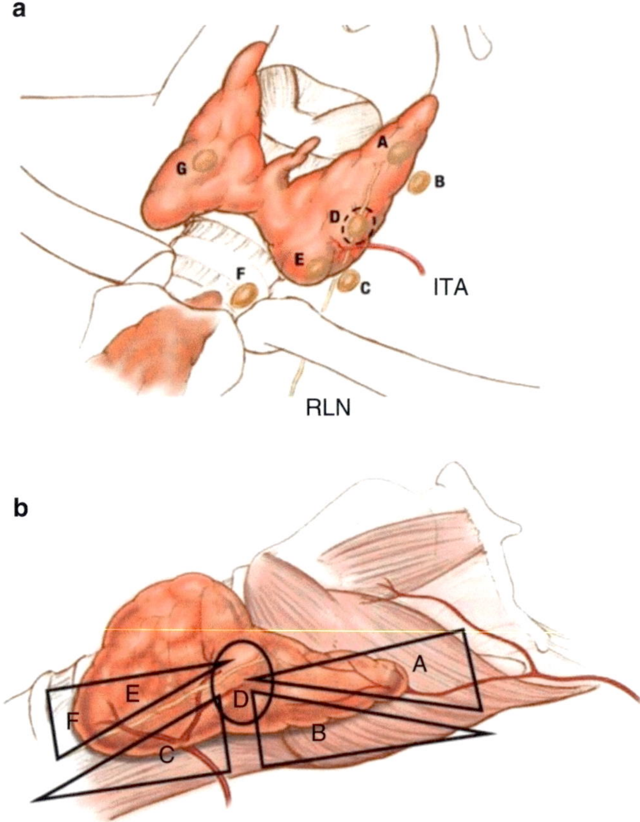

Fig. 2.1 (**a**) Anterior view displaying nomenclature of possible locations of parathyroid adenomas. *A*: Superior gland, in proximity of posterior surface of thyroid parenchyma, may be intracapsular/compressed. *B*: Superior gland, fallen posteriorly into tracheoesphageal groove, no contact with posterior surface of thyroid tissue in the cranio-caudal confines of thyroid lobe. *C*: Superior gland, fallen posteriorly into tracheoesphageal groove, no contact with posterior surface of thyroid tissue and is caudal/inferior to cranio-caudal confines of thyroid lobe. *D*: Superior or inferior gland, in mid region of posterior surface of thyroid parenchyma near junction of RLN and inferior thyroidal artery. *E*: Inferior gland, in region inferior to thyroid parenchyma, anterior to trachea. *F*: Inferior gland, descended into thyrothymic ligament or superior thymus and may appear in mediastinum. *G*: Intrathyroidal parathyroid. (**b**) Lateral view

"easiest" to remove. The type F gland is an inferior gland that has descended into the thyrothymic ligament or superior thymus. It may appear to be "ectopic" or within the mediastinum. An anterior-posterior view shows the type F gland to be anterior to and near the trachea. Finally, the type G gland is a rare intrathyroidal parathyroid gland.

Once familiar with the nomenclature, radiologists can more easily and concisely communicate with parathyroid surgeons the precise location of diseased glands.

The nomenclature allows a universal language among the multidisciplinary team, including radiologists, surgeons, anesthesiologists, endocrinologists, and pathologists. At our institution, we use the alphabet reference in approximately 90% of our preoperative imaging reports and operative records.

Preoperative Planning

Preoperative differentiation of an adenoma as superior or inferior allows the surgeon to plan the incision site and minimize both dissection and operative time. Superior glands are excised with a lateral approach, whereas inferior glands are often more easily excised with an anterior approach (Fig. 2.2). The surgical approach for a suspected superior parathyroid gland is a 2-cm incision made at the lateral extent of the marked 5-cm standard Kocher incision. The anterior border of the sternocleidomastoid muscle is identified and retracted laterally. The sternothyroid and sternothyroid muscles (the strap muscles) are separated longitudinally and retracted medially. The thyroid gland is retracted medially and the thyroid bed is inspected with fine dissection. Once identified, the enlarged parathyroid gland is removed after securing its vascular pedicle with small hemoclips. The surgical approach for a suspected inferior gland is a 2-cm incision made toward the ipsilateral side from the midline (Fig. 2.2). The strap muscles are identified, separated

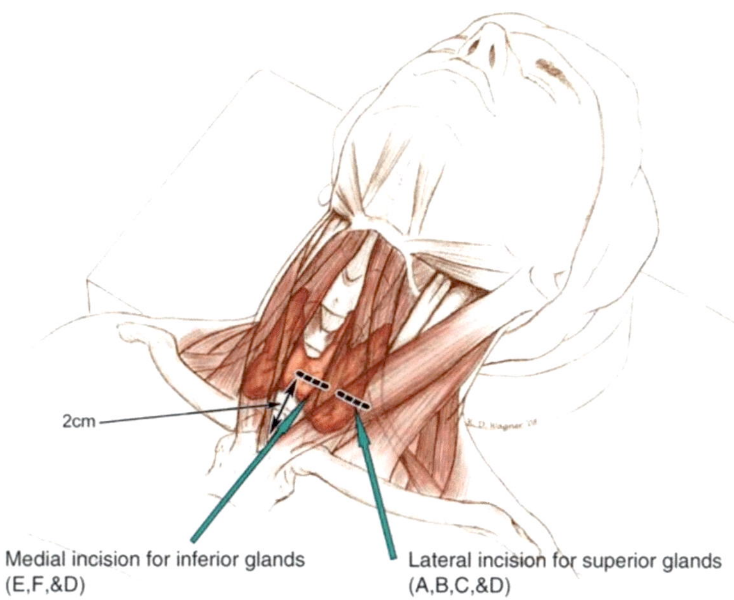

Fig. 2.2 Illustration of medial and lateral incisions for directed parathyroidectomy

longitudinally, and retracted laterally. The inferior pole of the thyroid is retracted medially. Gentle and meticulous dissection of the dorsal side of the gland and the superior thyrothymic ligament is performed in search of the adenoma.

Because of the differences in these two approaches, it is of utmost importance that the surgeon and the radiologists have excellent communication and that the surgeon reviews all images prior to surgical intervention.

Description of Imaging Modalities

Ultrasound

The goal of ultrasound (US) evaluation of the soft tissues of the neck in patients with PHPT is to identify potential parathyroid adenomas, alert the surgeon to the presence of reactive or malignant lymph nodes or nodules that could be misinterpreted as parathyroid adenomata, and identify concomitant thyroid disease. Because of the limited dissection associated with DP, the thyroid parenchyma is unable to be adequately palpated and inspected. Therefore, preoperative ultrasonographic (US) evaluation of the thyroid and regional lymph nodes for coexisting concomitant pathology is important when planning this procedure [4].

The effectiveness of ultrasound and US-guided fine-needle aspiration biopsy (FNAB) of the soft tissues of the neck is highly dependent on the expertise of the operator [5]. The successful usage of US is directly related to the skill level and experience of the ultrasound technologist and the radiologist, endocrinologist or surgeon performing the examination [6, 7]. A systematic US examination of the soft tissues of the neck includes a focused evaluation of the thyroid and nodal basins, including the jugular territories, paratracheal, submandibular, supraclavicular, and suprasternal regions. In patients with PHPT, US imaging is also focused in the traditional locations of the parathyroid glands. These include the regions superior and inferior to the thyroid gland in the anterior and posterior locations.

US of the soft tissues of the neck is performed with the patient in the supine position with the neck hyperextended. The US examination is performed using a high-resolution scanner (such as the Proforma 5500, Aloka Tokyo, Japan), with color and power Doppler capability, equipped with commercially available high-frequency broadband (7–13 MHz) linear-array transducers. Color and power Doppler examination is an integral part of a US examination of the soft tissues of the neck [4, 8].

Sonography has proven to be highly sensitive in detecting minute (a few mm in size) nonpalpable masses in the thyroid and soft tissues of the neck [9]. Although the detection rate of focal abnormalities with sonography is high, specificity of sonographic images is often insufficient to provide a clinically useful characterization of a solid thyroid nodule, an intrathyroidal parathyroid, or to differentiate an abnormal parathyroid gland from a prominent central neck lymph node.

FNAB under US guidance preoperatively provides a reliable tissue diagnosis and can diagnose malignancy in small thyroid nodules and lymph nodes not detected by other methods. US-guided FNAB may be useful for differentiation of an intrathyroidal parathyroid gland from a thyroid nodule—particularly in the reoperative setting. However, it is important that the cytologist is alerted to the concern because parathyroid gland cannot be differentiated from thyroid tissue without specific staining. Specimen assessment for PTH is most useful and very accurate. Additionally, comparison with alternate imaging modalities, such as nuclear scan and 4D-CT, may allow differentiation of thyroid tissue from parathyroid gland.

Nuclear Medicine

Technetium-99 sestamibi (Tc-99m MIBI) imaging is a modality that has been widely adopted for preoperative parathyroid localization. This imaging modality is available at most institutions and is complementary to the US evaluation of the soft tissues of the neck [10, 11].

The Tc-99m MIBI imaging technique detects increased radiotracer uptake in the neck associated with a functionally active parathyroid gland or glands. Tc-99m MIBI is distributed in proportion to blood flow and is sequestrated intracellularly within the mitochondria. The large number of mitochondria present in the cells of most parathyroid adenomas, especially oxyphilic cells, may be responsible for the avid uptake and slow release of Tc-99m MIBI seen in many but certainly not all parathyroid adenomas compared to normal parathyroid glands and surrounding thyroid tissue. Physiological thyroid uptake of Tc-99m MIBI gradually washes out with a half-life of 60 min, whereas activity in parathyroid tumors is generally stable over 2 h, thus explaining the better visualization of parathyroid adenomas at 1.5–3 h postinjection.

Typically, Tc-99m MIBI parathyroid scintigraphy is performed as a double-phase study. Following intravenous injection of 740–925 MBq (20–25 mCi) Tc-99m MIBI, two sets of planar images of the neck and upper chest are obtained using a low-energy high-resolution collimator. Views should extend from the mandible to a level below the aortic arch. The initial set of images acquired at 30 min postinjection corresponds to the thyroid phase, and a second set of images obtained at 1.5–3 h postinjection corresponds to the parathyroid phase. A focal activity in the neck or mediastinum that either progressively increases over the duration of the study or persists on delayed imaging in contrast to the decreased thyroid activity is interpreted as differential washout consistent with parathyroid adenoma. This double-phase technique has been reported to be successful in 84% of patients with adenomas and 63% with hyperplasia [5].

A meta-analysis of 52 studies published in 2004 reported sensitivities of Tc-99m MIBI ranging from 40 to over 90% [12]. Possible effects explaining this wide variation include the biochemistry of the disease; higher preoperative calcium levels have been observed more often in patients with positive scans [13]. A significant correlation was seen between the uptake ratio and preoperative PTH levels and higher PTH levels were more likely to be observed in patients with positive scans [14–16]. Vitamin D deficiency may also be associated with scan positivity [17]. A limitation in Tc-99m MIBI scanning is the decreased ability to identify patients with multiglandular disease [18]. Patients with single adenomas have been found to have more true-positive scans than those with multiglandular disease [19]. Additionally, the accuracy in this technique to detect double adenomas was only 30% in a cohort of 287 PHPT patients [20].

Tc-99m MIBI does not provide detailed anatomic information about the diseased parathyroid glands and their relationship to other structures in the neck. In addition, parathyroid adenomas within the thyroid and thyroid adenomas both demonstrate focal increased activity on MIBI, and thus cannot be differentiated by this modality. The sensitivity of Tc-99m MIBI has been found to be lower in the presence of thyroid nodules [21–23]. Oblique and lateral views are critically necessary to define the anterior-posterior location of parathyroid glands. Planar views do not provide the detailed information to inform the surgeon of the depth of the adenoma. For such details, the use of SPECT/CT is helpful [24, 25]. SPECT/CT is obtained by using an integrated imaging system with 6–16 slices of CT and software to make iterative reconstruction of 3D images with 1–4-mm-thin slices. SPECT/CT is excellent because it provides a combination of anatomic and functional information. Parathyroid adenomas overlying thyroid tissue and thyroid adenoma can be separated by use of SPECT/CT. It can also help determine whether the parathyroid tumor is in the anterior, posterior, or middle mediastinum. Thyroid pathology and/or coexisting lymphadenopathy may contribute to false-positive findings without SPECT/CT fusion images.

Four-Dimensional Computed Tomography

Four-dimensional computed tomography (4D-CT) is a multiphase multidetector computed tomography (CT). Multidetector CT provides rapid volumetric acquisition and in-plane spatial resolution of 1 mm or better, allowing improved visualization of parathyroid glands. The multiphase technique allows visualization of the temporal changes of the parathyroid adenoma (i.e., early enhancement and early washout) compared to other structures in the neck. The images generated provide detailed anatomic information which serves as a roadmap for the operating surgeon.

Our examinations are performed using a 16 or 64 row multidetector CT scanner (General Electric, 16 Lightspeed or 64 Lightspeed Volume CT, Fairfield Connecticut). The scanning protocol consists of four identical helical scan phases obtained in an automated, predetermined, timed sequence from the carina to the mandibular teeth. The first phase is without contrast. Twenty-five seconds before the beginning of the second phase, injection of 120 mL of iodinated contrast is commenced at 4 mL/s This timing was chosen such that imaging through the neck occurs during maximum opacification of vascular and tumoral structures. Thirty seconds after the end of the second phase, the third phase commenced and 45 s after the end of the third phase, the fourth and final phase commences. The four phases are identified as pre-contrast, immediate, early-delayed, and late-delayed. The pre-contrast phase allows distinction between the iodine-rich thyroid and surrounding tissue. The three vascular phases distinguish the uptake and washout characteristics of contrast in highly vascular tissue such as a parathyroid adenoma from those seen in thyroid tissue and lymph nodes.

We previously reported the use of 4D-CT in the preoperative localization of parathyroid adenomas [26]. In an evaluation of 75 patients with PHPT, 4D-CT demonstrated improved sensitivity (88%) over Tc-99m MIBI imaging (65%) and ultrasonography (57%), when the imaging studies were used to lateralize hyperfunctioning parathyroid glands to one side of the neck. Moreover, when used to localize parathyroid tumors to the correct quadrant of the neck (i.e., right inferior, right superior, left inferior, or left superior), the sensitivity of 4D-CT (70%) was superior. These results require the presence of an experienced radiologist for optimal results. Therefore, the combination of providing improved sensitivity with detailed anatomy renders CT a robust modality compared to Tc-99m MIBI or ultrasonography in planning minimally invasive parathyroid operations. Furthermore, compared to nuclear imaging and ultrasonography, CT is quicker, does not require nuclear isotope preparation or handling, and is not user-dependent. Disadvantages include radiation dose, cost, and the injection of iodinated contrast which is a contraindication in patients with poor renal function. In addition, the contrast material, as with any medication, can rarely cause severe allergic reactions.

Case Presentations

Primary Hyperparathyroidism Treated with Minimally Invasive Parathyroidectomy, Type E Gland

A 52-year-old woman with a history of depression and insomnia was found to have hypercalcemia on routine physical examination. As part of an evaluation, review of symptoms was notable for fatigue, constipation, muscle weakness, and difficulty with sleep. Laboratory results included a calcium of 2.65 mmol/L or 10.6 mg/dL (reference range 8.4–10.2 mg/dL), an ionized calcium of 1.34 mmol/L (reference range 1.13–1.32 mmol/L), a phosphorus of 0.97 mmol/L or 3.0 mg/dL (reference range 2.5–4.5 mg/dL), and an intact PTH of 108 pg/mL (reference range 9–80 pg/mL). The patient's urinary calcium was elevated at 401 mg/24 h (<150). Bone densitometry demonstrated osteoporosis of the lumbar spine with a T-score of −2.52. A diagnosis of primary hyperparathyroidism was made and surgical intervention planned.

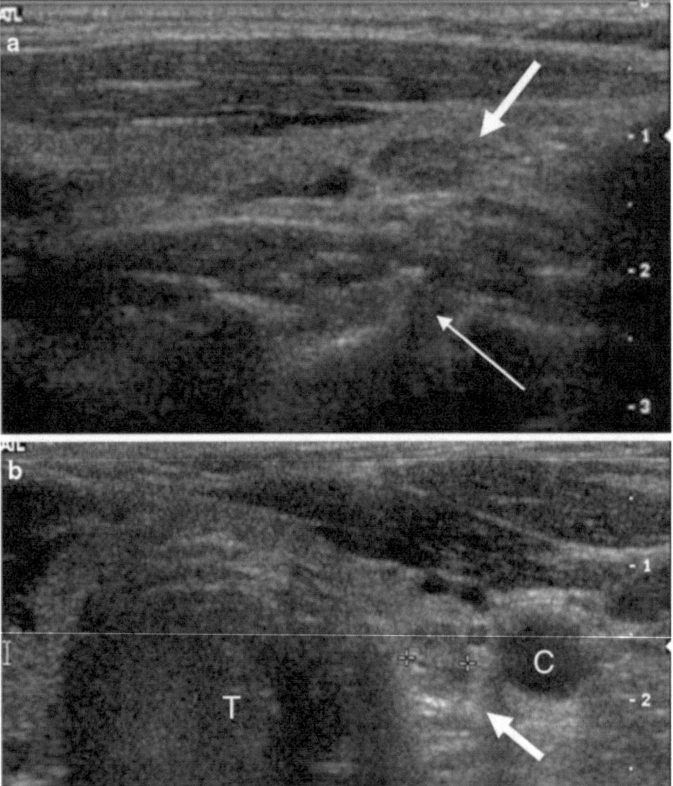

Fig. 2.3 Patient 1 ultrasound (US). (**a**) US image in the longitudinal plane, rotated clockwise 90° to match the CT sagittal reconstructed projection, demonstrates the parathyroid adenoma (1.1×0.5×0.5 cm) (*thick arrow*) along the inferior aspect of the left lobe of the thyroid (*thin arrow*). (**b**) US image in the transverse plane demonstrates the parathyroid adenoma (*arrow*) inferior to the left lobe of the thyroid lateral to the trachea (T) and medial to the carotid (C) that correlates with the position of the parathyroid adenoma documented on 4D-CT

Imaging Studies

Ultrasound

Ultrasound images performed in both the longitudinal and transverse plane demonstrated an unremarkable thyroid gland and a left nodule caudal to the inferior margin of the thyroid in the region of concern for a parathyroid adenoma (Fig. 2.3a, b). By US criteria, this nodule was considered nonspecific. Correlation with medical history and alternate imaging modalities suggested that this is an enlarged E type parathyroid adenoma.

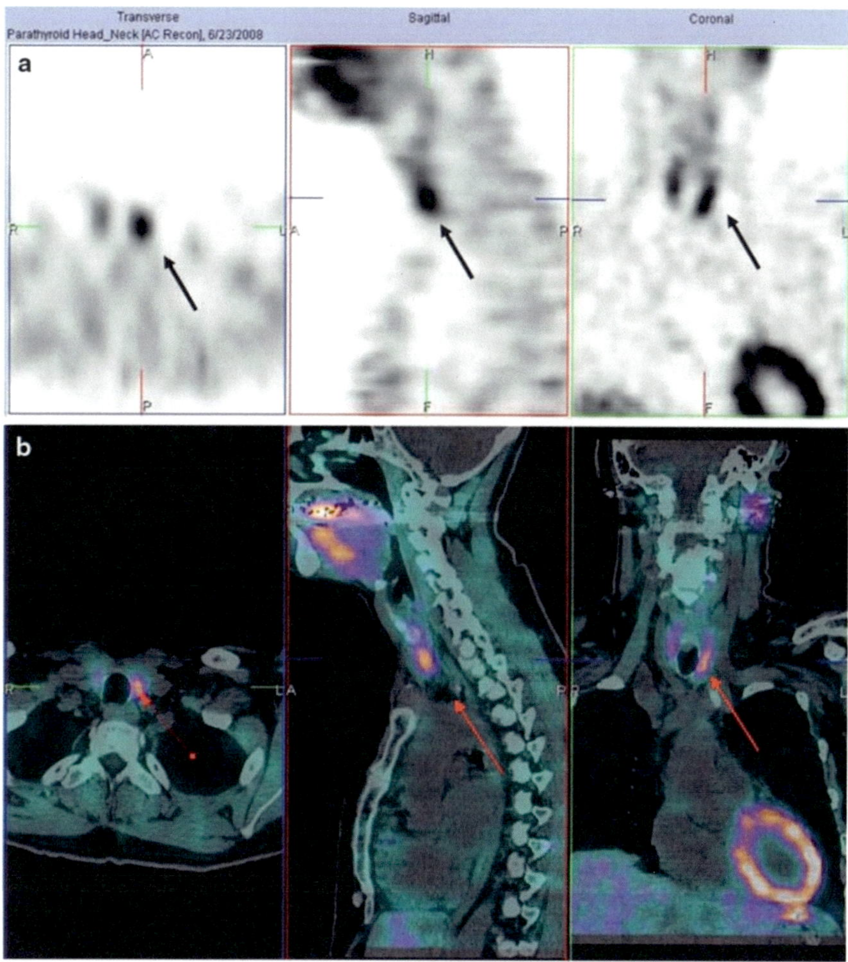

Fig. 2.4 Patient 1 technetium-99 m sestamibi (Tc-99 m MIBI). (**a**) Transverse, sagittal, and coronal static images of the neck and chest 30 min following the intravenous injection of 25 mCi of Tc-99 m MIBI demonstrate uptake in parathyroid adenoma (*black arrow*). (**b**) SPECT/CT images, obtained after the initial set of immediate postinjection images, demonstrate type E parathyroid gland (*red arrow*)

Nuclear Medicine

Routine serial static images as well as SPECT/CT of the neck and chest following the injection of 25 mCi Tc-99m MIBI demonstrated a focal area of slightly increased activity persistently in the left inferior thyroid bed on planar images (Fig. 2.4a). The SPECT/CT images demonstrated the increased activity corresponding to the small nodular density just behind or just below the inferior pole of the left thyroid lobe (Fig. 2.4b). These findings suggested a type E parathyroid gland.

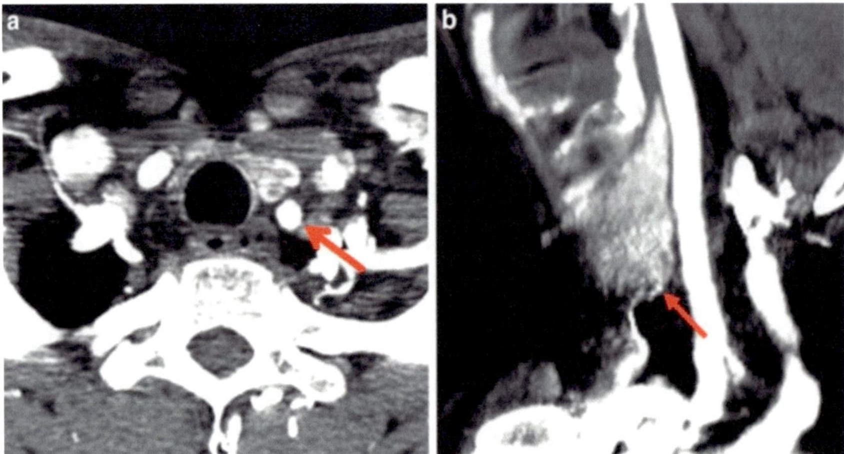

Fig. 2.5 Patient 1 4D-CT. (**a**) Axial postcontrast computed tomography (CT) scan reveals an enhancing parathyroid adenoma (0.8×0.5×0.9 cm) underlying the posterior surface of the left thyroid lobe (*arrow*). (**b**) Sagittal reconstructed maximal intensity projection (MIP) image demonstrates that the parathyroid adenoma is along the inferior aspect of the left thyroid lobe (*arrow*)

4D-CT

Postcontrast CT scan revealed an enhancing parathyroid adenoma underlying the posterior surface of the left thyroid lobe (Fig. 2.5a). Sagittal imaging demonstrated that the parathyroid adenoma was located along the inferior aspect of the left thyroid lobe consistent with a type E parathyroid adenoma (Fig. 2.5b).

Surgical Procedure

Combining the data from all the studies, this lesion was found to be a type E gland. Both the CT and sestamibi studies helped demonstrate the anterior location of the adenoma. Directed parathyroidectomy was performed as an outpatient procedure under local anesthesia with intravenous sedation. A 2-cm incision was made just to the left of midline, and the left strap muscles were retracted laterally. An enlarged and hypercellular left inferior parathyroid gland was identified in the E position and removed. Five and ten minutes following parathyroidectomy, the intraoperative PTH level fell 80 and 83%, respectfully, and into the normal range. The patient experienced an uneventful recovery. Following parathyroidectomy, the patient's calcium (2.33 mmol/L or 9.3 mg/dL), phosphorus (1.23 mmol/L or 3.8 mg/dL), and PTH (35 pg/mL) returned to within normal limits. Her constitutional symptoms improved.

Comment

This patient has biochemical evidence of primary hyperparathyroidism. The combination of constitutional symptoms and the presence of osteoporosis are indications for parathyroidectomy. As illustrated here, the majority of patients with primary hyperparathyroidism can undergo a directed, anatomic, unilateral operation with a high degree of success and low morbidity using a combination of preoperative imaging. Rapid intraoperative assay for intact PTH can be used to suggest when to stop the operation. In patients with excellent preoperative localization, parathyroidectomy can usually be successfully completed using local anesthesia with intravenous sedation in the outpatient setting. Advantages of this approach include improved patient comfort and rapid recovery.

Primary Hyperparathyroidism, Type C Gland

A 54-year-old woman with a history of recurrent nephrolithiasis was found to have biochemical evidence for primary hyperparathyroidism, with a calcium of 3.13 mmol/L or 12.5 mg/dL (reference range: 8.4–10.2 mg/dL), an ionized calcium of 1.64 mmol/L (reference range: 1.13–1.32 mmol/L), a phosphorus of 0.52 mmol/L or 1.6 mg/dL(reference range: 2.5–4.5 mg/dL), and an intact PTH of 435 pg/mL (reference range: 9–80 pg/mL). She was hospitalized, given intravenous fluid resuscitation, and referred for surgical consultation.

Imaging Studies

Ultrasound

Real-time sonographic examination demonstrated a nodule in the left paraesophageal region posterior to the left lobe of the thyroid and extending inferiorly (Fig. 2.6a). Correlation with 4D-CT and nuclear scanned confirmed that this represented a parathyroid adenoma. The sonographic evaluation also demonstrated a multinodular thyroid gland. The dominant nodules in the right and left lobe (Fig. 2.6b) were documented as benign colloid nodules by US-guided FNA.

Nuclear Medicine

There was avid focal tracer accumulation in a 3×1-cm soft tissue mass seen in the left paraesophageal region in the tracheoesophageal groove, extending from the lower pole of the left thyroid lobe to below the thyroid gland on both planar images and SPECT/CT (Fig. 2.7a, b). This finding was consistent with a large parathyroid adenoma in the C location.

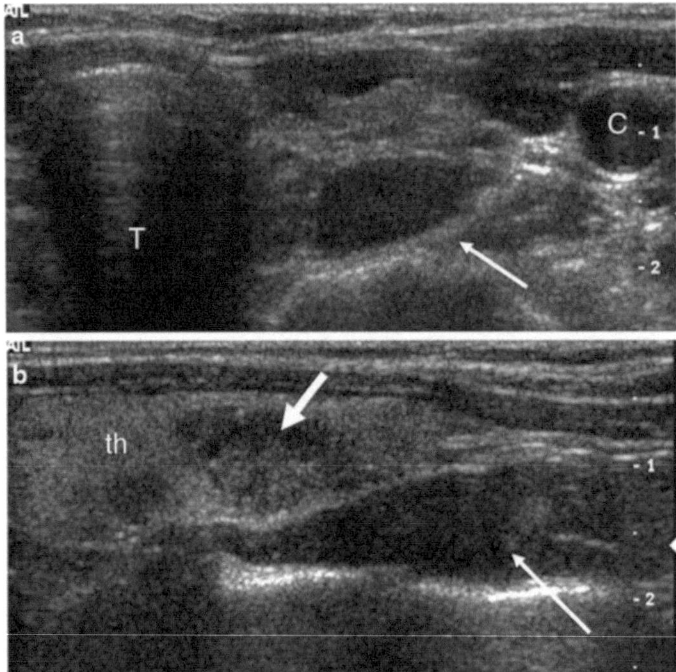

Fig. 2.6 Patient 2 US. (**a**) US image in the transverse plane demonstrates a parathyroid adenoma (3.2×1.3×0.9 cm) (*arrow*) in the paraesophageal region inferior to the left thyroid lobe lateral to the trachea (T) and medial to the carotid (C) that correlates with the position of the parathyroid adenoma documented on 4D-CT. (**b**) US image in the longitudinal plane demonstrates the parathyroid adenoma (*thin arrow*) inferior and posterior to the left thyroid (*th*). Incidental note is made of a multinodular thyroid. The dominant nodules in the right (0.8 cm) and left lobe of the thyroid (1.4 cm) (*thick arrows*) were documented as colloid nodules on US-guided biopsy prior to the MIP

Four-Dimensional Computed Tomography

Axial noncontrast CT showed a soft tissue attenuation parathyroid adenoma (3.4×1.4×0.9 cm) separate and posterior to the left thyroid lobe (Fig. 2.8a) along the paraesophageal region. Notice that the adenoma was lower in density relative to the thyroid gland. Following contrast administration, the parathyroid adenoma enhanced avidly during the arterial phase of the contrast bolus, almost the same attenuation as the thyroid gland (Fig. 2.8b). However, on the later phase of the study, contrast had washed out quickly from the adenomatous parathyroid and it was lower in attenuation relative to the thyroid gland (Fig. 2.8c). This is the characteristic enhancement pattern that we look for in a hyperfunctioning parathyroid gland. Coronal and sagittal reconstructed MIP images nicely demonstrated the parathyroid adenoma relative to the thyroid gland and adjacent structures (Fig. 2.8d, e). With the reconstructed images, the parathyroid adenoma was identified in all three planes.

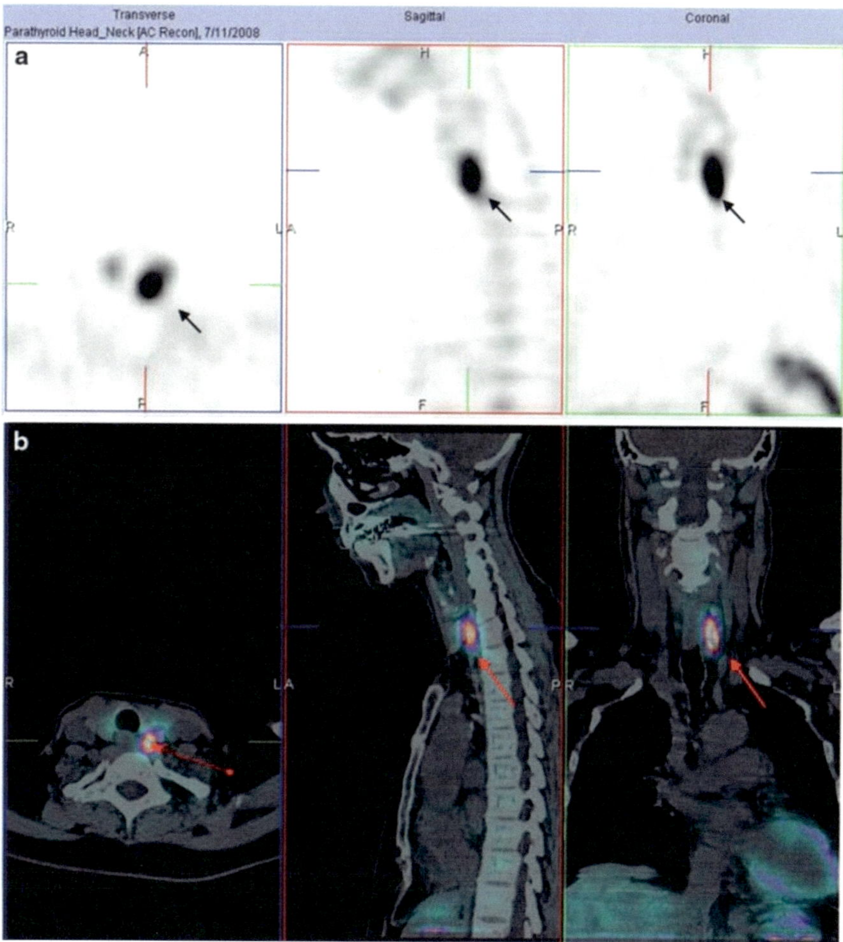

Fig. 2.7 Patient 2 technetium-99 m sestamibi (Tc-99 m MIBI). (**a**) Transverse, sagittal, and coronal static images of the neck and chest 30 min following the intravenous injection of 30 mCi of Tc-99 m MIBI demonstrate avid focal tracer in left paraesophageal region in the tracheoesophageal groove (*arrow*). (**b**) SPECT/CT images, obtained after the initial set of immediate postinjection images, demonstrate type C parathyroid adenoma (*red arrow*)

Surgical Intervention

Combining the data from all the studies, this lesion was thought to be a type C gland and the identified thyroid nodules were known to be benign by FNA. A DP was an appropriate option and the planned approach was a left lateral 2-cm incision with the focal area of interest posterior and inferior in the tracheoesophageal groove. At operation, an enlarged left superior parathyroid gland was identified in

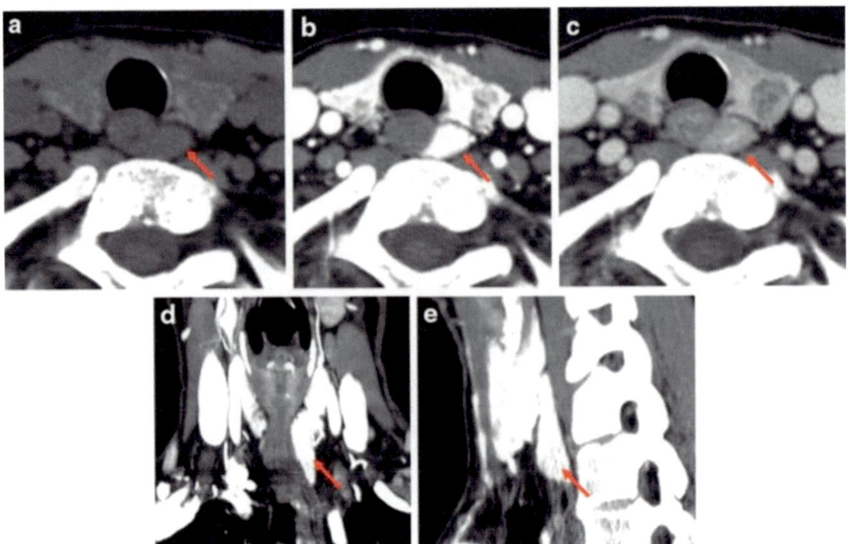

Fig. 2.8 Patient 2 CT. (**a**) Axial noncontrast CT shows a soft tissue attenuation parathyroid adenoma separate and posterior to the left thyroid lobe (*arrow*) along the paraesophageal region. (**b**) Following contrast administration, the parathyroid adenoma enhances avidly during the arterial phase of the contrast bolus. (**c**) On the later phase of the study, contrast has washed out quickly from the adenomatous parathyroid (*arrow*). (**d**) Coronal reconstructed MIP images demonstrate the parathyroid adenoma relative to the thyroid gland and adjacent structures. (**e**) Sagittal reconstructed MIP images demonstrate the parathyroid adenoma relative to the thyroid gland and adjacent structures

the tracheoesophageal groove at the cranial-caudal level of the inferior thyroid pole (Fig. 2.9). A nodular thyroid was encountered without obvious cancer. Following excision of the right superior parathyroid gland, the intraoperative PTH level fell 78 and 85% and into the normal range, 5 and 10 min, respectively.

Comment

Patients with advanced hypercalcemia require medical intervention. Medical management for severe hypercalcemic situations (usually defined as serum calcium >14.0 mg/dL) includes vigorous hydration and salt loading. These correct the initial crisis, but parathyroidectomy is the definitive cure. In this case, the ultrasonographic finding of a multinodular thyroid required preoperative FNA to rule out concomitant thyroid cancer. Thyroid nodules are common in patients with hyperparathyroidism, with or without a history of neck irradiation. Preoperative ultrasound is usually superior to physical examination for definitive diagnosis of thyroid nodules. It allows for directed assessment via FNAB of dominant or suspicious nodules in the outpatient setting so that appropriate treatment planning can occur prior to surgical intervention [6, 7].

Fig. 2.9 Patient 2.
Parathyroid gland placed
on a template in the left C
position

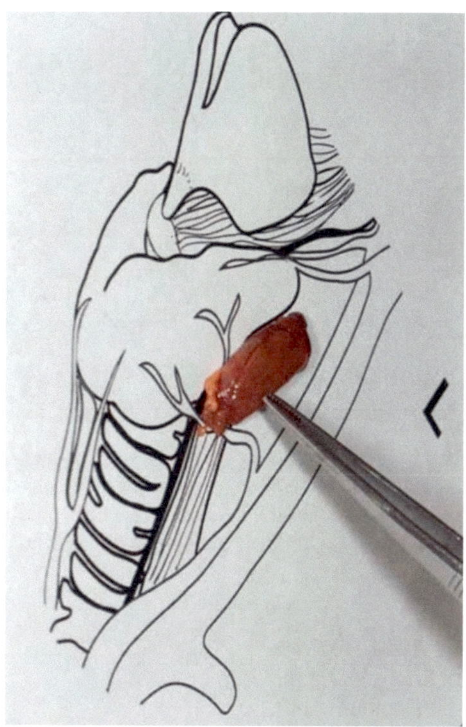

Primary Hyperparathyroidism and a Missing Parathyroid Gland, Type B Gland

An 83-year-old woman with hypertension, diabetes mellitus, and mild chronic renal insufficiency (blood urea nitrogen 11.78 mmol/L or 33 mg/dL [normal range 8–20 mg/dL], creatinine 114.39 μmol/L or 1.5 mg/dL [reference range: 0.8–1.5 mg/dL]) presented with biochemical evidence for primary hyperparathyroidism. The patient's calcium was 3 mmol/L or 12.0 mg/dL (reference range: 8.4–10.2 mg/dL), ionized calcium was 1.34 mmol/L(reference range: 1.13–1.32 mmol/L), phosphorus was 1.07 mmol/L or 3.3 mg/dL (reference range: 2.5–4.5 mg/dL), intact PTH was 133 pg/mL (reference range: 10–65 pg/mL), and urinary calcium was 200 mg/24 h (reference range: <150 mg/24 h). She had undergone prior cervical exploration with an inability to locate an enlarged parathyroid gland. She subsequently underwent a failed reoperative cervical exploration. She presented with biochemically proven persistent disease. Of note, she also had a remote history of thyroid gland ablation with radioiodine for thyrotoxicosis 45 years prior to this presentation. Given her prior cervical procedures, repeat imaging and video stroboscopy to evaluate vocal cord function were performed.

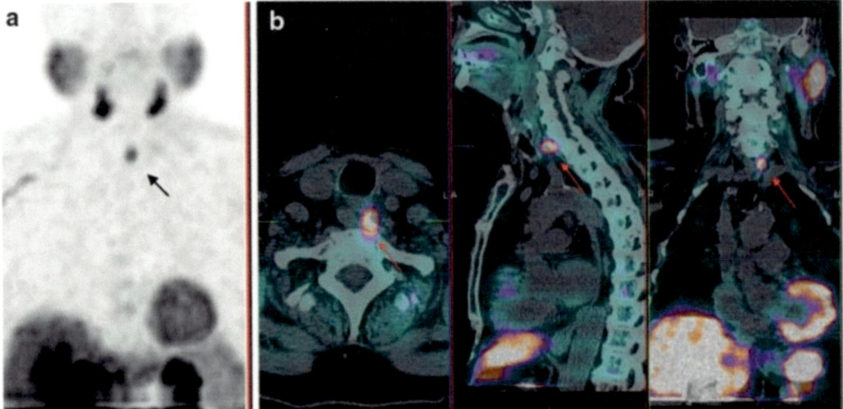

Fig. 2.10 (**a**) Patient 3 technetium-99 m sestamibi (Tc-99 m MIBI). On the planar transverse view, there is a focus of persistent Tc-99 m MIBI uptake in the lower thyroid bed region (*arrow*). (**b**) On the SPECT/CT images, the parathyroid gland is located immediately posterior to the esophagus, and, therefore, immediately anterior to the vertebral body (of T1 vertebra)

Imaging Studies

Ultrasound

Sonographic examination did not identify a parathyroid adenoma. The thyroid gland was unremarkable.

Nuclear Medicine

On the planar anterior view, there was a focus of persistent Tc-99 m MIBI uptake in the lower thyroid bed region (Fig. 2.10a). On the SPECT/CT images (Fig. 2.10b), the parathyroid gland was located immediately posterior to the esophagus, and, therefore, immediately anterior to the vertebral body (of T1 vertebra). This position was consistent with a type C gland. In addition, the right carotid artery was immediately lateral to the parathyroid adenoma.

4D-CT

Axial noncontrast CT showed a soft tissue attenuation parathyroid adenoma (0.9×0.5×1.9 cm) in the retroesophageal region (Fig. 2.11a). Of note was evidence of the previous total thyroidectomy. Following contrast administration, the parathyroid adenoma showed early enhancement (Fig. 2.11b) and early washout (Fig. 2.11c).

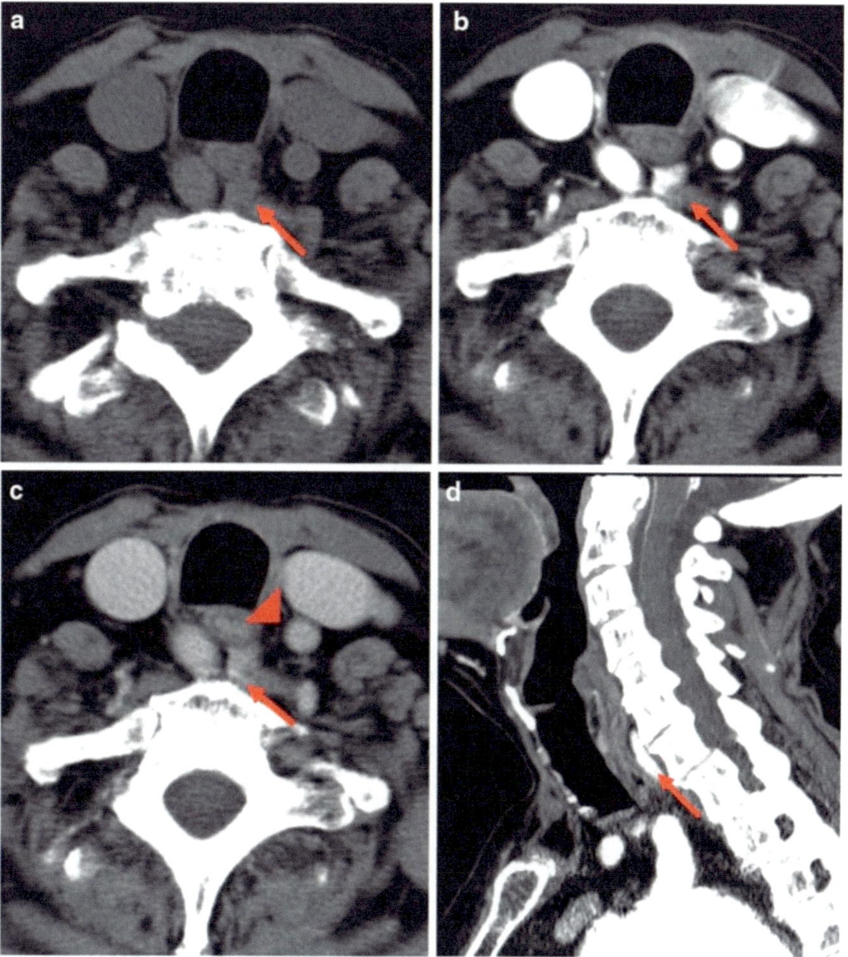

Fig. 2.11 Patient 3 CT. (**a**) Axial noncontrast CT shows a soft tissue attenuation parathyroid adenoma ($0.9 \times 0.5 \times 1.9$ cm) in the retroesophageal region (*arrow*). Note that the patient has had total thyroidectomy. (**b**) Following contrast administration, the parathyroid adenoma shows early enhancement (*arrow*). (**c**) Following contrast administration, the parathyroid adenoma shows early washout (*arrow*). Note the left common carotid artery (*arrowhead*). (**d**) Sagittal reconstructed MIP images demonstrate the parathyroid adenoma anterior to the C5 and C6 vertebral bodies (*arrow*)

This parathyroid adenoma was fairly deep in position, located posterior to the left common carotid artery and anterior to the vertebral body. Sagittal reconstructed MIP images demonstrated the parathyroid adenoma anterior to the C5 and C6 vertebral bodies (Fig. 2.11d).

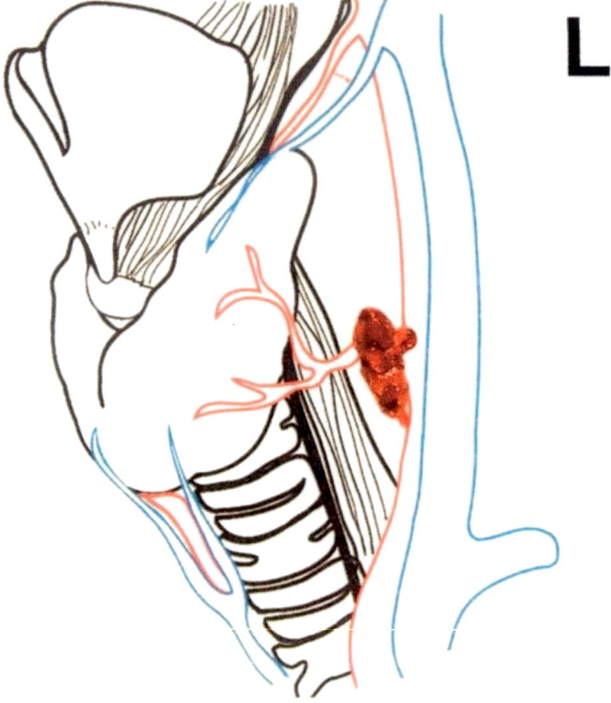

Fig. 2.12 Patient 3. Parathyroid gland placed on a template in the left B position

Surgical Intervention

In this case, the parathyroid adenoma was exceedingly posterior. This position was not capable of being visualized by ultrasonography. Both the 4D-CT and SPECT/CT helped localize this gland posterior to the esophagus in a type B position. A large, hypercellular parathyroid adenoma located posterior to the esophagus and immediately anterior to the cervical spine was resected via her previous Kocher collar incision. Her localizing studies were consistent with a type B gland (Fig. 2.12). PTH values dropped 77 and 86% and into the normal range, 5 and 10 min, respectively, following excision.

Comment

This case is an example of the value of being able to perform complimentary localization studies that are useful for surgical planning. Reoperative cases should have a minimum of two concomitant, concordant studies. The midline, posterior position of this gland was appreciated on both the 4D and SPECT/CT. In this reoperative setting, the clarity of the preoperative localization allowed for a direct approach with no unnecessary blind dissection amid intense scar tissue. We feel strongly that a thorough knowledge of the coexisting anatomy and precise gland localization is beneficial and cost-effective because it minimizes dissection, operative time, and hospital length of stay. Although difficult to quantify, each minute of dissection in the operating room with a patient under general anesthesia is costly. In addition, if a bilateral exploration is required, the necessary overnight observation as a caution against airway compromise from a postoperative bleed is an additional expense. This compares to accurate imaging and a directed approach which offer same day discharge. Actual billing and charges vary and are not easily trackable. Recent estimated costs of a cervical ultrasonographic examination is $300; Sestamibi scan $2,000, and 4D-CT $1,800. These may indeed be cheaper than the estimated $100 per minute of operating room costs if accurate imaging is not available and a more extensive dissection is necessary. In reoperations, the morbidity and the associated cost of managing aparathyroidism or RLN injury certainly supports concomitant concordant imaging to be cost-effective.

References

1. Adler JT, Sippel RS, Chen H. The Influence of surgical approach on quality of life after parathyroid surgery. Ann Surg Oncol. 2008;15(6):1559–65.
2. Chen H, Sokoll LJ, Udelsman R. Outpatient minimally invasive parathyroidectomy: a combination of sestamibi-SPECT localization, cervical block anesthesia, and intraoperative parathyroid hormone assay. Surgery. 1999;126(6):1016–21. discussion 1021–22.
3. Wang C. The anatomic basis of parathyroid surgery. Ann Surg. 1976;183(3):271–5.
4. Monroe DP, Edeiken-Monroe BS, Lee JE, Evans DB, Perrier ND. Impact of preoperative thyroid ultrasonography on the surgical management of primary hyperparathyroidism. Br J Surg. 2008;95(8):957–60.
5. Gilat H, Cohen M, Feinmesser R, et al. Minimally invasive procedure for resection of a parathyroid adenoma: the role of preoperative high-resolution ultrasonography. J Clin Ultrasound. 2005;33(6):283–7.
6. Lloyd MN, Lees WR, Milroy EJ. Pre-operative localisation in primary hyperparathyroidism. Clin Radiol. 1990;41(4):239–43.
7. Milas M, Stephen A, Berber E, Wagner K, Miskulin J, Siperstein A. Ultrasonography for the endocrine surgeon: a valuable clinical tool that enhances diagnostic and therapeutic outcomes. Surgery. 2005;138(6):1193–200. discussion 1200–1191.
8. Frates MC, Benson CB, Doubilet PM, Cibas ES, Marqusee E. Can color Doppler sonography aid in the prediction of malignancy of thyroid nodules? J Ultrasound Med. 2003;22(2):127–31. quiz 132–124.
9. Mazzaferri EL, Sipos J. Should all patients with subcentimeter thyroid nodules undergo fine-needle aspiration biopsy and preoperative neck ultrasonography to define the extent of tumor invasion? Thyroid. 2008;18(6):597–602.
10. Patel CN, Salahudeen HM, Lansdown M, Scarsbrook AF. Clinical utility of ultrasound and 99mTc sestamibi SPECT/CT for preoperative localization of parathyroid adenoma in patients with primary hyperparathyroidism. Clin Radiol. 2010;65(4):278–87.
11. Shah S, Win Z, Al-Nahhas A. Multimodality imaging of the parathyroid glands in primary hyperparathyroidism. Minerva Endocrinol. 2008;33(3):193–202.

12. Gotthardt M, Lohmann B, Behr TM, et al. Clinical value of parathyroid scintigraphy with technetium-99 m methoxyisobutylisonitrile: discrepancies in clinical data and a systematic metaanalysis of the literature. World J Surg. 2004;28(1):100–7.
13. Stawicki SP, Chaar ME, Baillie DR, Jaik NP, Estrada FP. Correlations between biochemical testing, pathology findings and preoperative sestamibi scans: a retrospective study of the minimally invasive radioguided parathyroidectomy (MIRP) approach. Nucl Med Rev Cent East Eur. 2007;10(2):82–6.
14. Calva-Cerqueira D, Smith BJ, Hostetler ML, et al. Minimally invasive parathyroidectomy and preoperative MIBI scans: correlation of gland weight and preoperative PTH. J Am Coll Surg. 2007;205(4 Suppl):S38–44.
15. Biertho LD, Kim C, Wu HS, Unger P, Inabnet WB. Relationship between sestamibi uptake, parathyroid hormone assay, and nuclear morphology in primary hyperparathyroidism. J Am Coll Surg. 2004;199(2):229–33.
16. Ugur O, Bozkurt MF, Hamaloglu E, et al. Clinicopathologic and radiopharmacokinetic factors affecting gamma probe-guided parathyroidectomy. Arch Surg. 2004;139(11):1175–9.
17. Schmidt M, Thoma N, Dietlein M, et al. 99mTc-MIBI SPECT in primary hyperparathyroidism influence of concomitant vitamin D deficiency for visualization of parathyroid adenomas. Nuklearmedizin. 2008;47(1):1–7.
18. Mihai R, Simon D, Hellman P. Imaging for primary hyperparathyroidism—an evidence-based analysis. Langenbecks Arch Surg. 2009;394(5):765–84.
19. Merlino JI, Ko K, Minotti A, McHenry CR. The false negative technetium-99 m-sestamibi scan in patients with primary hyperparathyroidism: correlation with clinical factors and operative findings. Am Surg. 2003;69(3):225–9. discussion 229–30.
20. Haciyanli M, Lal G, Morita E, Duh QY, Kebebew E, Clark OH. Accuracy of preoperative localization studies and intraoperative parathyroid hormone assay in patients with primary hyperparathyroidism and double adenoma. J Am Coll Surg. 2003;197(5):739–46.
21. Erbil Y, Barbaros U, Tukenmez M, et al. Impact of adenoma weight and ectopic location of parathyroid adenoma on localization study results. World J Surg. 2008;32(4):566–71.
22. Sukan A, Reyhan M, Aydin M, et al. Preoperative evaluation of hyperparathyroidism: the role of dual-phase parathyroid scintigraphy and ultrasound imaging. Ann Nucl Med. 2008;22(2):123–31.
23. Barczynski M, Golkowski F, Konturek A, et al. Technetium-99 m-sestamibi subtraction scintigraphy vs. ultrasonography combined with a rapid parathyroid hormone assay in parathyroid aspirates in preoperative localization of parathyroid adenomas and in directing surgical approach. Clin Endocrinol (Oxf). 2006;65(1):106–13.
24. Pata G, Casella C, Besuzio S, Mittempergher F, Salerni B. Clinical appraisal of (99 m)technetium-sestamibi SPECT/CT compared to conventional SPECT in patients with primary hyperparathyroidism and concomitant nodular goiter. Thyroid. 2010;20(10):1121–7.
25. Krausz Y, Bettman L, Guralnik L, et al. Technetium-99 m-MIBI SPECT/CT in primary hyperparathyroidism. World J Surg. 2006;30(1):76–83.
26. Rodgers SE, Hunter GJ, Hamberg LM, et al. Improved preoperative planning for directed parathyroidectomy with 4-dimensional computed tomography. Surgery. 2006;140(6):932–41.

Chapter 3
Primary and Secondary Hyperparathyroidism Testing and Assays

Jean-Hugues Brossard and Pierre D'Amour

Keywords Hypercalcemia • First-, second-, third-generation PTH assays • Serum and urinary calcium in diagnosis • Serum magnesium • Serum phosphate • Differential diagnosis of hypercalcemia • Polyclonal antibodies • Intact PTH assay • Whole PTH assay • Nichol's PTH assay • Normocalcemic hyperparathyroidism • Capture antibodies • N-PTH • Pseudohypoparathyroidism • PTH fragments • Osteocalcin • Alkaline phosphatase • Biomarkers of bone remodelling

Once considered rare disorders, primary (p) and secondary (s) hyperparathyroidism (HPT), are now frequently seen in all parts of the world in relation to the development of routine total calcium measurement and the availability of accurate parathyroid hormone (PTH) and 25-hydroxy-vitamin D (25(OH)D) assays. Both conditions can present with a very different biochemical profile, but normocalcemic primary HPT (pHPT) can also be very difficult to distinguish from mild sHPT. In the following chapter, we analyze which biochemical tests are best suited to investigate and diagnose these disorders.

J.-H. Brossard, M.D. (✉) • P. D'Amour, M.D.
Department of Medicine, Centre de recherche, Centre hospitalier de l'Université de Montréal (CHUM)-Hôpital Saint-Luc, Université de Montréal, Montreal, QC, Canada
e-mail: jean-hugues.brossard.chum@ssss.gouv.qc.ca

A.A. Khan and O.H. Clark (eds.), *Handbook of Parathyroid Diseases: A Case-Based Practical Guide*, DOI 10.1007/978-1-4614-2164-1_3,
© Springer Science+Business Media, LLC 2012

Primary Hyperparathyroidism

The essential biochemical measurements required to diagnose and differentiate pHPT from other hypercalcemic conditions include Ca_t and/or ionized calcium (Ca^{2+}), PTH levels and urinary calcium. In given circumstances, the level of serum magnesium, 25(OH)D and markers of bone turnover can also be useful.

Blood or Serum Calcium Measurements

In most cases, pHPT is first suspected with elevated total serum calcium (Ca_t) concentration, measured routinely in asymptomatic patients [1, 2]. Even if clinically suspected because of recurrent kidney stones, bone pain, pancreatitis or a positive familial history, the first step in the investigation is measurement of Ca_t concentration. The main differential diagnoses of hypercalcemia are outlined in Table 3.1, and a well-conducted history generally helps to orient the proper diagnosis.

Most laboratories have Ca_t values between 8.2 and 10.4 mg/dl (2.05 and 2.6 mmol/L). About 45% of Ca_t is bound to serum proteins, mainly albumin (31.5%), and it is usually necessary to measure albumin for the correct interpretation of Ca_t values. Correcting for albumin concentration usually adds very little to simple Ca_t measurement in patients with pHPT, but can be very useful for an adequate evaluation of cancer hypercalcemia [3]. Up to 20% of patients with pHPT may have a normal Ca_t concentration, usually at or near the upper limit of the normal Ca_t range. These patients have been more readily identified among renal stone patients with hypercalciuria [4–7] and among osteoporotic females [8]. Their Ca_t may always remain normal or fluctuate between high normal and slightly elevated values [9]. When their Ca_t is normal, they are picked up on abnormal PTH values and must be

Table 3.1 Differential diagnoses of hypercalcemia

Elevated or inappropriate PTH levels
Primary hyperparathyroidism (adenomatous, hyperplastic, cancer)
Tertiary hyperparathyroidism (developing on secondary hyperparathyroidism)
Hypocalciuric hypercalcemia (familial or autoimmune)
Lithium therapy
Ectopic production of PTH by cancers (rare)
Suppressed PTH levels
Malignancy-associated hypercalcemia (PTHrP, 1,25(OH)$_2$D, cytokines, etc.)
Vitamin D-related (vitamin D or 1,25(OH)$_2$D-induced, sarcoidosis and other granulomatous diseases)
Endocrine disorders (hyperthyroidism, Addison's disease)
Others (immobilization, thiazide diuretics, vitamin A intoxication, milk-alkali syndrome)

distinguished from patients with normocalcemic sHPT [4–8]. When possible, Ca^{2+} concentration should be measured in these patients because it more accurately detects milder cases of pHPT [8, 9], but pHPT patients with both normal Ca_t and Ca^{2+} have been described [10]. The NIH consensus panel on asymptomatic pHPT did not recommend routine Ca^{2+} measurement as most physicians cannot access a facility that can provide an accurate measurement [11]. Therefore, Ca_t is mostly used around the world despite its limitations.

PTH Measurements

Three generations of PTH assays have been developed over the last 40 years [12] to distinguish parathyroid from non-parathyroid causes of hypercalcemia. The latter causes (Table 3.1) present with suppressed PTH levels, whereas the former causes occur with elevated or inappropriate PTH concentrations for Ca_t or Ca^{2+} levels.

The first generation of mid or carboxyl-terminal (C) radioimmunoassays is rarely used today to measure circulating PTH. This is because they measure mainly PTH fragments that until recently were believed to be inactive [12] and thus unrelated to patient condition. Furthermore, when compared with the second generation of Intact (I) PTH radioimmunometric assays, they are less able to distinguish pHPT from non-parathyroid hypercalcemia [13, 14], even when a dynamic range of reference values is applied [15]. This is related to the fact that chronic non-parathyroid hypercalcemia enhances C-PTH fragment secretion [16].

I-PTH assays deploy polyclonal antibodies directed against region 39–84 of the human (h) PTH structure to capture circulating PTH molecular forms and 13-34-directed polyclonal antibodies to reveal hPTH(1–84). These assays do not react with hPTH(1–34) or C-PTH fragments, like hPTH(39–84) or (53–84) [17]. However, we demonstrated that they react with non-(1–84) PTH fragments, like hPTH(7–84) [18]. These represent 20% of I-PTH in a normal individual and up to 50% in advanced renal failure [18]. With most I-PTH assays, the normal range varies between 9–17.3 and 54–72 pg/ml (1–1.8 and 5.7–7.6 pmol/L) [19]. The non-suppressible fraction of I-PTH secretion at the upper limit of serum Ca_t concentration has been defined at 10.5 pg/ml (1.1 pmol/L) with Nichol's I-PTH IRMA in the presence of normal renal function [15]. Various degrees of renal failure increase I-PTH levels [20], and thus a value of 10.5 pg/ml to separate parathyroid from non-parathyroid hypercalcemia can only be used in the face of normal renal function and may vary from one commercial assay to another [19]. When a dynamic reference range is used all patients with pHPT have abnormally elevated I-PTH values [15], even if they are within the normal range [15]. Normocalcemic pHPT is also predictable with this dynamic reference range in patients with Ca_t levels between 9.2 and 10.4 mg/dl (2.3 and 2.6 mmol/L) and I-PTH concentrations between 10.5 and 50 pg/ml (1.1 and 5.2 pmol/L) or above [15]. Most patients with normocalcemic pHPT fit within these values which vary according to the PTH assay type [10, 21].

More recently, a third-generation PTH assay has been developed to avoid detection of non-(1–84) PTH fragments detected by I-PTH assays [18]. These assays incorporate the same capture antibodies as I-PTH assays, but reveal antibodies specific for region 1–6 of the hPTH structure. They react with hPTH(1–84) but not with hPTH(7–84) [22, 23]. They also recognize a new form of hPTH(1–84) which is post-translationally modified in region 15–20 and reacts poorly in I-PTH assays with a 13–20 epitope [24]. This new form of hPTH(1–84), called N-PTH, usually represents less than 10% of immunoreactive third-generation PTH in normal individuals and less than 15% in renal failure patients [25, 26] but can be overproduced in some patients with pHPT, mainly patients with parathyroid cancer and patients with severe forms of the disease [27, 28], although this may not always be the case [29]. All these patients have been identified because their third-generation PTH results were higher than their I-PTH results [27–29]. Usually, third-generation PTH results are lower than second-generation PTH values in normal individuals and renal failure patients [24–26]. The normal range is from 5 to 40 pg/ml (0.53 to 4.2 pmol/L) in the first assay developed [22, 23], but has varied between assays from different commercial sources [29]. One study found the first third-generation PTH assay to be more sensitive in detecting patients with mild pHPT [30], whereas another did not [31] discern any difference between third- and second-generation PTH results in this regard. A recent review on the subject concluded that third-generation PTH assays are not better than second-generation PTH assays in the diagnosis of pHPT [31]. A similar conclusion was also reached at the third International Workshop on asymptomatic pHPT [11, 32].

Familiarity with one well-known PTH assay is probably the best guarantee of appropriate interpretation of PTH results. We must remember that hypocalciuric hypercalcemia, lithium-induced hypercalcemia and ectopic PTH production by cancers of various origins cannot be distinguished from pHPT on the basis of serum PTH levels alone.

Urinary Calcium Measurement

The main utility of urinary calcium determination is to differentiate pHPT from familial or autoimmune hypocalciuric hypercalcemia. Urinary calcium excretion in patients with pHPT correlates with the degree of hypercalcemia and is inversely related to the degree of renal impairment [33]. In familial and autoimmune hypocalciuric hypercalcemia, the calciuria is reduced in the presence of an inactivating mutation [34] or autoimmune inactivation [35] of the renal calcium sensing receptor. Ca clearance/creatinine clearance is <0.01 in hypocalciuric hypercalcemia but higher in pHPT [36]. Lithium-treated patients can also present with hypercalcemia and hypocalciuria [37]. Like the direct effect of lithium on Ca receptor inactivation in the kidneys, it remains to be demonstrated to which extent the criteria of <0.01 also applies to these patients.

Other Tests

25(OH)D measurement: In patients with pHPT, there is an inverse relationship between 25(OH)D concentration and parathyroid tumour size [38]. There is also evidence of a decreased 25(OH)D levels in these patients [39], possibly in relation to increased clearance rate [39]. Severe vitamin D deficiency in pHPT may be associated with lower Ca_t values, osteomalacia and fractures, and greatly improves with 25(OH)D treatment [40]. Severe forms of primary hyperparathyroidism are more prevalent in developing countries and are associated with lower 25(OH)D levels [41]. Severe hypercalcemia in patients with more serious forms of pHPT also impairs $1,25(OH)_2D$ synthesis in the kidneys [42]. Decreasing serum calcium with an intravenous bisphosphonate in such patients, while supplementing them with vitamin D, can result in lower PTH levels and improved $1,25(OH)_2D$ synthesis, with amelioration of their bone disease prior to surgery and easier management of hungry bone disease after surgery [27, 42]. 25(OH)D measurement is always indicated in patients with severe pHPT and patients may benefit from vitamin D therapy prior to surgery. More recent data also suggest that replacement of vitamin D in pHPT patients with vitamin D insufficiency may improve PTH levels, markers of bone turnover, without increasing Ca_t concentration [43]. More studies are required before routine 25(OH)D measurement is recommended in pHPT. A good practice would be to measure it, at least in asymptomatic patients to be followed medically without surgery to ensure that adequate levels are present.

Magnesium measurement: Magnesium is mildly elevated in about 50% of patients with familial hypocalciuric hypercalcemia [44], and should be measured if this condition is suspected.

Serum markers of bone turnover measurement: In pHPT patients with severe hypercalcemia, it may be useful to measure at least bone alkaline phosphatase to detect active osteitis fibrosa cystica. Appropriate therapy of these patients with bisphosphonate IV and vitamin D replacement prior to surgery facilitates the treatment of hungry bone disease after surgery [27, 42].

Secondary Hyperparathyroidism

Secondary hyperparathyroidism (sHPT) is a PTH-mediated adaptative process of maintaining a normal Ca_t concentration in the presence of non-parathyroid clinical conditions which cause hypocalcemia. These conditions are best identified by measuring Ca_t and/or Ca^{2+} concentrations, PTH and 25(OH)D levels. Other tests, like serum phosphate, creatinine, magnesium, urinary calcium and markers of bone turnover, can also be helpful. A list of conditions associated with sHPT appears in Table 3.2. Vitamin D deficiency of any cause impairs Ca absorption and renal failure impairs $1,25(OH)_2D$ synthesis and these are the main causes of sHPT.

Table 3.2 Differential diagnoses of sHPT

Altered vitamin D status
Vitamin D deficiency (malabsorption, insufficient intake, lack of sunshine exposure)
Accelerate loss (impaired enterohepatic circulation, increased catabolism induced by phenobarbital, phenytoin)
Impaired 25-hydroxylation (congenital, isoniazid, terminal liver failure)
Impaired 1α-hydroxylation (renal failure, vitamin-dependent rickets-type I)
Peripheral resistance to $1,25(OH)_2D$ (vitamin D rickets-type II, phenytoin)
Excessive calcium deposition in the skeleton
Osteoblastic metastasis, hungry bone disease
Excessive calcium chelation
Rhabdomyolysis, chemotherapy
EDTA, citrate, phosphate infusion or therapy
Increased PTH resistance
Pseudohypoparathyroidism, magnesium deficiency

Blood or Serum Calcium Measurements

sHPT exists in both a compensated and non-compensated state. In the first situation, the rise in PTH concentration is sufficient to maintain normal Ca_t concentration, and the condition is usually identified by elevated PTH measurement which must be distinguished from normocalcemic pHPT. In the non-compensated state, the rise in PTH level is insufficient to maintain normal Ca_t or Ca^{2+} concentration and the patient is hypocalcemic. This usually reflects a longer clinical course, a more severe disease and osteomalacic bone with an impaired Ca_t or Ca^{2+} response to PTH.

PTH Measurements

PTH levels are expected to be elevated above the upper limit of the normal range in all patients with active sHPT independent of the PTH assay type used. We review data on the two main causes of sHPT, vitamin D deficiency and renal failure.

Vitamin D deficiency: Changes in PTH secretion associated with vitamin D deficiency have been well-studied in dogs [45] before and after vitamin D therapy. Over a 2-year period of calcium and vitamin D deficiency, there was a fivefold increase in parathyroid function measured by I-PTH assay and evidence of a decrease in C-PTH fragment secretion relative to hPTH(1–84) [45]. With vitamin D replacement therapy over 19 months, parathyroid function as measured by an I-PTH assay decreased by half while measured C-PTH assay did not change, resulting in a twofold higher C-PTH/I-PTH ratio than prior to vitamin D deficiency, as part of an adaptation to increased residual parathyroid gland mass [45]. This suggests that an increased C-PTH/I-PTH ratio in patients with elevated I-PTH levels and normocalcemia may be a reflection of pre-existing sHPT with adaptation to increased parathyroid tissue mass [46], particularly when 25(OH)D levels are normal or when

I-PTH levels do not decrease with vitamin D replacement therapy. Obviously, this condition must also be distinguished from normocalcemic pHPT, where the C-PTH/I-PTH ratio would be expected to be normal in the absence of renal failure [16]. The lack of commercially available C-PTH assays makes the verification of these data difficult. It is uncertain if combined I-PTH and third-generation PTH assay could achieve the same result, but this could be tested. Variation of PTH results with assays from different companies makes the task even more difficult [19].

Renal failure: The sHPT of renal failure has led to the evolution of PTH assays over the last 40 years [12]. C-PTH fragments, with or without a partially preserved aminoterminal structure, are mainly cleared by the kidneys and accumulate in renal failure [18]. This has, in part, greatly complicated PTH measurements with the first generation of mid or C-terminal PTH assays as these assays mainly detected fragments, until recently, believed to be inactive [12]. Furthermore, the biologic effects of C-PTH fragments are opposite to those of PTH(1–84) [47, 48] and contribute to the PTH resistance of renal failure [49]. It was initially believed that the poor correlations observed between mid or C-PTH results and the parameters of bone turnover or bone biopsy results were due to the measurement of inactive PTH molecular forms. This has led to the evolution of PTH assay towards an assay more specific for the bioactive form of PTH namely PTH(1–84) [50–52].

The second generation of PTH assay, I-PTH assays, were believed to react only with hPTH(1–84) until we demonstrated that they also react with non-(1–84) PTH fragments, like hPTH(7–84), which represent up to 50% of I-PTH in advanced renal failure [18]. Nonetheless, these assays proved easy to use, covered a large range of PTH values and generally improved the correlation between PTH results and the parameters of bone turnover and bone biopsy data in renal failure patients [50–52]. However, as the intact PTH assay also captures non-(1–84) PTH fragments this may reduce correlation with parameters of bone turnover. This lead to the development of a third generation of PTH assays with a specificity for region one to six of the hPTH(1–84) structure [23].

Third-generation PTH assays not only detect mainly hPTH(1–84), but also N-PTH which may represent up to 15% of immunoreactivity in renal failure patients. The biological potency of N-PTH relative to hPTH(1–84) is actually unknown. Comparison of the PTH results obtained with second- and third-generation PTH assays indicates that the former are generally about 35% higher than the latter [19]. But, contrary to what was initially expected, correlations between second- or third-generation PTH assay results and parameters of bone turnover or bone biopsy results are either neutral or slightly in favour of second-generation PTH values [53]. Measuring only one type of PTH may not be adequate as both hPTH(1–84) and C-PTH fragments appear to exert opposite biological effects via two different receptors [47, 48, 54–56]. Attempts to take this into consideration by measuring both hPTH(1–84) and large C-PTH fragments like hPTH(7–84) (by subtracting third-generation PTH data from second-generation PTH results) and calculating an hPTH(1–84)/non-(1–84) PTH ratio has improved the correlation between bone biopsy and PTH results in one study [57] but not in others [58, 59]. Again, these differences are related to the use of PTH assays from different companies, giving different values [60]. More studies looking at hPTH(1–84) bioactivity as a function of the C-PTH fragment/hPTH(1–84) ratio are going to be required to see if this approach improves the correlation between PTH results and phosphocalcic parameters in renal failure patients.

Serum 25(OH)D Measurement

Measuring of 25(OH)D and 1,25(OH)$_2$D levels with vitamin D supplementation in dogs helps us to understand the differences between compensated (normocalcemic) and non-compensated forms of vitamin D in adequacy. In the former condition, the progressive decrease in 25(OH)D from normal to deficient values is compensated by a progressive increase in 1,25(OH)$_2$D level well above the normal range in response to higher PTH concentrations, allowing maintenance of a normal calcium concentration [45]. But, at a certain point, 25(OH)D becomes too low and 1,25(OH)$_2$D starts to decrease within the normal range, despite the higher level of PTH and hypocalcemia follows [45]. These findings are pertinent to the human D deficiency model and indicate that 25(OH)D measurement is the best marker of the vitamin D status. From a practical point of view, adequate 25(OH)D levels have been defined in two different ways using either calcium absorption or PTH level as a criteria. There is a correlation between calcium absorption and 25(OH)D level for values up to 80 nmol/L (32 ng/ml), suggesting that optimal 25(OH)D concentration should be higher than 50 nmol/L (20 ng/ml) [61]. The relationship between PTH and 25(OH) D concentrations is not a simple one and is also affected by calcium concentration of the diet [62, 63]. Most studies suggest that, in the presence of normal calcium intake, the inverse linear relationship between PTH and 25(OH)D levels exists mainly for values < 50 nmol/L (20 ng/ml) of 25(OH)D [62–64], but values up to 80 nmol/L (32 ng/ml) have been reported [65]. D deficiencies, 25(OH)D < 25 nmol/L (10 ng/ml), D insufficiency, 25(OH)D > 25 and 50 nmol/L (>10 and <20 ng/ml), have been defined by such data. While the relationship between 25(OH)D and PTH is relatively well-established in normal individuals, it is less clear in renal failure patients who, despite deficient and insufficient vitamin D levels in a large proportion of patients, show less of a relationship to PTH levels in many studies [66–70]. This is probably related to the defect in 1,25(OH)$_2$D synthesis in these patients which directly affects PTH synthesis and secretion [71]. 25(OH)D should always be measured when sHPT is suspected as patients benefit from vitamin D replacement therapy.

Other Measurements

Serum Phosphate Measurement

In compensated sHPT, serum phosphate is reduced but may remain in the normal range [45]. When hypocalcemia is present, sHPT is more severe and serum phosphate is usually decreased [45] unless advanced renal failure is also present. A low phosphate concentration reflects the influence of increased PTH concentration on urinary phosphate excretion. In renal failure patients with stage I or II disease, serum phosphate can be normal or slightly decreased in relation to sHPT [20]. In more advanced stages, serum phosphate is either normal or increased, even in the presence of severe sHPT, because of the impaired capacity of the residual kidney to excrete phosphate [20]. High phosphate levels promote the development of sHPT by impairing PTH mRNA degradation [72].

Urinary Calcium Measurement

Urinary calcium is decreased in sHPT due to rises in PTH levels. It is also reduced in renal failure patients in response to higher PTH level and in proportion to the diminished glomerular filtration range [73, 74].

Serum Magnesium Measurement

Low magnesium levels cause PTH resistance and may affect PTH secretion when severe [75–78]. Even when magnesium concentration is normal, the retention of an intravenous magnesium load has been used to confirm magnesium deficiency with effects on PTH concentration [79]. It should be measured when deficiency is suspected clinically.

Serum Creatinine Measurement

Creatinine measurement is indicated to asses renal function.

Biochemical Markers of Bone Turnover

Measurement of bone alkaline phosphatase is helpful to have an idea of the extent of bone involvement in patients with hypocalcemia and sHPT. It is also useful to follow the response to treatment in these patients. Osteocalcin measurement and markers of bone resorption may serve the same purpose.

Conclusion

With the previously described tests, the causes of hypercalcemia or hypocalcemia are easily identified in most cases. Ectopic production of PTH by cancer will always remain a clinical challenge as will the distinction of normocalcemic pHPT from residual sHPT. Long-term follow-up, clinical expertise in depth knowledge regarding the utility of these laboratory tests enable us to address these clinical challenges.

References

1. Harrap JS, Barley JE, Woodhead JS. Incidence of hypercalcemia and primary hyperparathyroidism in relation to biochemical profile. J Clin Pathol. 1982;35:395–400.
2. Lafferty FW. Primary hyperparathyroidism. Changing clinical spectrum, prevalence of hypertension, and discriminant analysis of laboratory tests. Arch Intern Med. 1981;141:1761–6.
3. Lacher DA. Comparison of nonparametric recursive partitioning to parametric discriminant analyses in laboratory differentiation of hypercalcemia. Clin Chim Acta. 1991;204:199–208.
4. Gardin JP, Paillard M. Normocalcemic primary hyperparathyroidism: resistance to PTH effect on tubular reabsorption of calcium. Miner Electrolyte Metab. 1984;10:301–8.
5. Johansson H, Thorén L, Werner I, Grimelius L. Normocalcemic hyperparathyroidism, kidney stones, and idiopathic hypercalciuria. Surgery. 1975;77:691–6.
6. Maruani G, Hertig A, Paillard M, Houillier P. Normocalcemic primary hyperparathyroidism: evidence for a generalized target-tissue resistance to parathyroid hormone. J Clin Endocrinol Metab. 2003;88:4641–8.
7. Yang AH, Hsu CW, Chen JY, Tseng LM, Won GS, Lee CH. Normocalcemic primary hyperparathyroidism in patients with recurrent kidney stones: pathological analysis of parathyroid glands. Virchows Arch. 2006;449:62–8.
8. Monchik JM, Gorgin E. Normocalcemic hyperparathyroidism in patients with osteoporosis. Surgery. 2004;136:1242–6.
9. McLeod MK, Monchik JM, Martin HF. The role of ionized calcium in the diagnosis of subtle hypercalcemia in symptomatic primary hyperparathyroidism. Surgery. 1994;95:667–73.
10. Hagström E, Lundgren E, Rastad J, Hellman P. Metabolic abnormalities in patient with normocalcemic hyperparathyroidism detected at a population-based screening. Eur J Endocrinol. 2006;155:33–9.
11. Bilezikian JP, Khan A, Potts Jr JT. Guidelines for the management of asymptomatic primary hyperparathyroidism: summary statement from the third international workshop. J Clin Endocrinol Metab. 2009;94:335–9.
12. Gao P, D'Amour P. Evolution of the parathyroid hormone (PTH) assay. Importance of circulating PTH immunoheterogeneity and of its regulation. Clin Lab. 2005;51:21–9.
13. Hackeng WLH, Lips P, Netelenbos CJ. Clinical implications of estimation of intact parathyroid hormone (PTH) versus total immunoreactive PTH in normal subjects and hyperparathyroid patients. J Clin Endocrinol Metab. 1986;63:447–53.
14. St John A, Davies C, Riley WJ, Kent GN, Brown RC, Aston JP, Weeks I, Woodhead JS. Comparison of the performance and clinical utility of a carboxy-terminal assay and an intact assay for parathyroid hormone. Clin Chim Acta. 1988;178:215–23.
15. Lepage R, Whittom S, Bertrand S, Bahsali G, D'Amour P. Superiority of dynamic over static reference intervals for intact, midmolecule, and C-terminal parathyrin in evaluating calcemic disorders. Clin Chem. 1992;38:2129–35.
16. Brossard JH, Whittom S, Lepage R, D'Amour P. Carboxyl-terminal fragments of parathyroid hormone are not secreted preferentially in primary hyperparathyroidism as they are in other causes of hypercalcemia. J Clin Endocrinol Metab. 1993;77:413–9.
17. Nussbaum SR, Zahradnik RJ, Lavigne JR, Brennan GL, Nozawa-Ung K, Kim LY, Keutmann HT, Wang CA, Potts Jr JT, Segre GV. Highly sensitive two-site immunoradiometric assay of parathyrin, and its clinical utility in evaluating patients with hypercalcemia. Clin Chem. 1987;33:1365–7.
18. Brossard JH, Cloutier M, Roy L, Lepage R, D'Amour P. Accumulation of non-(1–84) molecular form of parathyroid hormone (PTH) detected by intact PTH assay in renal failure: importance in the interpretation of PTH values. J Clin Endocrinol Metab. 1996;81:3923–9.

19. Souberbielle JC, Boutten A, Carlier MC, Chevenne D, Coumaros G, Lawson-Body E, Massart C, Monge M, Myara J, Parent X, Plouvier E, Houillier P. Inter-method variability in PTH measurement: implication for the care of CKD patients. Kidney Int. 2006;70:345–50.
20. Brossard JH, Cardinal H, Roy L, Lepage R, Rousseau L, Dorais C, D'Amour P. Influence of glomerular filtration rate on intact parathyroid hormone levels in renal failure patients: role of non-(1–84) PTH detected by intact PTH assays. Clin Chem. 2000;46:697–703.
21. Lowe H, McMahon DJ, Rubin MR, Bilezikian JP, Silverberg SJ. Normocalcemic primary hyperparathyroidism: further characterization of a new clinical phenotype. J Clin Endocrinol Metab. 2007;92:3001–5.
22. John MR, Goodman WG, Gao P, Cantor TL, Salusky IB, Jüppner H. A novel immunoradiometric assay detects full-length human PTH but not amino-terminally truncated fragments: implications for PTH measurements in renal failure. J Clin Endocrinol Metab. 1999;84: 4287–90.
23. Gao P, Scheibel S, D'Amour P, John MR, Rao SD, Schmidt-Gayk H, Cantor TL. Development of a novel immunoradiometric assay exclusively for biologically active whole parathyroid hormone 1–84: implications for improvement of accurate assessment of parathyroid function. J Bone Miner Res. 2001;16:605–14.
24. D'Amour P, Brossard JH, Rousseau L, Roy L, Gao P, Cantor T. Amino-terminal form of parathyroid hormone (PTH) with immunologic similarities to hPTH(1–84) is overproduced in primary and secondary hyperparathyroidism. Clin Chem. 2003;49:2037–44.
25. D'Amour P, Brossard JH, Rousseau L, Nguyen-Yamamoto L, Nassif E, Lazure C, Gauthier D, Lavigne JR, Zahradnik RJ. Structure of non-(1–84) PTH fragments secreted by parathyroid glands in primary and secondary hyperparathyroidism. Kidney Int. 2005;68:998–1007.
26. D'Amour P, Räkel A, Brossard JH, Rousseau L, Albert C, Cantor T. Acute regulation of circulating parathyroid hormone (PTH) molecular forms by calcium: utility of PTH fragments/ PTH(1–84) ratios derived from three generations of PTH assays. J Clin Endocrinol Metab. 2006;91:283–9.
27. Räkel A, Brossard JH, Patenaude JV, Albert C, Nassif E, Cantor T, Rousseau L, D'Amour P. Overproduction of an amino-terminal form of PTH distinct from human PTH(1–84) in a case of severe primary hyperparathyroidism: influence of medical treatment and surgery. Clin Endocrinol. 2005;62:721–7.
28. Rubin MR, Silverberg SJ, D'Amour P, Brossard JH, Rousseau L, Sliney Jr J, Cantor T, Bilezikian JP. An N-terminal molecular form of parathyroid hormone (PTH) distinct from hPTH(1 84) is overproduced in parathyroid carcinoma. Clin Chem. 2007;53:1470–6.
29. Boudou P, Ibrahim F, Cormier C, Sarfati E, Souberbielle JC. Unexpected serum parathyroid hormone profiles in some patients with primary hyperparathyroidism. Clin Chem. 2006;52: 757–60.
30. Silverberg SJ, Gao P, Brown I, LoGerfo P, Cantor TL, Bilezikian JP. Clinical utility of an immunoradiometric assay for parathyroid hormone (1–84) in primary hyperparathyroidism. J Clin Endocrinol Metab. 2003;88:4725–30.
31. Souberbielle JC, Boudou F, Cormier C. Lessons from second- and third-generation parathyroid hormone assays in primary hyperparathyroidism. J Endocrinol Invest. 2008;31:463–9.
32. Eastell R, Arnold A, Brandi ML, Brown EM, D'Amour P, Hanley DA, Rao DS, Rubin MR, Goltzman D, Silverberg SJ, Marx SJ, Peacock M, Mosekilde L, Bouillon R, Lewiecki EM. Diagnosis of asymptomatic primary hyperparathyroidism: proceedings of the third international workshop. J Clin Endocrinol Metab. 2009;94:340–50.
33. Yamashita H, Noguchi S, Uchino S, Watanabe S, Murakami T, Ogawa T, Masatsugu T, Takamatsu Y, Miyatake E, Yamashita H. Influence of renal function on clinico-pathologic features of primary hyperparathyroidism. Eur J Endocrinol. 2003;148:597–602.
34. Pollak MR, Brown EM, Chou YH, Hebert SC, Marx SJ, Steinmann B, Levi T, Seidman CE, Seidman JG. Mutations in the human Ca(2+)-sensing receptor gene cause familial hypocalciuric hypercalcemia and neonatal severe hyperparathyroidism. Cell. 1993;75:1297–303.
35. Pallais JC, Kifor O, Chen YB, Slovik D, Brown EM. Acquired hypocalciuric hypercalcemia due to autoantibodies against the calcium-sensing receptor. N Engl J Med. 2004;351: 362–9.

36. Marx SJ, Attie MF, Levine MA, Spiegel AM, Downs RW, Lasker RD. The hypocalciuric or benign variant of familial hypercalcemia: clinical and biochemical features in fifteen kindreds. Medicine. 1981;60:397–412.
37. Miller PD, Dubovsky SL, Schrier RW, McDonald KM, Arnaud C. Hypocalciuric effect of lithium in man. Miner Electrolyte Metab. 1978;1:3–11.
38. Rao DS, Honasoge M, Divine GW, Phillips ER, Lee MW, Ansari MR, Talpos GB, Parfitt AM. Effect of vitamin D nutrition on parathyroid adenoma weight: pathogenetic and clinical implications. J Clin Endocrinol Metab. 2000;85:1054–8.
39. Clements MR, Davies M, Fraser DR, Lumb GA, Mawer EB, Adams PH. Metabolic inactivation of vitamin D is enhanced in primary hyperparathyroidism. Clin Sci. 1987;73:659–64.
40. Coen G, Bondatti F, de Matteis A, Ballanti P, Mazzaferro S, Sardella D, Smacchi A. Severe vitamin D deficiency in a case of primary hyperparathyroidism caused by parathyroid lipoadenoma, effect of 25OHD3 treatment. Miner Electrolyte Metab. 1989;15:332–7.
41. Mithal A, Bandeira F, Meng X, Silverberg SJ, Shi Y, Mishra SK, Griz L, Macedo G, Celdas G, Bandeira C, Bilezikian JB, Rao DS. Clinical presentation of primary hyperparathyroidism: India, Brazil and China. In: Bilezikian JP, Marcus R, Levine MA, editors. The parathyroids. London: Academic Press; 2001. p. 375–86. Chapter 22.
42. Brossard JH, Garon J, Lepage R, Gascon-Barré M, D'Amour P. Inhibition of 1,25(OH)$_2$D production by hypercalcemia in osteitis fibrosa cystica: influence on parathyroid hormone secretion and hungry bone disease. Bone Miner. 1993;23:15–26.
43. Grey A, Lucas J, Horne A, Gamble G, Davidson JS, Reid IR. Vitamin D repletion in patients with primary hyperparathyroidism and coexistent vitamin D insufficiency. J Clin Endocrinol Metab. 2005;90:2122–6.
44. Heath III H. Familial benign hypocalciuric hypercalcemia. Endocrinol Metab Clin North Am. 1989;18:723–40.
45. Cloutier M, Gagnon Y, Brossard JH, Gascon-Barré M, D'Amour P. Adaptation of parathyroid function to IV 1,25-dihydroxyvitamin D$_3$ or partial parathyroidectomy in normal dogs. J Endocrinol. 1997;155:133–41.
46. D'Amour P, Faughnan M, Paradis E, Lepage R, Ste-Marie LG, Brossard JH. An increased C-PTH level in a normocalcemic individual may reflect an adaptation to an increased parathyroid function. J Bone Miner Res. 1996;11(suppl 1: S493):T7361. Abstract.
47. Nguyen-Yamamoto L, Rousseau L, Brossard JH, Lepage R, D'Amour P. Synthetic carboxyl-terminal fragments of PTH decrease ionized calcium concentration in rats by acting on a receptor different from the PTH/PTHrP receptor. Endocrinology. 2001;142:1386–92.
48. Usatii M, Rousseau L, Demers C, Petit JL, Brossard JH, Gascon-Barré M, Lavigne JR, Zahradnik RJ, Nemeth EF, D'Amour P. Parathyroid hormone fragments inhibit active hormone and hypocalcemia-induced 1,25(OH)$_2$D synthesis. Kidney Int. 2007;72:1330–5.
49. Slatopolsky E, Finch J, Clay P, Martin D, Sicard G, Singera G, Gao P, Cantor T, Dusso A. A novel mechanism for skeletal resistance in uremia. Kidney Int. 2000;58:753–61.
50. Andress DL, Endres DB, Maloney NA, Kopp JB, Coburn JW, Sherrard DJ. Comparison of parathyroid hormone assays with bone histomorphometry in renal osteodystrophy. J Clin Endocrinol Metab. 1986;63:1163–9.
51. Cohen Solal Me, Sebert JL, Boudailliez B, Marie A, Moriniere P, Gueris J, Bouillon R, Fournier A. Comparison of intact, midregion and carboxy terminal assays of parathyroid hormone for the diagnosis of bone disease in hemodialyzed patients. J Clin Endocrinol Metab. 1991;73:516–24.
52. Coen G, Mazzaferro S, Ballanti P, Bonucci E, Cinotti GA, Fondi G, Manni M, Pasguali M, Perruzza I, Sardella D, Faggi F. Two-site immunoradiometric intact parathyroid hormone assay versus C-terminal parathyroid hormone in predicting osteodystrophic bone lesions in predialysis chronic renal failure. J Lab Clin Med. 1993;122:103–9.
53. D'Amour P. Lessons from second- and third-generation PTH assays in renal failure patients. J Endocrinol Invest. 2008;31:459–62.
54. Murray TM, Rao LG, Divieti P, Bringhurst FR. Parathyroid hormone secretion and action: evidence for discrete receptors for the carboxyl-terminal region and related biological actions of carboxyl-terminal ligands. Endocrine Rev. 2005;26:78–113.

55. Divieti P, John MR, Juppner H, Bringhurst FR. Human PTH-(7–84) inhibits bone resorption in vitro via actions independent of the type 1 PTH/PTHrP receptor. Endocrinology. 2002;143: 171–6.
56. Divieti P, Geller AI, Suliman G, Juppner H, Bringhurst FR. Receptors specific for the carboxyl-terminal region of parathyroid hormone on bone-derived cells: determinants of ligand binding and bioactivity. Endocrinology. 2005;146:1863–70.
57. Monier-Faugère MC, Geng Z, Mawad H, Friedler RM, Gao P, Cantor TL, Malluche HH. Improved assessment of bone turnover by the PTH-(1–84)/large C-PTH fragments ratio in ESRD patients. Kidney Int. 2001;60:1460–8.
58. Coen G, Bonucci E, Ballanti P, Balducci A, Calabria S, Nicolai GA, Fischer MS, Lifrieri F, Manni M, Morosetti M, Moscaritolo E, Sardella D. PTH 1–84 and PTH(7–84) in the non-invasive diagnosis of renal bone disease. Am J Kidney Dis. 2002;40:348–54.
59. Salusky IB, Goodman WG, Kuizon BD, Lavigne JR, Zalvranik RJ, Gales B, Wang JH, Elashaff RM, Juppner H. Similar predictive value of bone turnover using first- and second-generation immunometric PTH assays in pediatric patients treated with peritoneal dialysis. Kidney Int. 2003;63:1801–8.
60. Kollar H, Zitt E, Staudacher G, Neyer U, Mayer G, Rosenkranz AR. Variable parathyroid hormone(1–84)/carboxyl-terminal PTH ratios detected by 4 novel parathyroid hormone assays. Clin Nephrol. 2004;61:337–43.
61. Heaney RP, Dowell MS, Hale CA, Bendich A. Calcium absorption varies within the reference range for serum 25-hydroxyvitamin D. J Am Coll Nutr. 2003;22:142–6.
62. Steingrimsdottir L, Gunnarsson O, Indridason OS, Franzson L, Sigurdsson G. Relationship between serum parathyroid hormone levels, vitamin D sufficiency and calcium intake. J Am Med Assoc. 2005;294:2336–41.
63. Adami S, Viapiana O, Gatti D, Idolazzi L, Rossini M. Relationship between serum parathyroid hormone, vitamin D sufficiency, age, and calcium intake. Bone. 2008;42:267–70.
64. Souberbielle JC, Cormier C, Kindermans C, Gao P, Cantor T, Forette F, Baulieu EE. Vitamin D status and redefining serum parathyroid hormone reference range in the elderly. J Clin Endocrinol Metab. 2001;86:3086–90.
65. Lips P, Pluijm SMF, Smit JH, Van Schoor NM. Vitamin D status and the threshold for secondary hyperparathyroidism in the longitudinal aging study Amsterdam (LASA). Bone. 2005;36(suppl):S141. Abstract.
66. González EA, Sachdeva A, Oliver DA, Martin KJ. Vitamin D insufficiency and deficiency in chronic kidney disease. Am J Nephrol. 2004;24:503–10.
67. Mucsi I, Almási C, Deák G, Marton A, Ambrus C, Berta K, Lakatos P, Szabó A, Horváth C. Serum 25(OH)-vitamin D levels and bone metabolism in patients on maintenance hemodialysis. Clin Nephrol. 2005;64:288–94.
68. Taskapan H, Ersoy FF, Passadakis PS. Severe vitamin D deficiency in chronic renal failure patients on peritoneal dialysis. Clin Nephrol. 2006;66:247–55.
69. Zehnder D, Landray MJ, Wheeler DC, Fraser W, Blackwell L, Nuttall S, Hughes SV, Townend J, Ferro C, Baigent C, Hewison M. Cross-sectional analysis of abnormalities of mineral homeostasis, vitamin D and parathyroid hormone in a cohort of pre-dialysis patients. The chronic renal impairment in Birmingham (CRIB) study. Nephron Clin Pract. 2007;107:C109–16.
70. Saclier DM, Magee CC. Prevalence of 25(OH) vitamin D (calcidiol) deficiency at time of renal transplantation: a prospective study. Clin Transplant. 2007;21:683–8.
71. Naveh-Many T, Friedlaender MM, Mayer H, Silver J. Calcium regulates parathyroid hormone messenger ribonucleic acid (mRNA), but not calcitonin mRNA in vivo in the rat. Dominant role of 1,25-dihydroxyvitamin D. Endocrinology. 1989;125:275–80.
72. Moallem E, Kilav R, Silver J, Naveh-Many T. RNA-protein binding and post-transcriptional regulation of parathyroid hormone gene expression by calcium and phosphate. J Biol Chem. 1998;273:5253–9.
73. Robertson WG. Urinary excretion of calcium phosphorus and magnesium. In: Nordin BEC, editor. Calcium phosphate and magnesium metabolism. Clinical physiology and diagnostic procedures. Edinburgh: Churchill Livingstone; 1976. p. 120. Chapter 3.

74. Bringhurst FR. Physiologic actions of PTH and PTHrP. II. Renal actions. In: Bilezikian JP, Marcus R, Levine MA, editors. The parathyroids: basic and clinical concepts. San Diego, USA: Academic Press; 2001. p. 227–44. Chapter 14.
75. Estep H, Shaw WA, Watlington C, Hobe R, Holland W, Tucker SG. Hypocalcemia due to hypomagnesemia and reversible parathyroid hormone unresponsiveness. J Clin Endocrinol Metab. 1969;29:842–8.
76. Suh SM, Tashjian Jr AH, Matsuo N, Parkinson DK, Fraser D. Pathogenesis of hypocalcemia in primary hypomagnesemia: normal end-organ responsiveness to parathyroid hormone, impaired parathyroid gland function. J Clin Invest. 1973;52:153–60.
77. Anast CS, Winnacker JL, Forte LR, Burns TW. Impaired release of parathyroid hormone in magnesium deficiency. J Clin Endocrinol Metab. 1976;42:707–17.
78. Rude RK, Oldham SB, Sharp Jr CF, Singer FR. Parathyroid hormone secretion in magnesium deficiency. J Clin Endocrinol Metab. 1978;47:800–6.
79. Sahota O, Mundey MK, San P, Godber IM, Hosking DJ. Vitamin D insufficiency and the blunted PTH response in established osteoporosis: the role of magnesium deficiency. Osteoporos Int. 2006;17:1013–21.

Chapter 4
Symptomatic Primary Hyperparathyroidism Medical Therapy

Ghada El-Hajj Fuleihan

Keywords Hypercalcemic crisis • Acute management • Volume and sodium repletion • IV bisphosphonates • Calcitonin • Oral antiresorptive therapy • Medical parathyroidectomy • Phosphate therapy • Furosemide • Calcitriol • Pamidronate • Zoledronate • Thiazide • Lithium • Estrogen • Raloxifene • Clodronate • Etidronate • Residronate • Calcimimetics • Calcium-sensing receptor agonists • Cinacalcet • Angiographic ablation of parathyroid adenoma • Ethanol ablation • Nephrocalcinosis • Stone disease • Hyperparathyroidism

Introduction

The oldest published case of primary hyperparathyroidism is a woman who lived in what is now Germany, in the early Neolithic period, around 7,000 years ago [1]. Her skeleton showed pathognomonic skeletal lesions of symptomatic hyperparathyroidism, namely, generalized bone demineralization, scalloping of the phalanges, and "salt pepper" appearance of the skull, and histology revealed enhanced endosteal resorption. In 1948, Albright and Reifenstein described the clinical findings in symptomatic primary hyperparathyroidism dividing them into three categories: those due to bone disease detailed above, those due to diseases of the urinary tract, and those due to hypercalcemia per se [2]. The urinary tract abnormalities include a concentrating defect, nephrolithiasis, and nephrocalcinosis, and clinical findings due to hypercalcemia included loss of muscle tone, constipation, poor appetite, and weight loss [2]. The above classical manifestations of symptomatic hyperparathyroidism,

G. El-Hajj Fuleihan, MD, MPH (✉)
Calcium Metabolism and Osteoporosis Program, WHO Collaborating Center
for Metabolic Bone Disorders, Department of Medicine, American University
of Beirut-Medical Center, Riad El Solh, Beirut, Lebanon
e-mail: gf01@aub.edu.lb

A.A. Khan and O.H. Clark (eds.), *Handbook of Parathyroid Diseases:
A Case-Based Practical Guide*, DOI 10.1007/978-1-4614-2164-1_4,
© Springer Science+Business Media, LLC 2012

known as the "Bones, Stones, and Moans," reflected the severity of the hypercalcemia which went undetected until the development of these complications.

Due to the availability of routine, automated serum chemistries, the clinical profile of primary hyperparathyroidism in developed countries is that of an asymptomatic disease in the majority of patients. Some patients may suffer from neuropsychiatric, cardiovascular, and metabolic complications; however, their causal link to hyperparathyroidism is unclear, and the best therapy thus undefined. The management of such patients is discussed in the previous chapter. Currently, it is estimated that about 20% of patients from Western countries have symptoms; such patients usually have persistent elevations in their serum calcium level above 12 mg/dl [3]. Conversely, in many developing countries, where vitamin D deficiency is common and routine calcium testing is unavailable, classical symptomatic disease continues to predominate [3]. Indeed, in the two most recent series of patients with primary hyperparathyroidism from India, 50–80% of patients had bony pain [4, 5], fatigue, or proximal myopathy; Brown tumors were present in 58% [4], fractures in 23% [5], renal calculi in 42%, and nephrolithiasis in 12% [4].

Whereas the management of asymptomatic hyperparathyroidism continues to evolve [6–9], the optimal treatment of symptomatic disease with its classical complications is straightforward and has always been parathyroidectomy [2, 10–12]. However, few patients may present in hypercalcemic crisis, previously known as parathyroid poisoning [2], a life-threatening condition with very high serum calcium levels (usually, above 14 mg/dl) necessitating immediate medical intervention prior to parathyroidectomy (Box 1, [13]). In others, surgery may not be possible or desirable due to patient refusal, previous parathyroidectomy and persistent or recurrent hyperparathyroidism, or concomitant medical problems that increase the risk of parathyroidectomy.

In this chapter, we review medical therapies for symptomatic hyperparathyroidism, that is, treatment of symptomatic hypercalcemia in the acute setting, and then treatment of symptomatic hyperparathyroidism to prevent complications of the disease in the chronic setting. To date, no drug has been approved by the Food and Drug Administration (FDA) for use in primary hyperparathyroidism.

The Case

A 65-year-old woman presented to the emergency room because of anorexia, low grade fever, and constipation of few days duration. Her workup in the emergency room revealed a normal WBC count with a left shift; urinalysis was positive for many WBC, gram stain revealed gram-negative bacteria, and the urine culture 2 days later was positive for *E coli*. Her serum calcium was 13 mg/dl (3.25 mmol/L) with a normal albumin, phosphate of 1.8 mg/dl, serum BUN was 34 mg/dl, and creatinine was 0.9 mg/dl. CT evaluation of abdomen and pelvis revealed no kidney obstruction or kidney stones. She had a reported history of hip fracture with a fall from a standing height 3 years prior to presentation, and her BMD at the time revealed a T-score of −4 at the femoral neck and forearm. She also reported a history of hypertension, coronary artery disease status post coronary artery bypass grafting, and a history of recurrent urinary tract infections. Her medications on admission included allopurinol, zocor, lipanthyl, and hydrochlorthiazide. Her physical examination was remarkable for an intact mental status, positive orthostasis with a 15-mm drop in BP, tachycardia 100 beats/min, and dry mucous membranes. Additional studies revealed a serum-ionized calcium of 1.67 mmol/L (normal: 1.13–1.40 mmol/L), a serum-intact PTH level of 258 pg/ml (normal 10–76 pg/ml), and a serum 25-hydroxyvitamin D (25-OHD) of 8 ng/ml (desirable level >25 ng/ml); there was no shortening of the QT interval by electrocardiogram. Alkaline phosphatase was 145 IU/L. In summary, this woman presented with hypercalcemia due to hyperparathyroidism, dehydration possibly precipitated by anorexia (due to hypercalcemia), thiazide therapy, and pyelonephritis, in the setting of vitamin D deficiency. The thiazide was discontinued, and the patient was given antibiotics, intravenous fluids with 3 L of normal saline/24 h, and subcutaneous calcitonin at a dose of 4 units/kg every 12 h for the first 48 h; and oral phosphate was given as potassium phosphate at a dose of 450 mg tid for the first 5 days. She was also given vitamin D, as 10,000 IU of vitamin D_3 once weekly, when her vitamin D level became available 2 days post admission. On day 4 of her admission, her serum albumin-corrected calcium was 11 mg/dl (2.75 mmol/L) and her serum phosphate was 2.4 mg/dl. Therapy with intravenous zoledronate was considered on admission but deferred due to the hypophosphatemia and hypovitaminosis D, and then in view of the improvement in her serum calcium level with initial therapy. It was left to be considered as a future therapy depending on her serum calcium as an outpatient and once her vitamin D and serum phosphate levels normalized (to avoid severe hypocalcemia).

Medical Intervention in the Acute Setting Aiming at Lowering Serum Calcium Levels

The urgency to treat hypercalcemia is dictated by the severity of the hypercalcemia, the rapidity with which it developed, and ultimately the presence of symptoms, the latter being related to both parameters [10]. Symptoms of hypercalcemia include varying levels of altered mental status, coma, dry mouth, polyuria, constipation, and myopathy. In the case described above, the moderately severe hypercalcemia and dehydration, in an elderly woman with an acute infection, were indications to immediately lower the serum calcium relatively aggressively.

(a) *Volume and sodium repletion*: The calcium-sensing receptor (CaSR) is the key regulator of calcium homeostasis on a minute-to-minute basis, responding to increments in serum-ionized calcium by suppressing parathyroid hormone (PTH) secretion and enhancing urinary calcium excretion. Although the molecular basis of primary hyperparathyroidism is not secondary to mutations in the CaSR, direct or indirect stimulation of the receptor could be used to control the hypercalcemia. This receptor plays a key role not only in calcium, but also in water metabolism. Both hypercalcemia and hypercalciuria can cause a decrease in urinary concentrating capacity, which in some cases progresses to frank nephrogenic diabetes insipidus [14]. It is present in two nephron segments, the medullary thick ascending loop (MTAL) and the intermedullary collecting duct (IMCD). Its activation by hypercalcemia reversibly diminishes vasopressin-activated water flow by 30–40% in perfused IMCD tubules, and also directly reduces the expression of the aquaporin-2 water channel protein, thus further decreasing vasopressin-elicited water reabsorption in MTAL and IMCD. Furthermore, Ca stimulated CaSR-mediated diminution in NaCl reabsorption in the MTAL by reducing the medullary countercurrent gradient, further decreasing the kidney's urinary concentrating power during hypercalcemia [15]. Finally, the above vicious cycle is perpetuated by a decrease in the oral intake of fluids due to anorexia precipitated by hypercalcemia. The acute treatment of severe hypercalcemia, regardless of its etiology, therefore, consists of correction of the dehydration and total body sodium depletion with the administration of intravenous normal saline, and not half-normal saline. The total volume of saline used and the rate of its administration, in part, depend on the severity of the calcium elevation and are tempered by the cardiac and pulmonary status of the patient. Volume repletion with 3–4 L of normal saline in 24 h is not unusual, and in one series of eight cases of acute parathyroid crisis with a serum calcium between 14 and 18 mg/dl (3.5 and 4.5 mmol/L) patients received a mean of 16±6 L of intravenous isotonic saline [13]. Rehydration partially corrects serum calcium, depending on the degree to which the patient is dehydrated, and decrements of 1–2 mg/dl are not unusual within 24–48 h. Additional medical therapy (see below) would complement hydration to achieve and maintain normocalcemia. Although the use of furosemide along with hydration has been part of recommended algorithms to treat hypercalcemia in many reference textbooks and manuals, its efficacy in the management of acute hypercalcemia is not established due to the lack of randomized trials, and is unlikely in view of the pathophysiology outlined above. Indeed, such practice has been questioned by LeGrand et al. in a review of 9 articles describing the treatment of 39 hypercalcemic episodes in 37 patients using furosemide intravenously or orally, at doses varying between 240 and 2,400 mg/24 h and a mean dose of 1,120 mg/day [16]. The review revealed no consistent rapid effect with furosemide treatment [16]. The only study using oral furosemide at a dose of 40–60 mg/day failed to normalize serum calcium after 12 days [16]. In view of the above findings, loop diuretics should be reserved for subjects with or at risk for developing congestive heart failure while receiving intravenous saline infusions.

(b) *Phosphate therapy*: The pathophysiology of hypercalcemia and hypercalciuria in primary hyperparathyroidism is in part secondary to elevations in serum levels of $1, 25(OH)_2$ vitamin D. Hypophosphatemia is a well-recognized stimulus for elevated levels of calcitriol, and phosphate therapy may thus be a possible means to correct the above abnormality. Older studies using intravenous phosphate therapy have reported several serious adverse events, such as acute decreases in serum calcium, increases in serum creatinine, and extraskeletal calcifications, thus rendering its use unadvisable [17]. The latest detailed study, using oral phosphate therapy at a dose of 1 g/day for 1 year in ten patients with primary hyperparathyroidism and elevated calcitriol levels, revealed a reduction in mean serum calcium level from 11.7 mg/dl (2.75 mmol/L) to 10.7 mg/dl (2.62 mmol/L), a rise in serum PTH level (measured with a mid-region assay) from 243 to 497 nleq/ml, a mild but significant decrease in serum phosphorus from 2.8 to 2.5 mg/dl, a decrease in calcitriol level from 84 to 56 pg/ml, and a drop in 24-h calcium excretion on both a 400- and a 1,000-mg calcium diet, without any change in creatinine clearance [18]. Histomorphometric parameters showed a trend for a reduction in bone remodeling, but due to the wide variation in this parameter, it did not reach significance. Although no adverse events were noted in the above study, the very modest decrease in mean serum calcium level and the lack of information on long-term effects of such therapy on skeletal homeostasis render the use of oral phosphate therapy limited to select cases of severe hyperparathyroidism. These include cases with severe hypophosphatemia ($SPO_4 < 2$ mg/dl), possibly compounded by vitamin D deficiency, such as the case in our patient, and when used requires careful monitoring of serum calcium, phosphorus, and creatinine levels, aiming at avoiding reaching a $Ca \times PO_4$ product exceeding 60–65.

(c) *Intravenous bisphosphonates*: This family of compounds represents the gold standard therapy for hypercalcemia of malignancy and would be anticipated to have similar efficacy in severe hypercalcemia due to hyperparathyroidism. However, the experience with the use of intravenous bisphosphonates in primary hyperparathyroidism is limited. In a small series of nine patients with hyperparathyroidism and a mean serum calcium of 12.4 mg/dl (3.1 mmol/L), a single infusion of pamidronate at doses of 15–60 mg, normalized mean serum calcium levels by day 4 post infusion, and monthly pamidronate infusions for 6 and 9 months kept serum calcium levels at the upper limit of normal in two patients prior to reoperation [19]. In another report of two patients with hyperparathyroidsm, 90 mg of pamidronate decreased serum calcium by 4 mg/dl, where it remained normal for 10 days, and retreatment with 60 mg 2 months later again normalized serum calcium for a week [20]. Similarly, treatment of the second patient with two doses of pamidronate of 60–90 mg 2 weeks apart helped achieve near-normal calcium levels while awaiting surgery [20]. Two small studies using alendronate intravenously at doses of 2.5 mg daily for 5 days or 5 mg once showed modest decrements in serum calcium levels of 1.2 and 0.7 mg/dl, respectively [21]. Intravenous bisphosphonate therapy resulted in decrements in urinary calcium excretion, probably secondary to the decrements in serum calcium levels, and no change or modest increments in serum PTH levels [21]. There are no studies reporting on the use of zoledronate in primary hyperparathyroidism. A systematic review of 26 articles using bisphosphonates in the setting of hypercalcemia of malignancy revealed normalization of serum calcium in 70% of the patients, with a mean time to normocalcemia of 2–6 days [22]. Zoledronate, the most potent currently available bisphosphonate, was more effective than pamidronate in terms of proportion of subjects reaching normocalcemia and in doubling the median time to relapse from 18 days for pamidronate at a dose of 90 mg to 32 days for zoledronate at a dose of 4 mg [23]. In such patients, zoledronate at a dose of 4 mg would result in an average serum decrease in serum calcium of 3 mg/dl (0.75 mmol/L) 4 days post infusion and of 4 mg/dl (1 mmol/L) at 10 days [23]. Thus, a single dose of pamidronate 90 mg, or zoledronate 4 mg (extrapolating from the data in hypercalcemia of malignancy), would effectively lower serum calcium level by 2–4 mg/dl (0.5–1 mmol/L) in patients with symptomatic primary hyperparathyroidism. The onset of the drug effect starts 48 h post infusion, the nadir is 5–7 days later, with a possible need to retreat to maintain normocalcemia 2–4 weeks later. Zoledronate is readily available in many countries, can be administered over 15–30 min, and may have the added benefit of an anticipated maintenance or modest increments in bone mass and decrements in fracture risk, as would be relevant for our case, and had been demonstrated in women with postmenopausal osteoporosis ([24], Box 3).

(d) *Systemic calcitonin*: The onset of the antiresorptive effect of nasal calcitonin is more rapid than that of intravenous bisphosphonates, occurring as early as within 2 h of therapy [25]. Such therapy had been used concomitantly with bisphosphonates in malignant hypercalcemia to bridge the time between volume expansion and the onset of effect of intravenous bisphophonates, i.e., 1–2 days after which it is stopped [25–27]. Two small studies have used calcitonin in patients with primary hyperparathyroidism with a mean serum calcium level between 11 and 12 mg/dl (2.75–3 mmol/L) [28, 29]. The first study compared the efficacy of a single dose of salmon calcitonin given as 100 IU intramuscularly or intranasally at doses of 110, 200, or 400 IU to 12 patients, with monitoring for 24 h and a 3-day washout period between doses. Only the intramuscular dose lowered serum-ionized calcium, by 0.1 mmol/L (0.4 mg/dl), and resulted in a decrease in the area under the curve of that parameter, with a nadir at 8–12 h and a return toward baseline by 24 h post injection [28]. In the second study, a single dose of calcitonin 100 IU given intramuscularly was compared to the same dose used continuously as a 5-day infusion in 20 patients with hyperparathyroidism and a serum calcium level of 11.4 mg/dl (2.85 mmol/L). The peak and overall hypocalcemic response were greater with the continuous infusion, with a peak reduction on day 2 at 8 am, a reduction that was attenuated thereafter possibly due to tachyphylaxis [29]. Calcitonin at doses of 4–6 IU/kg given subcutaneously or intramuscularly every 6–12 h is approved for use in patients with hypercalcemia of malignancy, and results in a lowering of serum calcium by 1–2 mg/dl (0.25–0.5 mmol/L) beginning 4–6 h post infusion, an effect that is usually short-lived ([25], Box 4). Calcitonin can, thus, be used along with intravenous hydration and intravenous bisphoshonates for the initiation of a rapid reduction in serum calcium that can later be sustained with the delayed onset of the bisphosphonate effect.

Medical Intervention in the Chronic Setting

(a) Ruling out concomitant conditions causing hypercalcemia.

The evaluation of a patient with hyperparathyroidism and severe or worsening hypercalcemia includes ruling out concurrent conditions that could elevate serum calcium levels further (see Box 2), and treatment of these conditions would improve the hypercalcemia [30, 31]. Data from the Swedish registry revealed that patients with primary hyperparathyroidism are at increased risk of developing malignancies, with a reported standardized incidence ratio of 1.43[CI 1.35–1.52]; breast cancer accounted for one-quarter of the incidence in women, and colon, kidney, and squamous cell cancers were reported in both genders [30]. Similarly, a thorough review of the patient's medications is indicated. Subjects with normal PTH dynamics do not develop hypercalcemia on the daily replacement doses of calcium, i.e., 1,500 mg, used for the prevention or treatment of osteoporosis [32]. Those who do are likely to have an underlying abnormality in calcium homeostasis, such as hyperparathyroidism. Indeed, although the abnormal parathyroid gland(s) in hyperparathyroidism is (are) not totally autonomous [32], its physiologic response to an oral calcium load is partially blunted, resulting in higher serum calcium and PTH levels than in normal controls [33]. Drugs that may commonly unmask or worsen hypercalcemia in patients with hyperparathyroidism are thiazide diuretics or lithium.

Thiazide therapy: Although thiazides are less frequently used in the treatment of hypertension nowadays, they are present in several preparations in combination with ACE inhibitors or ARII blockers. Thiazide diuretics reduce urinary calcium excretion and have been associated with mild hypercalcemia (up to 11.5 mg/dL (2.875 mmol/L)). In a population-based study of residents of Olmsted County, Minnesota, the annual age and gender-adjusted annual incidence of thiazide-associated hypercalcemia were 7.7/100,000 [34]. The hypercalcemia was detected on the average 6 years after thiazide initiation, and was identified in 33 patients and persisted in 21 who discontinued the thiazide, 18 of whom were diagnosed with primary hyperparathyroidism [34]. Thiazides can, thus, unmask primary hyperparathyroidism; the latter is more likely when the initial serum calcium value is above 12 mg/dL (4 mmol/L), as was the case in our patient, or when the hypercalcemia persists after drug withdrawal [35].

Lithium therapy: Lithium is the drug of choice for bipolar disorders. It interferes with CaSR signaling, probably downstream of the receptor, altering calcium–PTH dynamics, but its precise mechanism of action is unknown [36, 37]. It, therefore, increases serum total and ionized calcium, serum magnesium, and intact PTH levels within weeks, but these remain within the normal range in most subjects [37]. Even in the absence of hypercalcemia, lithium can induce a defect in calcium–PTH regulation, raising serum PTH concentrations slightly and increasing parathyroid gland volume [37]. Ten to twenty percent of patients taking lithium develop hypercalcemia and hypocalciuria, and a smaller percentage have high serum PTH concentrations [37]. In a study of 142 patients on lithium for at least 15 years, the overall prevalence of hypercalcemia was 3.6%, and of surgically verified HPTH 2.7%, approximately 8 times that expected in the general Swedish population [38]. It appears that lithium therapy may unmask adenomas in patients with preexisting parathyroid lesions, if the hypercalcemia is diagnosed within few years of the start of therapy, whereas it may induce four gland hyperplasia with more chronic use [39]. If the lithium can be stopped without exacerbating the psychiatric condition, the hypercalcemia may resolve. Normalization of serum calcium is more likely to occur 1–4 weeks post lithium withdrawal in patients with a relatively short duration of lithium use (less than a few years), and is less likely in patients receiving lithium for more than 10 years [39]. In some patients, the serum calcium concentration may not fall for 1–4 months after lithium is discontinued [37].

In summary, if a patient develops hypercalcemia while on lithium or thiazide therapy, the drug should be discontinued and replaced by alternative therapy whenever possible. If the serum calcium level does not normalize several weeks post discontinuation, the patient is likely to have hyperparathyroidism and should be evaluated and treated accordingly.

(b) *Oral antiresorptive drugs*: The efficacy of oral antiresorptive drugs has been exclusively evaluated in patients with mild hyperparathyroidism, who were in large part asymptomatic, as detailed in the previous chapter. The results of such studies may, therefore, not apply to the symptomatic patient with more severe disease. Furthermore, these studies were unable to ascertain the efficacy of the intervention on hard outcomes of the disease due to the relatively small number of patients and short study duration.

Estrogen and estrogen-like therapies have been evaluated in postmenopausal women [21]. Ethinyl estradiol at doses of 30–50 µg/day for up to 20 months and conjugated equine estrogens in doses between 0.3 and 2.5 mg/day for up to 2 years have been shown to decrease serum calcium by 0.1–1 mg/dl, reduce urinary calcium excretion and bone turnover markers, increase PTH levels in some studies, and in the case of conjugated estrogens increase bone mineral density at the spine and hip in two trials [21]. Raloxifene at doses of 60–120 mg may reduce serum calcium slightly by 0.4–0.6 mg and reduce bone remodeling, but its positive effects on bone mineral density 1 year post therapy have been demonstrated in only three patients [21]. The increased risk of thromboembolic events and stroke with hormonal therapy and raloxifene, and of breast cancer and cardiovascular disease with combination hormonal therapy, renders such interventions suboptimal in older postmenopausal women with hyperparathyroidism.

Oral bisphosphonates, including clodronate, etidronate, residronate, and alendronate, have been used in patients with hyperparathyroidism, and have been shown to decrease serum calcium levels by 0.1–1 mg/dl (0.025–0.25 mmol/L), and increase PTH levels albeit transiently. Increments in bone mass at the spine and total body have been reported in one study using cyclical etidronate 400 mg, and at the spine and hip in several studies using alendronate at a daily dose of 10 mg for 1–2 years [21]. Although oral bisphosphonates may maintain bone mass, surgical intervention was more efficacious in reducing serum calcium, increasing bone density, reducing fractures, and improving survival in a prospective study of 33 high-risk patients with primary hyperparathyroidism [40].

(c) *Replacement of vitamin D in hypovitaminosis D*: Hypovitaminosis D is common in patients with primary hyperparathyroidism and patients with the lowest vitamin D levels are more likely to have higher serum levels of PTH, higher bone remodeling parameters biochemically and histomorphometrically, lower bone mineral density, and may be at higher risk for fractures [41–44]. In a recent review of this topic, Michail reported four studies, from Denmark, France, and the USA, that revealed a prevalence of hypovitaminosis D varying between 53 and 93%, a proportion that exceeded that of controls and varied depending on the country and cutoff used (20 vs. 25 ng/ml [45]). In a study of 124 patients with mild primary hyperparathyroidism from New York, 33% had a serum 25-OHD level less than 16 ng/ml and 66% had a level below 23 ng/ml [43], whereas only 13% of 39 patients from India had levels above 20 ng/ml [4]. The Panel of the Third International Workshop on Asymptomatic Hyperparathyroidism recommended the measurement of serum concentrations of 25-OHD in all patients with suspected primary hyperparathyroidism and initiation of vitamin D supplementation for a 25-OHD that is below 20 ng/ml [46]. Indeed, untreated hypovitaminosis D may have deleterious consequences to the skeleton.

It may be associated with a worsening of their hyperparathyroidism due to loss of the inhibitory effect of 1,25-dihydroxyvitamin D on PTH secretion and gene expression. Furthermore, in a retrospective study from India, the subset of patients who remained vitamin D deficient post parathyroidectomy were more likely to have delayed bone recovery, as assessed through improvements in symptoms or increments in bone mass [47]. Finally, it was recently demonstrated in a histomorphometric study of 30 subjects with mild primary hyperparathyroidism that low 25-OHD levels are associated with higher concentrations of PTH levels, greater catabolic effects on cortical bone, and anabolic effects on trabecular bone [48].

Caution against efforts to correct this deficiency using vitamin D doses that exceeds 400 IU/day has been recommended to avoid rendering the hypercalcemia and/or hypercalciuria worse [3]. However, a literature review up to July 2010 revealed that five studies reported on vitamin D supplementation in patients with concomitant primary hyperparathyroidism and vitamin D deficiency [45]. Three were prospective studies of 25–57 subjects, lasting 34–52 weeks, and two of which used oral doses of vitamin D of 50,000 IU/week for the first 4–8 weeks followed by various titration regimens. Vitamin D supplementation was in general safe, resulting in a mild decrease in serum PTH level with mean decrements of 3–25%. Notable side effects included hypercalcemia that occurred in less than 5% of subjects, and an increase in mean serum calcium in 2/5 studies [45]. It is worthwhile to note that patients in these trials had mild hypercalcemia (serum Ca < 12 mg/dl) and the studies lacked randomization and appropriate controls.

Therefore, in patients with primary hyperparathyroidism and concomitant vitamin D deficiency, it seems prudent to recommend an oral daily intake of elemental calcium that does not exceed 1,000 mg, and vitamin D at doses of 400 to 1,000–2,000 IU/day, depending on the baseline serum calcium and 25-OHD, with periodic monitoring of serum calcium and 24-h urinary calcium values. The efficacy of such therapy in increasing BMD and decreasing fractures, whether these patients are continued to be treated medically or surgically, is however not established. The recommended daily allowance of vitamin D estimated to cover the needs of ≥97.5% of the population is estimated by the National Institute of Medicine to be 600 IU in adults and 800 IU in the elderly [49]. Conversely, the Endocrine Society Practice Guidelines Committee recommendations for patients at risk for vitamin D deficiency varies between 1,500 and 2,000 IU/day daily [50]. Similarly, the recommended target desirable levels differ [49, 50], and none of these recommendations apply to patients with primary hyperparathyroidism.

(d) *Calcimimetics*: These are small hydrophobic molecules, allosteric activators of the CaSR that increase its affinity for ionized calcium through interactions distal to the cell surface domain of the receptor, and result in decrements in serum calcium and PTH levels [51–53]. Because of their reliance on the presence of ionized calcium for receptor activation, they are known as "modulators" rather than "agonists" of the CaSR. In patients with mild hyperparathyroidism, cinacalcet has been shown to reduce serum-ionized calcium level modestly by 0.05 mmol/L (0.2 mg/dl) and to reduce serum-intact PTH levels in a dose-dependant manner, with a reduction by 50% at the highest dose of 160 mg [54]. It was also shown to normalize serum calcium and result in similar decrements in PTH levels 4 h post dosing in a 2-week study at the highest dose of 50 mg bid [55]. In a multicenter randomized trial of 78 patients with primary hyperparathyroidism, cinacalcet at doses of 30–50 mg bid normalized serum calcium in over two-third of subjects and resulted in a 7% drop in intact PTH levels [56]. However, the lack of fracture efficacy and improvements in bone mass [56] has held its approval by the FDA for use in such patients. It is, however, approved for use in patients with stage 5 chronic kidney disease (i.e., with GFR <15 ml/min, who are generally on dialysis), as well as those with parathyroid cancer. In such patients, cinacalcet titrated to doses of 90 mg four times daily was shown to decrease serum calcium from 14.1 to 12.4 mg/dl (3.525–3.1 mmol/L) in the overall group and from 15 to 11.2 mg/dl in responders, without causing any major changes in intact PTH levels [57]. Cinacalcet is approved for use in primary hyperparathyroidism in Canada and by the European Medicine Agency in several European countries. It has also been shown to be effective across a wide spectrum of disease severity in patients with primary hyperparathyroidism [58]. Therefore, cinacalcet could be used to lower serum calcium acutely in patients with symptomatic hyperparathyroidism, but its effect on bone disease and stone disease in such patients is unknown. Indeed, when used at lower doses in patients with mild primary hyperparathyroidism, there was no evidence for a beneficial effect on these outcomes [56].

Medical Parathyroidectomy

Few studies have reported successful ablation of pathologic parathyroid gland(s) using the percutaneous angiographic approach with embolization or using ethanol. Angiographic ablation of a parathyroid adenoma has been used as of the mid-seventies to treat mediatinal adenomas medically, thus avoiding a sternotomy. It is conducted using ionic contrast material under sedation, only after confirmation of the pathologic mediastinal lesion by a combination of localization tests [58]. In a report of four patients with severe hypercalcemia and persistent hyperparathyroidism, angiographic parathyroid ablation of a single feeding vessel of the parathyroid adenoma resulted in a cure in all patients 22–68 months post intervention [58]. The most extensive experience with angiographic ablation of a parathyroid adenoma comes from a report of 23 cases of persistent hyperparathyroidism treated at the National Institutes of Health, where a success rate of 83% was reported at 1 month and of 71% at 9 years [59]. Similarly, angiographic ablation in 18 patients with symptomatic disease normalized calcium within 48 h, and resulted in a cure rate of 67% of patients, at a mean follow-up of 35 months [59].

Ethanol ablation was initially introduced for the management of parathyroid hyperplasia in the 1980s [60]. The original series of ethanol ablation in primary hyperparathyroidism was implemented in 36 patients at the Mayo Clinic because of high surgical risk from medical comorbidities, persistent disease post parathyroidectomy, or patients' choice [61]. Most patients had symptomatic disease and a baseline serum calcium between 10.3 and 13.4 mg/dl (2.575–3.35 mmol/L). They underwent ablation under ultrasound guidance, with one to three injections 1 week apart (mean 2), using a 25-gauge needle attached to a 2-ml syringe containing 95% ethanol; the volume of ethanol per treatment was between 50 and 70% of the gland volume (0.1–1.25 ml [61]). One-third of patients were normocalcemic at a median follow-up of 16 months post ablation, and 5.5% had recurrent laryngeal nerve palsy [61]. Failures occurred in patients where the nonpathologic gland was injected, in patients with multiglandular disease, and in those with an incompletely treated gland due to large size and spread of ethanol into the surrounding tissues. Thus, adequate preoperative localization, confirmation of parathyroid pathology of the suspicious gland by fine needle aspirate and PTH assay, and avoidance of ethanol extravasation are essential prerequisites for the success of such intervention. A modified, percutaneous, ultrasound-guided two-step procedure was recently described in two patients [62]. The first step was meant to create solid fibrosis around the capsule of the adenoma using 0.5 ml of 95% ethanol, being first performed in the posterior section of the adenoma, and then repeated five to seven times around the perimeter of the lesion at 10-day intervals. The second step was performed 2 weeks after completing the first step by injecting 95% ethanol at the center of the lesion using 80–85% of the volume of the lesion. In the first patient, serum calcium decreased from 10.4 to 8.0 mg/dl (2.6–2 mmol/L) at 1 month and remained at that level 45 months post ablation, and significant increments in bone mass were noted at the spine and hip. In the second patient, serum calcium decreased from 12.6 to 8.4 mg/dl (3.15–2.1 mmol/L) 17 months post ablation [62]. Although the experience with percutaneous parathyroid ablation using angiographic or ethanol is most abundant in patients with failed parathyroidectomies, it may be an acceptable first alternative in high-risk selected patients, provided it is conducted in centers with expertise in localization and ablation techniques.

Minimally invasive parathyroidectomy performed under local anesthesia may render surgical intervention an acceptable option even in high-risk patients due to its low surgical risks. Indeed, it was superior to medical therapy in a recent prospective nonrandomized controlled study of 33 high-risk patients in reducing hypercalcemic episodes, preserving renal function, reducing fractures, and improving the overall survival [40].

Conclusion

Symptomatic hyperparathyroidism is uncommon in developed countries but continues to predominate in regions, where routine biochemical screen is unavailable and vitamin D deficiency common, such as Asian countries. An evaluation to rule out concurrent conditions or drugs that can contribute to the hypercalcemia is important. Parathyroidectomy is the optimal therapeutic option in symptomatic disease because it decreases the risk of recurrent stones, increases bone mass, and may possibly reduce the risk of fractures. However, in patients who cannot or refuse surgical intervention, management in the acute setting includes volume repletion and high-dose systemic calcitonin the first 24–48 h, along with an intravenous infusion of zoledronate. This efficaciously reduces serum calcium by 2–4 mg/dl for 2–4 weeks, and would improve impaired neurocognitive function. Judicious replacement of vitamin D in patients with hypovitaminosis D is safe and probably beneficial. Medical interventions in the chronic setting have been evaluated almost exclusively in patients with mild disease who were in large part asymptomatic. These include antiresorptive drugs that could prevent the skeletal complications of the disease or drugs that lower PTH levels and have the potential to prevent both skeletal and renal complications of the disease. Antiresorptive drugs, such as hormone therapy, raloxifene, and bisphosphonates, for which the evidence is most abundant, may reduce serum calcium slightly and for some only transiently, reduce bone remodeling, and maintain bone mass. The calcimimetic cinacalcet is approved by the FDA for use in parathyroid carcinoma, but not in primary hyperparathyroidism due to lack of a demonstrable beneficial effect on bone mass, as demonstrated in trials conducted in patients with mild disease.

There is no evidence to date for efficacy of any of the medical interventions outlined above in improving classical outcomes of the disease, such as stone disease, nephrocalcinosis, or fractures, or any of its nonclassical outcomes. Therefore, parathyroidectomy remains the treatment of choice in symptomatic hyperparathyroidism, as outlined in the following chapter/section.

Box 1 Characteristic Features of Hypercalcemic Crisis (Ref. 13)

Biochemistries: Serum Ca > 14 mg/dl (3.5 mmol/L) and PTH levels several hundreds picogram/milliliter

Pathology: >80% of cases a single adenoma with degenerative changes/hemorrhage

Risk factors:

Concommittant infection
Pregnancy, hyperemesis gravidarum
Acute pancreatitis
Thyrotoxicosis
Thiazide therapy

Others: Postcoronary artery bypass surgery, herpes zoster, breast carcinoma, and schizophrenia

---

Box 2 Conditions to Be Ruled Out in a Patient with Hyperparathyroidism and Worsening or Severe Hypercalcemia*

Hypercalcemic crisis (see Box 1)

Concurrent Medical Illnesses:

Adrenal insufficiency
Pheocromocytoma
Hyperthyroidism
Milk alkali syndrome
Pancreatitis

Drugs

Thiazides
Lithium
Milk alkali
Parathyroid hormone
Intravenous theophylline
Tamoxifen flare
Vitamin A intoxication

(continued)

Box 2 (continued)

Vitamin D-mediated hypercalcemia:

Granulomatous diseases: Sarcoidosis, silicosis, tuberculosis, candidiasis, etc.
Exogenous vitamin D therapy
Some malignancies (see below)

*Malignancies***

PTHrP mediated: Squamous cell carcinoma
Calcitriol mediated: Malignant lymphoproliferative disorders
Local osteolytic metastases: Producing cytokines, e.g., multiple myeloma

*Overlap may exist between major categories: For example, thiazides are listed under drugs but are also a risk factor for hypercalcemic crisis
**Patients with malignancies are usually known to have the disease by the time the worsening hypercalcemia occurs

Box 3 Intravenous Zoledronate in the Acute Management of Hypercalcemia in Hyperparathyroidism (*Adapted from Product Drug Information from Lexicomp-UpToDate Version 16.3*)

(A) *Dose*: Zoledronate 4 mg in 100 cc over 30 min, can be repeated every 2–4 weeks.

(B) *Adverse reactions: Reporting those with a frequency > 1%*
Up to 44% acute-phase reaction (arthralgia, fever, myalgias, flu-like symptoms) usually resolves within 3–4 days, may take up to 14 days, pretreatment with acetaminophen prior to and for 72 h may decrease incidence; incidence decreases with repeated infusions.

FDA warning: Severe incapacitating musculoskeletal pain, different from acute-phase reaction above, occurring within days, months, or years after starting a bisphosphonate. Pain may completely resolve after stopping bisphosphonate or may resolve slowly or incompletely. Risk factors are unknown (http://www.fda.gov/medwatch/safety/2008/safety08.htm#Bisphosphonates).

Greater than 10%: Hypotension or edema, headache, dizziness, anxiety, depression, agitation, confusion, dermatitis, alopecia, hypophosphatemia, hypokalemia, hypomagnesemia, anorexia, nausea, vomiting, constipation, diarrhea, abdominal pain, urinary tract infection, anemia, neutropenia, neuromuscular symptoms as described above, renal deterioration (in up to 40% of patients with abnormal baseline creatinine), dyspnea, and cough.

(continued)

Box 3 (continued)

One to ten percent: Chest pain, somnolence, hypocalcemia, dysphagia, dyspepsia, mucositis, stomatitis, pancytopenia, pleural effusion, and respiratory tract infection.

(C) *Warnings*:

1. Concerns related to adverse events: Bone/joint and muscle pain, osteonecrosis of the jaw (<1%) mostly seen in cancer patients, less frequently with oral bisphoshonate use, renal deterioration.
2. Disease-related concern: Aspirin-sensitive asthma may cause bronchoconstriction, if hepatic impairment use with caution, hypocalcemia, renal impairment. In cancer patients, renal toxicity is more likely with doses exceeding 4 mg or when infused in 15 min.
3. Special populations: Use with caution in elderly, advise women of childbearing age against getting pregnant, not approved for use in children.

(D) *Contraindications*:

Intravenous zoledronate: Hypersensitivity to zoledronate or other bisphosphonates or any component of the formulation; hypocalcemia; not recommended in patients with SCr > 3 mg/dl and bone metastases; use in hypercalcemia of malignancy; no dose adjustment needed in mild–moderate renal failure; in cases of severe renal impairment (SCr > 4.5 mg/dl), use is recommended only if benefits exceed risk.

(E) *Approval for use*:

Zoledronate is not approved by the FDA for use in primary hyperparathyroidism; recommendation is, therefore, based on its efficacy and approval for use in hypercalcemia of malignancy.

Box 4 Calcitonin in the Acute Management of Hypercalcemia in Hyperparathyroidism (*Adapted from Product Drug Information from Lexicomp-UpToDate Version 16.3*)

(A) *Dose*:

Intramuscular or subcutaneous calcitonin, 4–6 U/kg every 8–12 h for 48 h

(B) *Adverse reactions*: *Reporting those with a frequency > 1%*

10%: Local reaction and nausea

1–5%: Flushing, rash

(continued)

Box 4 (continued)

1–3: Myalgias, arthralgias, hypertension, angina, dizziness, gastrointestinal, fatigue, depression, cystitis, conjunctivitis, bronchospasm.

(C) *Warnings*:
Hypersensitivity to salmon products; safety not established in children.

(D) *Contraindications*:
Hypersensitivity to salmon calcitonin.

(E) *Approval for use*:
Calcitonin is not approved by the FDA for use in primary hyperparathyroidism; recommendation is, therefore, based on its efficacy and approval for use in hypercalcemia of malignancy.

Acknowledgments The author would like to thank Ms Aida Farha for retrieving articles that were not available online, Mr Ghassan Baliki and Ms Tala Ghalayini for PubMed searches and article retrieval, and Ms Rola El-Rassi for assisting in manuscript preparation. This work was in part supported by an Institutional grant from the American University of Beirut and the Lebanese National Council for Scientific Research.

References

1. Zink AR, Panzer S, Fesq-Martin M, Burger-Heinrich E, Wahl J, Nerlich AG. Evidence for a 7000-year-old case of primary hyperparathyroidism [letter]. JAMA. 2005;293:40–2.
2. Albright F, Reifenstein E. The parathyroid glands and metabolic bone disease. Baltimore: Williams & Wilkins; 1948.
3. Bilezikian JP, Silverberg SJ. Asymptomatic primary hyperparathyroidism. N Engl J Med. 2004;530:1746–51.
4. Priya G, Jyotsna VP, Chumber S, Bal CS, Karak AK, Seth A, et al. Clinical and laboratory profile of primary hyperparathyroidism in India. Postgrad Med J. 2008;84:34–9.
5. Muthukrishnan J, Jha S, Modi KD, Jha R, Kumar J, Verma A, et al. Symptomatic primary hyperparathyroidism: a retrospective analysis of fifty one cases from a single centre. J Assoc Physicians India. 2008;56:503–7.
6. Silverberg SJ, Shane E, Jacobs TP, Siris E, Bilezikian JP. A 10-year prospective study of primary hyperparathyroidism with or without parathyroid surgery. N Engl J Med. 1999;341:1249–55.
7. Utiger RD. Treatment of primary hyperparathyroidism. N Engl J Med. 1999;341:1301–2.
8. Rubin MR, Bilezikian JP, McMahon DJ, Jacobs T, Shane E, Siris E, et al. The natural history of primary hyperparathyroidism with or without parathyroid surgery after 15 years. J Clin Endocrinol Metab. 2008;93:3462–70.
9. El-Hajj Fuleihan G. Hyperparathyroidism: time to reconsider current clinical decision paradigms? Editorial. J Clin Endocrinol Metab. 2008;93:3302–304.

10. Bilezikian JP. Drug therapy: management of acute hypercalcemia. N Engl J Med. 1992; 326:1196.
11. Potts JT Jr, Fradkin JE, Aurbach GD, Bilezikian JP, Raisz LG, editors. Proceedings of the NIH consensus development conference on the diagnosis and management of asymptomatic primary hyperparathyroidism. J Bone Miner Res. 1991;6 Suppl 2.
12. Bilezikian JP, Potts JT, El-Hajj Fuleihan G, Kleerekoper M, Neer R, Peacock M, et al. Summary statement from a workshop on asymptomatic hyperparathyroidism: a perspective for the 21st century. J Clin Endocrinol Metab. 2002;87:5353–61.
13. Phitayakorn R, McHenry CR. Hyperparathyroid crisis: use of bisphosphonates as a bridge to parathyroidectomy. J Am Coll Surg. 2008;206:1106–15.
14. Brown EM, Pollak M, Seidman CE, Seidman JG, Chou YH, Riccardi D, et al. Calcium-ion-sensing cell-surface receptors. N Engl J Med. 1995;333:234–40.
15. Chattopadhyay N, Brown EM. Role of calcium-sensing receptor in mineral ion metabolism and inherited disorders of calcium-sensing. Mol Genet Metab. 2006;89:189–202.
16. LeGrand SB, Leskuski D, Zama I. Narrative review: furosemide for hypercalcemia: an unproven yet common practice. Ann Intern Med. 2008;118:1966–9.
17. Shackney S, Hasson J. Precipitous fall in serum calcium, hypotension, and acute renal failure after intravenous phosphate therapy for hypercalcemia. Report of two cases. Ann Intern Med. 1967;66:906–16.
18. Broadus AE, Magee JS, Mallette LE, Horst RL, Lang R, Jensen PS, et al. A detailed evaluation of oral phosphate therapy in selected patients with primary hyperparathyroidism. J Clin Endocrinol Metab. 1983;56:953–61.
19. Jansson S, Tisell LE, Lindstedt G, Lundberg PA. Disodium pamidronate in the preoperative treatment of hypercalcemia in patients with primary hyperparathyroidism. Surgery. 1991;110:480–6.
20. Tal A, Graves L. Intravenous pamidronate for hypercalcemia of primary hyperparathyroidism. South Med J. 1996;89:637–40.
21. Vestergaard P. Current pharmacological options for the management of primary hyperparathyroidism. Drugs. 2006;66:2189–211.
22. Saunders Y, Ross JR, Broadley KE, Edmonds PM, Patel S, Steering Group. Systematic review of bisphosphonates for hypercalcaemia of malignancy. Palliat Med. 2004;18:418–31.
23. Major P, Lortholary A, Hon J, Abdi E, Mills G, Menssen HD, et al. Zoledronic acid is superior to pamidronate in the treatment of hypercalcemia of malignancy: a pooled analysis of two randomized, controlled clinical trials. J Clin Oncol. 2001;19:558–67.
24. Black DM, Delmas PD, Eastell R, Reid IR, Boonen S, Cauley JA, et al. Once-yearly zoledronic acid for treatment of postmenopausal osteoporosis. N Engl J Med. 2007;356:1809–22.
25. Wisneski LA. Salmon calcitonin in the acute management of hypercalcemia. Calcif Tissue Int. 1990;46(Suppl):S26–30.
26. Sekine M, Takami H. Combination of calcitonin and pamidronate for emergency treatment of malignant hypercalcemia. Oncol Rep. 1998;5:197–9.
27. Thiébaud D, Jacquet AF, Burckhardt P. Fast and effective treatment of malignant hypercalcemia. Combination of suppositories of calcitonin and a single infusion of 3-amino 1-hydroxy-propylidene-1-bisphosphonate. Arch Intern Med. 1990;150:2125–8.
28. Tørring O, Bucht E, Sjöstedt U, Sjöberg HE. Salmon calcitonin treatment by nasal spray in primary hyperparathyroidism. Bone. 1991;12:311–6.
29. Stone MD, Marshall DH, Hosking DJ, Garcia-Himmelstine C, White DA, Worth HG. Comparison of low-dose intramuscular and intravenous salcatonin in the treatment of primary hyperparathyroidism. Bone. 1992;13:265–71.
30. Nilsson I, Zedenius J, Yin L, Ekbom A. The association between primary hyperparathyroidism and malignancy: nationwide cohort analysis on cancer incidence after parathyroidectomy. Endocr Relat Cancer. 2007;14:135–40.
31. Yoshida T, Iwasaki Y, Kagawa T, Sasaoka A, Horino T, Morita T, et al. Coexisting primary hyperparathyroidism and sarcoidosis in a patient with severe hypercalcemia. Endocr J. 2008;55:391–5.

32. Insogna KL, Mitnick ME, Stewart AF, Burtis WJ, Mallette LE, Broadus AE. Sensitivity of the parathyroid hormone-1,25-dihydroxyvitamin D axis to variations in calcium intake in patients with primary hyperparathyroidism. N Engl J Med. 1985;313:1126–30.
33. Tohme JF, Bilezikian JP, Clemens TL, Silverberg SJ, Shane E, Lindsay R. Suppression of parathyroid hormone secretion with oral calcium in normal subjects and patients with primary hyperparathyroidism. J Clin Endocrinol Metab. 1990;70:951–6.
34. Wermers RA, Kearns AE, Jenkins GD, Melton 3rd LJ. Incidence and clinical spectrum of thiazide-associated hypercalcemia. Am J Med. 2007;120:911–5.
35. Christensson T, Hellström K, Wengle B. Hypercalcemia and primary hyperparathyroidism. Prevalence in patients receiving thiazides as detected in a health screen. Arch Intern Med. 1977;137:1138–42.
36. Haden ST, Stoll AL, McCormick S, Scott J, El-Hajj Fuleihan G. Alterations in parathyroid dynamics in lithium-treated subjects. J Clin Endocrinol Metab. 1997;82:2844–8.
37. Khairallah W, Fawaz A, Brown EM, El-Hajj Fuleihan G. Hypercalcemia and diabetes insipidus in a patient previously treated with lithium. Nat Clin Pract Nephrol. 2007;3:397–404.
38. Bendz H, Sjodin I, Toss G, Berglund K. Hyperparathyroidism and long-term lithium therapy – a cross-sectional study and the effect of lithium withdrawal. J Intern Med. 1996;240:357–65.
39. Nordenstrom J, Strigard K, Perbeck L, Willems J, Bagedahl-Strindlund M, Linder J. Hyperparathyroidism associated with treatment of manic-depressive disorders by lithium. Eur J Surg. 1992;158:207–11.
40. Fang WL, Tseng LM, Chen JY, Chiout SY, Chout YH, Wu CW, et al. The management of high-risk patients with primary hyperparathyroidism-minimally invasive parathyroidectomy vs. medical treatment. Clin Endocrinol. 2008;68:520–8.
41. Inoue Y, Kaji H, Hisa I, Tabimatsu T, Naito J, Iu M, et al. Vitamin D status affects osteopenia in postmenopausal patients with primary hyperparathyroidism. Endocr J. 2008;55:57–65.
42. Rao DS, Agarwal G, Talpos GB, Phillips ER, Bandeira F, Mishra SK, et al. Role of vitamin D and calcium nutrition in disease expression and parathyroid tumor growth in primary hyperparathyroidism: a global perspective. J Bone Miner Res. 2002;17 Suppl 2:N75–80.
43. Silverberg SJ, Shane E, Dempster DW, Bilezikian JP. The effects of vitamin D insufficiency in patients with primary hyperparathyroidism. Am J Med. 1999;107:561–7.
44. Nordenström E, Westerdahl J, Lindergård B, Lindblom P, Bergenfelz A. Multifactorial risk profile for bone fractures in primary hyperparathyroidism. World J Surg. 2002;26:1463–7.
45. Michail N. Clinical significance of vitamin D deficiency in primary hyperparathyroidism, and safety of vitamin D therapy. South Med J. 2011;104(1):29–33.
46. Eastell R, Arnold A, Brandi ML, et al. Diagnosis of asymptomatic primary hyperparathyroidism; proceedings of the third international workshop. J Clin Endocrinol Metab. 2009;94: 340–50.
47. Pradeep PV, Mishra A, Agarwal G, Agarwal A, Verma AK, Mishra SK. Long-term outcome after parathyroidectomy in patients with advanced primary hyperparathyroidism and associated vitamin D deficiency. World J Surg. 2008;32(5):829–35.
48. Stein EM, Dempster DW, Udesky J, et al. Vitamin D deficiency influences histomorphometric features of bone in primary hyperparathyroidism. Bone. 2011;48:557–61.
49. Ross AC, Manson JAE, Abrams SA, et al. The 2011 report on dietary reference intakes for calcium and vitamin D from the Institute of Medicine: what clinicians need to know. J Clin Endocrinol Metab. 2011;96:53–8.
50. Holick MF, Binkley NC, Bischoff-Ferrari H, et al. Evaluation, treatment, and prevention of vitamin D deficiency: an Endocrine Society Clinical Practice Guideline. J Clin Endocrinol Metabol. 2011. doi:10.1210/jc.2011.
51. Nemeth EF. Calcimimetic and calcilytic drugs: just for parathyroid cells? Cell Calcium. 2004;35:283–9.
52. Wuthrich RP, Martin D, Bilezikian JP. The role of calcimimetics in the treatment of hyperparathyroidism. Eur J Clin Invest. 2007;37:1113–5.

53. Steddon SJ, Cunningham J. Calcimimetics and calcilytics – fooling the calcium receptor. Lancet. 2005;365:2237–9.
54. Silverberg SJ, Bone 3rd HG, Marriott TB, Locker FG, Thys-Jacobs S, Dziem G, et al. Short-term inhibition of parathyroid hormone secretion by a calcium-receptor agonist in patients with primary hyperparathyroidism. N Engl J Med. 1997;337:1506–10.
55. Shoback DM, Bilezikian JP, Turner SA, McCary LC, Guo MD, Peacock M. The calcimimetic cinacalcet normalizes serum calcium in subjects with primary hyperparathyroidism. J Clin Endocrinol Metab. 2003;88:5644–9.
56. Peacock M, Bilezikian JP, Klassen PS, Guo MD, Turner SA, Shoback D. Cinacalcet hydrochloride maintains long-term normocalcemia in patients with primary hyperparathyroidism. J Clin Endocrinol Metab. 2005;90:135–41.
57. Silverberg SJ, Rubin MR, Faiman C, Peacock M, Shoback DM, Smallridge RC, et al. Cinacalcet hydrochloride reduces the serum calcium concentration in inoperable parathyroid carcinoma. J Clin Endocrinol Metab. 2007;92:3803–8.
58. Peacock M, Bilezekian JP, Bolognese MA, et al. Cinacalcet HCl reduces hypercalcemia in primary hyperparathyroidism across a wide spectrum of disease severity. J Clin Endocrinol Metab. 2011;96:E8–19.
59. Heller HJ, Miller GL, Erdman WA, Snyder 3rd WH, Breslau NA. Angiographic ablation of mediastinal parathyroid adenomas: local experience and review of the literature. Am J Med. 1994;97:529–34.
60. Miller DL, Doppman JL, Chang R, Simmons JT, O'Leary TJ, Norton JA, et al. Angiographic ablation of parathyroid adenomas: lessons from a 10-year experience. Radiology. 1987;165:601–7.
61. Pallotta JA, Ba S, Moller DE, Eisenberg H. Arteriographic ablation of cervical adenomas. J Clin Endocrinol Metab. 1989;69:1249–55.
62. Harman R, Grant CS, Hay ID, Hurley DL, Van Heerden JA, Thompson GB, et al. Indications, technique, and efficacy of alcohol injection of enlarged parathyroid glands in patients with primary hyperparathyroidism. Surgery. 1998;124:1011–20.
63. Cappelli C, Pelizzari G, Pirola I, Gandossi E, De Martino E, Delbarba A, et al. Modified percutaneous ethanol injection of parathyroid adenoma in primary hyperparathyroidism. QJM. 2008;101:657–62.

Chapter 5
Surgical Management of Primary Hyperparathyroidism

Meei J. Yeung and Janice L. Pasieka

Keywords Parathyroidectomy • Surgical indication • Parathyroid cancer • Hungry bone disease • Hyperparathyroidism • Osteitis fibrosa cystica • Nephrolithiasis • Hypercalcemic crisis • Quality of life outcomes • Psychiatric assessment tools • Surgical approaches • Embryology • Anatomy • Thymus • Neck exploration—unilateral • Bilateral • Parathyroid carcinoma • Parathyroid hyperplasia • Resection • Multi-gland disease • Preoperative imaging • Minimally invasive parathyroidectomy • Image-directed parathyroidectomy • Intra-operative PTH assays • Miami criterion • Surgical success rates • Radio-guided parathyroidectomy • Gramma probe • Endoscopic parathyroidectomy • Video-assisted parathyroidectomy • Hungry bone syndrome • Recurrent disease • Persistent disease

Primary hyperparathyroidism (PHPT) is a disease that affects calcium metabolism leading to elevated serum calcium in the presence of an inappropriately normal or high parathyroid hormone (PTH) level. It is a relatively common condition, with prevalence rates reported to be about 1–4 per 1,000 with a female:male ratio of 3:1 and as frequent as 1 in every 500 women over the age of 50 years [1–3]. PHPT is most commonly due to a single parathyroid adenoma (80–85% of cases), but may also be attributable to the presence of multiple adenomas, hyperplasia or malignancy.

M.J. Yeung, MD, FRACS
Department of Surgery, Monash University Endocrine Surgery Unit, Melbourne, Australia

J.L. Pasieka, MD, FRCSC, FACS (⊠)
Department of Surgery and Oncology, Divisions of General Surgery and Surgical Oncology,
University of Calgary, North Tower, Foothills Medical Center, 1403 29th Street NW,
Calgary, AB, Canada T2N 2T9
e-mail: janice.pasieka@albertahealthservices.ca

A.A. Khan and O.H. Clark (eds.), *Handbook of Parathyroid Diseases:
A Case-Based Practical Guide*, DOI 10.1007/978-1-4614-2164-1_5,
© Springer Science+Business Media, LLC 2012

The first successful parathyroidectomy for PHPT was performed by Felix Mandl in 1925. He removed a parathyroid adenoma in a patient with von Recklinghausen's bone disease (osteitis fibrosa cystica) [4]. Hyperparathyroidism was only diagnosed in patients with osteitis fibrosa cystica until the 1930s when Albright noted that 80% of patients diagnosed and treated on the finding of osteitis fibrosa cystica also had nephrolithiasis or nephrocalcinosis [2]. Following that time, patients typically presented with these classical symptoms of PHPT. However, with the introduction of routine calcium screening and the use of multi-channel biochemical testing in the early 1970s, the majority of patients had a diagnosis of PHPT made at a much earlier stage, thereby avoiding the overt manifestations of PHPT [5]. Today, fewer than 20% of patients with PHPT present with nephrolithiasis and fewer than 3% in developed counties have osteitis fibrosa cystica [6, 7]. Surgical removal of abnormal parathyroid tissue is the only curative treatment for PHPT.

The classic symptoms and metabolic complications of PHPT that warrant surgery include:

- Osteitis fibrosa cystica
- Decreased renal function
- Nephrolithiasis or nephrocalcinosis
- Significant myopathy and weakness
- Osteoporosis and fractures
- Hypercalcaemic crisis

However, with the change in presentation of PHPT from overt complications of the end-organ damage to more subtle symptomatology, the National Institutes of Health (NIH) sponsored a Consensus Conference in 1990 to develop guidelines for the surgical management of patients with PHPT [8]. A decade later, the NIH reconvened in 2002 to update its guidelines [9]. In 2009, in the most recent consensus, the panel recommended parathyroidectomy for all symptomatic patients and for asymptomatic patients with the following [10]:

- Hypercalcemia—serum calcium >0.25 mmol/L or 1 mg/dL above the normal reference range
- Hypercalciuria—a 24-h urinary calcium level >0.01 mmol/kg/day or 400 mg/24 h (optional)
- Renal impairment—elevated creatinine
- BMD > 2.5 standard deviations below peak bone mass (T score < −2.5)
- <50 years old
- Patients who could not participate in appropriate follow-up [34]

Rationale for Surgical Intervention

Although 20% of patients display the classical symptoms and an additional 31% meet at least one of the NIH criteria for surgical intervention, there is increasing evidence that many of the remaining 49% of patients benefit from surgical intervention [11–14]. Vague non-specific symptom, such as fatigue, irritability and depression, have been recognized as consistent manifestations of PHTP. With a greater appreciation of the significance of subjective symptoms associated with PHPT, in 2005 and again in 2009, the American Association of Clinical Endocrinologists and the American Association of Endocrine Surgeons released a position statement that concluded, "operative management should be considered and recommended for all 'asymptomatic' patients with PHPT who have a reasonable life expectancy and are suitable operative candidates" [13, 15].

Quality of Life

A clear definition of "asymptomatic" PHPT remains controversial. There is a growing body of evidence that supports the opinion that the majority of the so-called asymptomatic patients are in reality symptomatic [5, 7, 12–14, 16–24]. A large part of the debate over the definition is due to the fact that many of the subjective symptoms, including weakness, fatigue, mood swings and malaise, have previously been difficult to quantify. These are in contrast to the objective parameters in NIH guidelines, which are easily measurable.

Despite the difficulty in measuring these vague, non-specific symptoms, a number of quality of life (QoL) and psychiatric assessment measurement tools have been utilized in an attempt to quantify them [16, 25, 26]. Burney et al. used a Short Form 36 item (SF-36) health status questionnaire that was originally developed as part of a Medical Outcomes Study which looks at eight domains of health status that are predictive of the patients' QoL [17]. The Michigan group was able to demonstrate that surgical correction of PHPT substantially improved six of the eight SF-36 domains at 2 months following surgery, particularly in the areas resulting from emotional problems and bodily pain [17]. It went on to demonstrate that these findings were independent of the degree of hypercalcemia [16]. In a study by Talpos et al., the SF-36 Health Survey was used in a randomized trial of parathyroidectomy versus observation in patients with confirmed "asymptomatic" mild PHPT [20]. They demonstrated a statistically significant improvement in two domains in the surgically managed group compared with those undergoing medical surveillance. Similar results demonstrating the benefit of surgical intervention on improving QoL have been shown by other authors [18, 22, 25, 27]. However, two additional randomized trials failed to demonstrate a significant improvement in the surgically treated patients' QoL, despite demonstrating a lower QoL than a normal population preoperatively [28, 29]. A potential weakness in these studies is in the generic nature of the assessment tools that have been used. Consequently, a disease-specific outcome tool has been developed and validated by Pasieka et al. [21, 26]. This instrument includes both classic and non-classic symptoms, assessing 13 disease-specific items. The patients' symptoms were documented using a visual analogue scale allowing a quantitative measurement of their symptoms, termed Parathyroidectomy Assessment of Symptoms (PAS) scores. The preoperative PAS scores were significantly higher compared to the comparison group of non-toxic thyroidectomy patients. Following successful surgical intervention, the PHPT patients reported a significant improvement in their PAS scores that persisted at 1-year follow-up. At 1 year, the PHPT patients reported a significant improvement in their self-rated health and an improved QoL. These findings were substantiated in a multi-centre trial utilizing this disease-specific tool, further illustrating that the majority of PHPT patients suffer from vague non-specific symptoms that are improved following successful surgery [21]. The 10-year follow-up data demonstrated that this significant reduction in the PAS scores in the PHPT patients persists and that these patients reported a significantly improved QoL at 10 years compared to their preoperative state ($p < 0.05$) [30].

Bone Disease

Early reports of PHPT often involved patients with severe bone disease as the primary presentation [4]. Although conditions such as osteitis fibrosa cystica are rarely seen in developed countries today, skeletal involvement in the mildly symptomatic or apparently "asymptomatic" patient is still demonstrable with the use of bone mineral densitometry and bone biopsy with histomorphometric analysis [31]. Bone mineral density (BMD) is an important marker in the prediction of increased fracture risk [32]. PHPT is associated with a reduction in BMD [1]. The effect on bone of PTH excess appears to be catabolic at cortical sites (e.g. radius) and relatively sparing or even anabolic at cancellous bone sites (e.g. spine) [1, 31]. Studies have clearly demonstrated that parathyroidectomy in symptomatic patients experience sustained increases in their BMD, particularly at the lumbar spine and femoral neck [31, 33–36]. There were also increases in BMD at the radius, although this was less dramatic. Some authors have suggested that vertebral osteopenia to be considered as another indication for parathyroidectomy, as this is the site most likely to improve following surgery [34]. A recent prospective randomized study by Almqvist et al. demonstrated that early parathyroidectomy is preferable to reduce the risk of fractures, especially in the hip [35]. They were able to show that patients with mild PHPT who underwent parathyroidectomy at the time of diagnosis had significant increases in hip BMD that did not occur in patients who had surgery delayed for a year after diagnosis. There are now two randomized trials that have demonstrated an improvement in BMD in the surgically treated arm [28, 29].

Nephrolithiasis

It is now unusual to see overt renal complications of hypercalcemia, such as nephrolithiasis or nephrocalcinosis. The prevalence of stone disease as an indication for surgery has steadily decreased from 60–80% of cases in the 1960s down to 7–15% in more recent series [3, 37]. In patients who present with renal stones, it is estimated that 3–8% will have PHPT [38, 39]. The formation of renal calculi is multifactorial and its exact pathogenesis is still somewhat unclear. There is currently no defined biochemical abnormality that separates patients with PHPT who develop stones and those that do not [38]. The presence of nephrolithiasis or nephrocalcinosis in the presence of PHPT is a clear indication for parathyroidectomy. The development of new renal stones is reduced by 90% after parathyroidectomy and patients with PHPT who do not undergo surgery are at increased risk of developing kidney stones [33, 40].

Surgical Approaches to Primary Hyperparathyroidism

Surgery is the only definitive treatment for PHPT [8]. The aim of parathyroidectomy is to remove all hyperfunctioning parathyroid tissue. Traditionally, an open, bilateral neck exploration (BNE) with identification of all four glands was performed. However, with advances of more accurate preoperative localization techniques and the utilization of intra-operative PTH (iPTH), we have seen the evolution to a focused or minimal access parathyroidectomy.

Embryology and Anatomy

A comprehensive understanding of the embryology and anatomy is vital for successful parathyroid surgery. The superior parathyroid glands originate from the dorsal wing of the fourth branchial pouch and descend with the thyroid gland to rest at the upper pole of the thyroid gland. Approximately 80% are found within 1 cm above the intersection of the recurrent laryngeal nerve and the inferior thyroid artery [41]. When enlarged, a superior thyroid gland may descend posteriorly under the inferior thyroid artery along the tracheal-esophageal groove. Due to their longer pathway of descent, the inferior parathyroid glands have a higher variability of location compared to the superior parathyroid glands. The inferior parathyroid glands arise from the dorsal aspect of the third branchial pouch and the thymus arises from the ventral aspect. During foetal development, the inferior parathyroids migrate caudally and usually dissociate from the thymus to come to rest at the posterolateral aspect of the inferior pole of the thyroid gland, where about 60% are found. If they fail to dissociate, the inferior glands may be located within the thymus in the antero-superior mediastinum. In the absence of descent, suggested by the lack of thymic tissue caudal to the thyroid gland, the inferior parathyroid glands may be found at the superior pole of the thyroid or at the carotid bulb (undescended parathyroid), imitating a superior parathyroid gland. Since the third branchial arch gives rise to the carotid, ectopic inferior glands can be found in the carotid sheath. The majority of patients have four glands (84% of cases) with only three glands being present in 3% [41]. Supernumerary glands are rare and have been reported in 0.7% of cases [42]. Parathyroid glands are usually spherical, bean shaped or spherical in shape, with an average size of $5 \times 3 \times 1$ mm and weight of 35–40 mg [41]. In adults, they tend to have a brownish-tan colour. In PHPT, a solitary adenoma is found in about 80–85% of patients, with double adenomas being present in 5%. About 15% of patients have hyperplastic glands [41].

Bilateral Neck Exploration

BNE with morphological evaluation of all four glands is the traditional and gold standard procedure in the surgical management of PHPT. This technique relies on the experience of the surgeon to be able to distinguish solitary disease from multiglandular disease based on the morphological appearance of the glands. When an experienced endocrine surgeon performs this technique, the cure rates exceed 95% [2, 3, 43, 44]. The operation is performed under general anaesthetic through an anterior, transverse neck incision placed approximately 2 cm above the sternal notch. Once the recurrent laryngeal nerves and all four parathyroid glands have been identified, the morphological abnormal parathyroid gland or glands are removed. In patients who have parathyroid hyperplasia, either a subtotal parathyroidectomy should be performed—where three and a half glands are removed—or a total parathyroidectomy with autotransplantation of parathyroid tissue into the forearm. If all four glands are not found in their usual locations, a systematic exploration of the neck, including the tracheal-oesophageal groove and posterior mediastinum for the missing superior gland; the thymus, anterior mediastinum and the carotid sheath in search of a missing inferior gland. Intra-thyroidal parathyroid glands have been reported in about 3% of patients and are often identified on preoperative ultrasound.

Parathyroid carcinoma is a rare cause of PHPT. If it is suspected prior to surgery because of profound hypercalcemia or a palpable parathyroid tumour, a BNE or access to adjuncts, such as iPTH, should be utilized since up to 25% of parathyroid carcinomas are associated with coexisting parathyroid hyperplasia. Parathyroid carcinoma occurs more often in patients with isolated familial PHPT and jaw tumour syndrome. Intra-operatively, parathyroid carcinomas are usually large, firm, pale or whitish tumours that may be invading local structures. The treatment is an en bloc resection of the involved parathyroid gland with the ipsilateral thyroid lobe and central nodal compartment. The ipsilateral normal parathyroid gland should also be identified and removed in order to remove all parathyroid tissue from the affected side.

Unilateral Neck Exploration

Unilateral neck exploration (UNE) relies on positive preoperative localizing studies and the morphological appearance of the parathyroid glands. It is commenced in the same manner as a BNE; however, only one side of the neck is exposed and explored with the contralateral side left undisturbed if the surgeon is able to identify one abnormal and one normal parathyroid gland. This technique was developed in the 1970s by Drs. C. A. Wang and Sten Tibblin, based on the premise that parathyroid adenomas are solitary in up to 85% of cases, and once an abnormal gland and a normal appearing gland were identified on one side the likelihood of multi-gland disease was low. However, failure to find one normal and one abnormal gland on the same side necessitates exploration of the contralateral side. There is evidence that has shown patients who underwent UNE had less post-operative hypocalcaemia and a significantly shorter mean operating time compared to patients who had BNE [45]. The choice of which side to commence the neck exploration was initially arbitrary but was later aided by preoperative imaging modalities. At that time, radionuclide scans were only able to localize approximately 53% of parathyroid adenomas and as a consequence this technique did not gain much support [46]. Nonetheless, in one of the largest reported series of patients to have undergone UNE, the permanent cure rates were shown to be comparable to those of a BNE at 98.4% [47]. It is important to recognize that for all comers in which the intent was a UNE, in up to 32% of cases the contralateral side requires exploration as the surgeon was unable to identify one normal and one abnormal gland on the initial side [47]. iPTH has increasingly played a role in this approach by confirming solitary gland disease when the second gland on that side is not well-seen or the surgeon is unsure if it is normal on morphological examination. However, iPTH is not necessary for a UNE as long as the surgeon is able to identify both parathyroid glands.

Image-Directed Parathyroidectomy

Image-directed exploration (IDP), also known as minimal access or minimally invasive parathyroidectomy, involves a focused approach to the single abnormal parathyroid gland seen on preoperative imaging [48–52]. The procedure may be performed under general or local anaesthetic with sedation. The preoperative imaging directs the surgeon through a small 2–2.5-cm incision to the abnormal gland either anteriorly or through a lateral incision. It has surpassed UNE and BNE as the procedure of choice. The evolution of IDP has relied upon two important developments: the refinement of accurate preoperative localization techniques and the introduction of iPTH measurements.

In 1989, the introduction of a new isotope, technetium 99 m-labelled sestamibi, for parathyroid imaging was described [53]. This is now the most widely used agent for parathyroid scintigraphy and has reported sensitivities for detecting adenomas ranging from 65 to 85% [43]. Unfortunately, sestamibi scans do not appear to be as accurate when multi-gland disease is present. In only one-third of the time the sestamibi scan demonstrates multi-gland disease; the remaining scan is either misleading (showing solitary disease) or has non-visualization. Therefore, further confirmation of solitary disease increases the sensitivity of this modality. Ultrasonography is a non-invasive, readily available and relatively inexpensive imaging modality.

Its sensitivity in detecting parathyroid adenomas is reported to be in the order of up to 80% but is highly user dependent and not good at localizing ectopic glands [48]. When both ultrasound and technetium 99 m sestamibi scanning are concordant, localization of a solitary parathyroid adenoma is accurate in over 90% of cases [48, 54]. With this information, it is therefore possible to be guided to not only the side, but also position of the abnormal parathyroid gland. However, IDP does not allow examination of any other parathyroid glands and theoretically up to 15% of patients have double adenomas or hyperplastic glands that are missed. Despite this observation, the rate of persistent hypercalcaemia does not seem to have been affected thus far, though this may simply be a reflection of lack of long-term follow-up [48].

Without the evaluation of the remaining parathyroid glands, the presence of multi-gland disease is unknown; many surgeons, therefore, use iPTH to document when all of these hyperfunctioning parathyroid glands have been removed. Intact PTH has a half-life of about 3 min, so once a diseased gland is resected the PTH levels should fall by 50% or more from the highest pre-removal level at 10 min following removal of all hyperfunctioning tissue [55, 56]. This criterion, known as the Miami Criterion, has been shown to have an accuracy of 97% in predicting post-operative normocalcaemia [55]. Proponents of iPTH feel that it is an important adjunct in IDP. In reality, the absolute necessity and cost-effectiveness of iPTH in IDP have been questioned [49, 54, 57]. A recent article by Stalberg et al. showed that iPTH did not substantially add value to decision making and its success rate would have been changed from 98 to 99% with the use of iPTH [54]. To date, success rates of up to 99% with IDP have been comparable to those seen with BNE [44]. If a solitary adenoma is not found at the position where it had been localized preoperatively or the iPTH does not fall by more than 50%, the procedure will need to be converted to a BNE. IDP is not suitable for patients with known hyperplasia or parathyroid carcinoma.

Besides the focused approach where the incision is placed to allow direct assess to the involved pararthyroid, other techniques have been adopted by surgeons, including radio-guided parathyroidectomy and endoscopic and video-assisted pararthyroidectomy [50–52]. Radio-guided parathyroidectomy is a minimal access operation, whereby a gamma probe is used to guide the surgeon to the site of the abnormal parathyroid gland and is utilized to confirm removal of all abnormal glands. Patients are injected intravenously with Technetium 99 m sestamibi 2–4 h prior to surgery. Intra-operatively, a handheld gamma probe measures gamma counts in the four quadrants and directs the surgeon to the diseased gland. Once removed, ex vivo counts confirm the removal of the imaged abnormality as well as confirm the absence of other hyperfunctioning glands that are still present [52]. This technique does not require iPTH or the use of frozen sections to confirm removal of the abnormal hyperfunctioning gland. Radio-guided parathyroidectomy, however, has not been universal adopted by the endocrine surgical community, since it requires an additional sestamibi scan to localize the already observed abnormal parathyroid gland. It can, however, be helpful in the setting of re-operative cases, where scar tissue can impair the surgeon's ability to find the gland.

Endoscopic parathyroidectomy, as the name suggests, is a technique that uses endoscopic equipment to remove abnormal parathyroid glands. A number of different approaches have been described, including anterior video-assisted [50] and a lateral approach [51]. These operations provide excellent exposure through small incisions and can be done safely in experienced hands. The reason that these techniques have not gained wide utilization is likely due to the ease to with the focused approach can be adapted by endocrine surgeons and achieve success without the need for a general anaesthetic and specialized equipment.

Clinical Scenarios that the Surgeon Must Be Aware of

Case 1: Hungry Bones

Seen more commonly when patients with PHPT had symptomatic bone disease (osteitis fibrosa cystica) and chronic increase in bone resorption

Preoperative clues

- Elevated alkaline phosphatase
- Older
- Elevated blood urea nitrogen
- Preop calcium and PTH not predictive
- Significant osteoporosis
- Histomorphological bone assessment
- Subperiosteal resorption on industrial grade hand films

Intra-operative clues

- Large-volume adenoma, 5 ml

Pathogenesis

- Increased PTH

    - Increased bone turnover with increases in both resorption and mineral apposition
    - Overall resorption greater

- Abrupt drop in PTH

    - Increased bone mineralization using Ca, PO_4, Mg
    - Therefore, significant drops of these values with nadir at day 2 or 3

Clinical picture

- Well-defined clinical criteria for the diagnosis are lacking
- Hypocalcaemia

    - Dominates
    - May be associated with tetany and seizures

- Hypophosphataemia + hypomagnesaemia

    - Due to decreased bone resorption and increased bone formation

Post-op management

- Dependent of severity of symptoms
- Calcium replacement

    - Oral 4–6 g of elemental calcium daily in divided doses
    - Intravenous

        (a) Calcium gluconate infusion—titrated to effect

    - Vitamin D

        (a) 1 mcg/day

        (b) 1,25 hydroxy Vitamin D (Rocaltrol® 0.5 mg BID)

- Magnesium

    - Hypomagnesia may contribute to hypocalcaemia by decreasing PTH secretion
    - Replace as necessary

- Phosphate

    - Serum phosphate should be measured as may drop post op and oral calcium intake will add to this decline
    - Intravenous replacement should be avoided

Case 2: *Parathyroid Carcinoma*

Parathyroid carcinoma occurs in 1–2% of all PHPT patients. It has equal *in common in men and women* and is usually found in patients *older* than 50 years of age. If not recognized at the time of surgery, there is a high *risk of local recurrence*.

Preoperative clues

- Significant manifestations of hypercalcaemia (myopathy, coma, osteitis fibrosis cystica)
- Hoarse voice
- Palpable mass
- Marked hypercalcaemia (>14 mg/dL or >3.50 mmol/L)
- Markedly elevated PTH levels: three to ten times above normal range
- Raised serum alkaline phosphatase
- Brown tumours (Fig. 5.1)

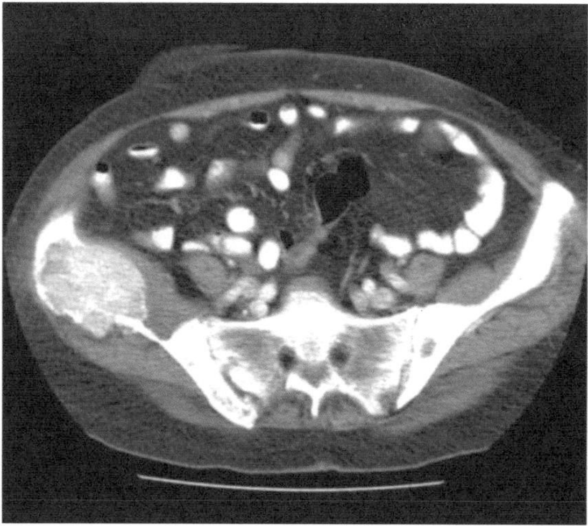

Fig. 5.1 Brown tumour of the pelvis in a patient with parathyroid carcinoma

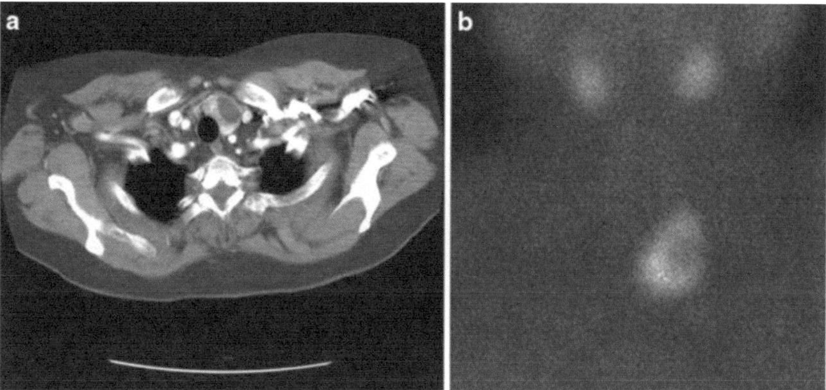

Fig. 5.2 (**a**) CT scan of a left superior parathyroid carcinoma. The tumour has a necrotic centre and is displacing the trachea to the right. (**b**) The corresponding sestamibi scan demonstrating a large left parathyroid gland at 2 h

Diagnosis

- Ultrasound features of large lesion +/− invasion
- CXR—metastasis
- CAT—invasive mass (Fig. 5.2)

Intra-operative clues

- Firm, hard, whitish grey-lobulated mass with a dense fibrous capsule.
- Local infiltration
- Occasionally enlarged lymph nodes

Surgery

- Four gland exploration or unilateral exploration with iPTH to rule out hyperplasia
- En bloc resection ipsilateral thyroid lobectomy
- Including ipsilateral normal parathyroid and thymus to remove all functioning parathyroid tissue on this side in case of recurrence
- Therapeutic ipsilateral central and lateral neck dissection if obvious enlarged nodes
- High rate of recurrence (>50%) when carcinoma not suspected at initial surgery because of failure to adequately remove all malignant tissue

Post-op management

- Higher risk of hungry bones (see case 1)

Management of recurrence (see case 3 and/or 4)

- Recur locally and distally to bones, lungs, liver and visceral organs
- Surgical resection to reduce tumour load and hypercalcaemia

Case 3: Hypercalcaemic Crisis

Regardless of cause, aims of initial management are the same:

1. Hydrate

    (a) Aggressive volume replacement with intravenous normal saline
    (b) 1-L normal saline bolus, then 200–300 ml/h
    (c) Goal is to hydrate to about 8 L/day, urine output > 100 cc/h

2. Increase renal excretion of calcium

    (a) Add loop diuretic (e.g. Furosemide) once adequate hydration
    (b) May be able to drop serum calcium by 1.5–2.0 mg/dL in 24–48 h
    (c) Avoid thiazide diuretics as they increase distal tubular resorption of calcium

3. Decrease bone resorption of calcium with inhibitors of osteoclast activity

    (a) Bisphosphonates
    (b) Cinacalcet
    (c) Calcitonin
    (d) Gallium nitrate
    (e) Glucocorticoids

Bisphosphonates

- Drugs that are incorporated into bony matrix
- Directly inhibit osteoclast function

- Given intravenously
- For example, pamidronate 60–90 mg over 2–4 h
- Effect seen in 24 h

Cinacalcet

- Calcimimetic agent
- Binds to calcium-sensing receptor on parathyroid cells, increasing sensitivity to extracellular calcium, therefore reducing secretion of PTH
- Given orally 30–60 mg once daily

Calcitonin

- Potent inhibitor of osteroclastic born resorption and promotes calciuresis
- Rapid onset of action (within 2 h)
- Given intramuscularly or subcutaneously 3–6 iU/kg
- Best used as adjunctive agent

Gallium nitrate

- Inhibits osteoclast activity (is rarely used)

Glucocorticoids

- Increase urinary excretion of calcium and decrease intestinal absorption
- For example, hydrocortisone 200–300 mg/day (not used very often for parathyroid crisis; most useful in sarcoidosis (Dent's Sign))

Case 4: Recurrent/Persistent Hyperpcalcaemia

Recurrent—hypercalcaemia developing after 6 months of normocalcaemia following parathyroidectomy

Persistent—hypercalcaemia recurring within 6 months of surgery

Causes

- Incorrect diagnosis 2–10%
- Inexperienced surgeon
- Undetected enlarged gland
- Multiple gland disease 37%
- Failure to locate ectopic gland
- Supernumerary glands
- PTH carcinoma
- Parathyromatosis

Management

- Confirm diagnosis—repeat Ca, PTH, exclude other causes (BFHH, sarcoidosis, etc.)
- Review previous operation report and histology

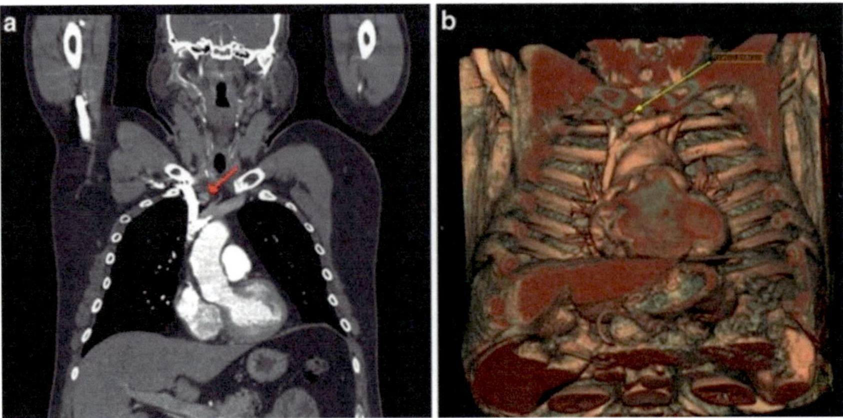

Fig. 5.3 (**a**) Following a failed operation, a CT of the mediastinum reveals an Rt-inferior parathyroid adenoma between the innominate vein and brachiocephalic artery (*arrow*) (**b**) 3-D recontractions can help aid in the surgical planning

- Localization studies—requires both functional and anatomical imaging

    - Anatomical—Ultrasound, CAT, MRI (Fig. 5.3)
    - Functional—Sestamibi (including fusion CT, Fig. 5.4), selective venous sampling

- Nasopharyngoscopy—assesses vocal cord function
- Operative strategies

    - If neck scarred, lateral approach
    - Sites of missing glands

        (a) Superior

            Medial to upper pole of thyroid
            Retro-oesophagus
            Undescended parathyroid at hyoid bone
            Intra-thyroidal
            Posterior mediastinum

        (b) Inferior

            Thymus
            Carotid sheath
            Anterior mediastinum
            Intra-thyroidal
            Undescended

- Consider cryopreservation of parathyroid tissue as the removed gland may be the only remaining parathyroid tissue
- Autotransplant parathyroid tissue when three parathyroid glands have been removed

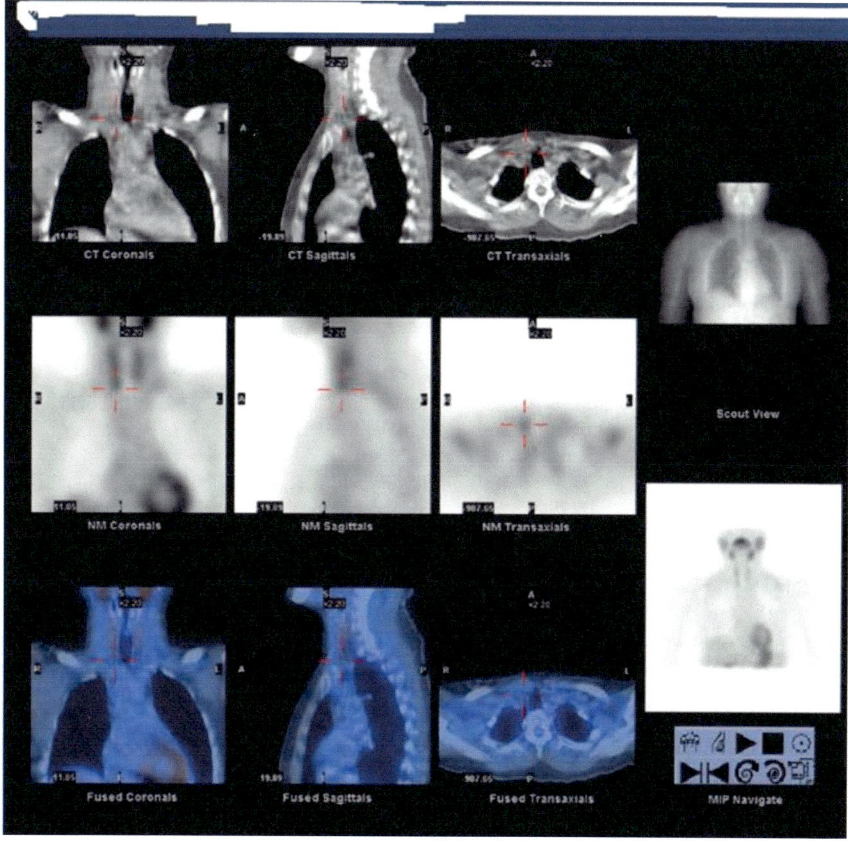

Fig. 5.4 Fusion sestamibi/CT imaging helps provide both anatomical and functional imaging. A right inferior parathyroid gland is identified

References

1. Khan A, Bilezikian J. Primary hyperparathyroidism: pathophysiology and impact on bone. CMAJ. 2000;163(2):184–7.
2. Eigelberger MS, Clark OH. Surgical approaches to primary hyperparathyroidism. Endocrinol Metab Clin North Am. 2000;29(3):479–502.
3. Delbridge LW, et al. Surgery for primary hyperparathyroidism 1962–1996: indications and outcomes. Med J Aust. 1998;168(4):153–6.
4. Hackett DA, Kauffman Jr GL. Historical perspective of parathyroid disease. Otolaryngol Clin North Am. 2004;37(4):689–700. vii.
5. Perrier ND. Asymptomatic hyperparathyroidism: a medical misnomer? Surgery. 2005;137(2):127–31.
6. Bilezikian JP, Silverberg SJ. Clinical practice. Asymptomatic primary hyperparathyroidism. N Engl J Med. 2004;350(17):1746–51.
7. Mack LA, Pasieka JL. Asymptomatic primary hyperparathyroidism: a surgical perspective. Surg Clin North Am. 2004;84(3):803–16.

8. NIH conference. Diagnosis and management of asymptomatic primary hyperparathyroidism: consensus development conference statement. Ann Intern Med. 1991;114(7):593–7.
9. Bilezikian JP, et al. Summary statement from a workshop on asymptomatic primary hyperparathyroidism: a perspective for the 21st century. J Bone Miner Res. 2002;17 Suppl 2:N2–11.
10. Silverberg SJ, et al. Presentation of asymptomatic primary hyperparathyroidism: proceedings of the third international workshop. J Clin Endocrinol Metab. 2009;94(2):351–65.
11. Silverberg SJ, Bilezikian JP. Primary hyperparathyroidism: still evolving? J Bone Miner Res. 1997;12(5):856–62.
12. Sywak MS, et al. Do the National Institutes of Health consensus guidelines for parathyroidectomy predict symptom severity and surgical outcome in patients with primary hyperparathyroidism? Surgery. 2002;132(6):1013–9. discussion 1019–20.
13. Udelsman R, et al. Surgery for asymptomatic primary hyperparathyroidism: proceedings of the third international workshop. J Clin Endocrinol Metab. 2009;94(2):366–72.
14. Caron NR, Pasieka JL. What symptom improvement can be expected after operation for primary hyperparathyroidism? World J Surg. 2009;33(11):2244–55.
15. The American Association of Clinical Endocrinologists and the American Association of Endocrine Surgeons position statement on the diagnosis and management of primary hyperparathyroidism. Endocr Pract. 2005;11(1):49–54.
16. Burney RE, et al. Health status improvement after surgical correction of primary hyperparathyroidism in patients with high and low preoperative calcium levels. Surgery. 1999;125(6):608–14.
17. Burney RE, et al. Surgical correction of primary hyperparathyroidism improves quality of life. Surgery. 1998;124(6):987–91. discussion 991–2.
18. Chan AK, et al. Clinical manifestations of primary hyperparathyroidism before and after parathyroidectomy. A case–control study. Ann Surg. 1995;222(3):402–12. discussion 412–4.
19. Lundgren E, et al. Case–control study on symptoms and signs of "asymptomatic" primary hyperparathyroidism. Surgery. 1998;124(6):980–5. discussion 985–6.
20. Talpos GB, et al. Randomized trial of parathyroidectomy in mild asymptomatic primary hyperparathyroidism: patient description and effects on the SF-36 health survey. Surgery. 2000;128(6):1013–20. discussion 1020–1.
21. Pasieka JL, et al. Patient-based surgical outcome tool demonstrating alleviation of symptoms following parathyroidectomy in patients with primary hyperparathyroidism. World J Surg. 2002;26(8):942–9.
22. Eigelberger MS, et al. The NIH criteria for parathyroidectomy in asymptomatic primary hyperparathyroidism: are they too limited? Ann Surg. 2004;239(4):528–35.
23. Prager G, et al. Parathyroidectomy improves concentration and retentiveness in patients with primary hyperparathyroidism. Surgery. 2002;132(6):930–5. discussion 935–6.
24. Mittendorf EA, et al. Improvement of sleep disturbance and neurocognitive function after parathyroidectomy in patients with primary hyperparathyroidism. Endocr Pract. 2007;13(4):338–44.
25. Quiros RM, et al. Health-related quality of life in hyperparathyroidism measurably improves after parathyroidectomy. Surgery. 2003;134(4):675–81. discussion 681–3.
26. Pasieka JL, Parsons LL. Prospective surgical outcome study of relief of symptoms following surgery in patients with primary hyperparathyroidism. World J Surg. 1998;22(6):513–8. discussion 518–9.
27. Mihai R, Sadler GP. Pasieka's parathyroid symptoms scores correlate with SF-36 scores in patients undergoing surgery for primary hyperparathyroidism. World J Surg. 2008;32(5):807–14.
28. Bollerslev J, et al. Medical observation, compared with parathyroidectomy, for asymptomatic primary hyperparathyroidism: a prospective, randomized trial. J Clin Endocrinol Metab. 2007;92(5):1687–92.
29. Ambrogini E, et al. Surgery or surveillance for mild asymptomatic primary hyperparathyroidism: a prospective, randomized clinical trial. J Clin Endocrinol Metab. 2007;92(8):3114–21.

30. Pasieka JL, Parsons L, Jones J. The long-term benefit of parathyroidectomy in primary hyperparathyroidism: a 10-year prospective surgical outcome study. Surgery. 2009;146(6): 1006–13.
31. Silverberg SJ, et al. Increased bone mineral density after parathyroidectomy in primary hyperparathyroidism. J Clin Endocrinol Metab. 1995;80(3):729–34.
32. Marshall D, Johnell O, Wedel H. Meta-analysis of how well measures of bone mineral density predict occurrence of osteoporotic fractures. BMJ. 1996;312(7041):1254–9.
33. Silverberg SJ, et al. A 10-year prospective study of primary hyperparathyroidism with or without parathyroid surgery. N Engl J Med. 1999;341(17):1249–55.
34. Silverberg SJ, Locker FG, Bilezikian JP. Vertebral osteopenia: a new indication for surgery in primary hyperparathyroidism. J Clin Endocrinol Metab. 1996;81(11):4007–12.
35. Almqvist EG, et al. Early parathyroidectomy increases bone mineral density in patients with mild primary hyperparathyroidism: a prospective and randomized study. Surgery. 2004;136(6): 1281–8.
36. Rubin MR, et al. Dynamic and structural properties of the skeleton in hypoparathyroidism. J Bone Miner Res. 2008;23(12):2018–24.
37. Mollerup CL, et al. Risk of renal stone events in primary hyperparathyroidism before and after parathyroid surgery: controlled retrospective follow up study. BMJ. 2002;325(7368):807.
38. Rodman JS, Mahler RJ. Kidney stones as a manifestation of hypercalcemic disorders. Hyperparathyroidism and sarcoidosis. Urol Clin North Am. 2000;27(2):275–85. viii.
39. Mollerup CL, Lindewald H. Renal stones and primary hyperparathyroidism: natural history of renal stone disease after successful parathyroidectomy. World J Surg. 1999;23(2):173–5. discussion 176.
40. Deaconson TF, Wilson SD, Lemann Jr J. The effect of parathyroidectomy on the recurrence of nephrolithiasis. Surgery. 1987;102(6):910–3.
41. Akerstrom G, Malmaeus J, Bergstrom R. Surgical anatomy of human parathyroid glands. Surgery. 1984;95(1):14–21.
42. Russell CF, Grant CS, van Heerden JA. Hyperfunctioning supernumerary parathyroid glands. An occasional cause of hyperparathyroidism. Mayo Clin Proc. 1982;57(2):121–4.
43. Suliburk JW, Perrier ND. Primary hyperparathyroidism. Oncologist. 2007;12(6):644–53.
44. Udelsman R. Six hundred fifty-six consecutive explorations for primary hyperparathyroidism. Ann Surg. 2002;235(5):665–70. discussion 670–2.
45. Tibblin S, Bondeson AG, Ljungberg O. Unilateral parathyroidectomy in hyperparathyroidism due to single adenoma. Ann Surg. 1982;195(3):245–52.
46. Russell C. Unilateral neck exploration for primary hyperparathyroidism. Surg Clin North Am. 2004;84(3):705–16.
47. Sidhu S, Neill AK, Russell CF. Long-term outcome of unilateral parathyroid exploration for primary hyperparathyroidism due to presumed solitary adenoma. World J Surg. 2003;27(3): 339–42.
48. Palazzo FF, Delbridge LW. Minimal-access/minimally invasive parathyroidectomy for primary hyperparathyroidism. Surg Clin North Am. 2004;84(3):717–34.
49. Gil-Cardenas A, et al. Is intraoperative parathyroid hormone assay mandatory for the success of targeted parathyroidectomy? J Am Coll Surg. 2007;204(2):286–90.
50. Miccoli P, et al. Results of video-assisted parathyroidectomy: single institution's six-year experience. World J Surg. 2004;28(12):1216–8.
51. Henry JF, et al. Indications and results of video-assisted parathyroidectomy by a lateral approach in patients with primary hyperparathyroidism. Surgery. 2001;130(6):999–1004.
52. Murphy C, Norman J. The 20% rule: a simple, instantaneous radioactivity measurement defines cure and allows elimination of frozen sections and hormone assays during parathyroidectomy. Surgery. 1999;126(6):1023–8. discussion 1028–9.
53. Coakley AJ, et al. 99Tcm sestamibi – a new agent for parathyroid imaging. Nucl Med Commun. 1989;10(11):791–4.
54. Stalberg P, et al. Intraoperative parathyroid hormone measurement during minimally invasive parathyroidectomy: does it "value-add" to decision-making? J Am Coll Surg. 2006;203(1):1–6.

55. Irvin 3rd GL, Carneiro DM. Intraoperative parathyroid hormone assay as a surgical adjunct in patients with sporadic primary hyperparathyroidism. In: Clark O, Duh QY, Kebebew E, editors. Textbook of endocrine surgery. Philadelphia: Elsevier Saunders; 2005. p. 472–80.
56. Carneiro DM, et al. Comparison of intraoperative iPTH assay (QPTH) criteria in guiding parathyroidectomy: which criterion is the most accurate? Surgery. 2003;134(6):973–9. discussion 979–81.
57. Gauger PG, et al. Intraoperative parathyroid hormone monitoring fails to detect double parathyroid adenomas: a 2-institution experience. Surgery. 2001;130(6):1005–10.

Chapter 6
Primary Hyperparathyroidism: Asymptomatic Medical Management

Aliya A. Khan

Keywords Asymptomatic pHPT • Estrogen therapy • Aminobisphosphonates • Alendronate • Risedronate • Zoledronate • Raloxifene • SERMs • Calcimimetics • Cinacalcet • Medical monitoring • Guidelines for surgery

Primary hyperparathyroidism (PHPT) is a relatively common endocrine condition being identified now in its early stages following introduction of multichannel biochemical screening and identification of hypercalcemia in those without signs or symptoms of its presence [1]. Previously, PHPT would present clinically with symptomatic hypercalcemia, renal stones, and skeletal complications, including osteitis fibrosa cystica characterized by Brown tumors of the long bones, tapering of the distal clavicles, a salt and pepper appearance of the skull, as well as subperiosteal bone resorption of the distal phalanges. The previous chapter addressed the management of classical PHPT with symptomatic disease. This chapter addresses asymptomatic PHPT characterized by mild hypercalcemia without signs or symptoms of its presence and without target organ complications of skeletal or renal disease.

The majority of individuals with asymptomatic PHPT are brought to medical attention following identification of hypercalcemia on routine biochemical screening or during the evaluation of other conditions, such as osteoporosis. These individuals may not have any specific signs or symptoms of their underlying PHPT. The clinical evaluation includes a comprehensive assessment with exclusion of other causes of hypercalemia, including familial hypocalciuric hypercalcemia (FHH). FHH is a rare condition transmitted in an autosomal dominant manner resulting from an inactivating mutation of the calcium-sensing receptor gene (discussed in Chap. 11). It also includes an assessment of potential target organ damage. Skeletal status and the presence of prior fragility fractures are evaluated as well an assessment of bone mineral

A.A. Khan, MD, FRCPC, FACP, FACE (⬚)
Department of Endocrinology and Metabolism, McMaster University, Hamilton, ON, Canada
e-mail: aliya@mcmaster.ca

A.A. Khan and O.H. Clark (eds.), *Handbook of Parathyroid Diseases: A Case-Based Practical Guide*, DOI 10.1007/978-1-4614-2164-1_6, © Springer Science+Business Media, LLC 2012 density and fracture risk. Bone scanning is appropriately completed in the presence of elevations in alkaline phosphatase. Biochemical markers of bone turnover are elevated in approximately 1/3 of those with PHPT reflecting increases in bone turnover. Renal function is evaluated and a baseline ultrasound of the kidneys is completed to ensure that occult nephrolithiasis is not present and to confirm that the patient is truly "asymptomatic" without overt bone or renal disease. Low bone density may be present and may be a reflection of bone loss in association with PHPT or due to other factors, such as postmenopausal bone loss.

Elevations of parathyroid hormone (PTH) in the presence of an elevated serum calcium provide the basis for diagnosis of PHPT. Other factors contributing to hypercalcemia should be excluded, such as the use of thiazide diuretics or lithium in which case these drugs should be discontinued and the biochemical assessment repeated in 3 months. Serum phosphorous is normal or low in PHPT. Elevations in serum chloride may be seen with a decrease in serum bicarbonate. Due to the effects of PTH on the kidney, approximately 30% of individuals have elevations in the 24-h urine calcium. 25-hydroxy vitamin D levels may be in the low range of normal or may be frankly low. Vitamin D insufficiency with levels of 25-hydroxy vitamin D < 50 nmol/L or 20 ng/mL has been reported in approximately 81% of patients with PHPT in comparison to the control population in whom it has been reported to be approximately 60% [2]. It is possible that in PHPT there is increased catabolism of 25-hydroxy vitamin D [3]. Vitamin D insufficiency has also been associated with increased weight of the parathyroid adenomas and in an increased severity of the condition [4, 5].

PTH can be evaluated by either the second- or the third-generation assays (discussed in detail in Chap. 3). The third-generation PTH assay provides results which are approximately 50% lower in individuals with chronic kidney disease in comparison to the second-generation assays. In normal individuals, the third-generation assay is approximately 20% lower in comparison to second-generation assays [6]. PTH values can also be affected by other factors, including race, gender, and age. Elevations in PTH have been noted in older individuals as well as in blacks in comparison to whites [7–9]. Low calcium intake is also associated with elevations in PTH [10]. As documented in the previous chapter, vitamin D insufficiency is associated with elevations in PTH. At the recent third international workshop on asymptomatic PHPT, it was recommended that all patients with vitamin D insufficiency be replaced with vitamin D supplementation with achievement of a 25-hydroxy vitamin D level of greater than 50 nmol/L [11].

Skeletal X-rays can be completed in the presence of bone pain. Spinal X-rays are of value in individuals with spinal deformity. Routine skeletal surveys, however, are not recommended in those with asymptomatic PHPT as the likelihood of identifying additional skeletal pathology is minimal. Dual-energy X-ray absorptiometry (DXA) assessment is of benefit in identifying the degree of demineralization present [12]. In PHPT, typically, the greatest impact with respect to decreases in bone density is noted at the distal 1/3 radial site with relatively well-maintained bone density at the lumbar spine and intermediate bone mineral density (BMD) values are noted at the hip [13]. Reductions in volumetric BMD evaluated by peripheral

Table 6.1 Comparison of new and old guidelines for parathyroid surgery in asymptomatic PHPT[a]

Measurement	1990	2002	2008
Serum calcium (>upper limit of normal)	1–1.6 mg/dL (0.25–0.4 mmol/L)	1.0 mg/dL (0.25 mmol/L)	1.0 mg/dL (0.25 mmol/L)
24-h urine for calcium	>400 mg/day (>10 mmol/day)	>400 mg/day (>10 mmol/day)	Not indicated[b]
Creative clearance (calculated)	Reduced by 30%	Reduced by 30%	Reduced to <60 mL/min
BMD	Z-score <−2.0 in forearm	T-score <−2.5 at any site[c]	T-score <−2.5 at any site[c] and/or previous fracture fragility[d]
Age (year)	<50	<50	<50

[a]Surgery is also indicated in patients for whom medical surveillance is neither desired nor possible
[b]Some physicians still regard 24-h urinary calcium excretion >400 mg as an indication for surgery
[c]Lumbar spine, total hip, femoral neck, or 33% radius (1/3 site). This recommendation is made recognizing that the other skeletal features may contribute to fracture risk in PHPT and that the validity of this cut-point for any site vis-à-vis fracture risk prediction has not been established in PHPT
[d]Consistent with the position established by the International Society for Clinical Densitometry, the use of Z-scores is recommended in evaluating BMD in premenopausal women and men younger than 50 years

quantitative computed tomography (pQCT) of the radius have shown a significant reduction in patients with PHPT in comparison to controls [14]. In this study, areal BMD was also evaluated by DXA and the PHPT population had comparable BMD at the lumbar spine with decreases at the 1/3 radial site in comparison to the control population [14]. The pQCT studies of the tibia have demonstrated catabolic effect on both trabecular and cortical skeletal sites in patients with PHPT in comparison to controls [15]. It appears in summary that different patterns of bone loss may occur. Catabolic effects at sites rich in trabecular bone with preservation of geometric properties as well as catabolic effects in sites rich in cortical bone with cortical thinning and endosteal resorption have been described [16].

Observational data over 15 years has demonstrated disease progression in approximately 1/3 of patients with mild PHPT. Parathyroidectomy, however, has been associated with improvements in BMD at both cortical and trabecular skeletal sites with reductions in bone turnover. At the third International workshop held in 2008, it was recommended to proceed with parathyroidectomy in the presence of low BMD with T-scores of −2.5 or less at the lumbar spine, femoral neck, total hip, or 1/3 distal radial sites in postmenopausal women and men aged 50 and older [11]. The revised recommendations for surgical intervention in those with asymptomatic PHPT are described in the Tables 6.1 and 6.2 [17]. Individuals under the age of 50 have demonstrated progressive bone loss in comparison to older individuals, with 65% of the younger individuals experiencing decreases in bone density in comparison to 23% of those over the age of 50. Those with asymptomatic PHPT who do not proceed with surgery should be closely followed. The revised recommendations for follow-up from the Third International workshop are listed below [11].

Table 6.2 Comparison of new and old management guidelines for patients with asymptomatic primary hyperparathyroidism who do not undergo parathyroid surgery

Measurement	1990	2002	2008
Serum calcium	Biannually	Biannually	Annually
24-h urinary calcium	Annually	Not recommended	Not recommended
Creatinine clearance (24-h urine collections)	Annually	Not recommended	Not recommended
Serum creatinine	Annually	Annually	Annually
Bone density	Annually (forearm)	Annually (3 sites)	Every 1–2 year (3 sites)[a]
Abdominal X-ray (±ultrasound)	Annually	Not recommended	Not recommended

[a]This recommendation acknowledges country-specific advisories as well as the need for more frequent monitoring if the clinical situation is appropriate

In those with stable disease, follow-up can be completed on an annual basis with monitoring of serum calcium and serum creatinine. BMD testing is recommended on a 1–2-year basis evaluating three skeletal sites, including assessment of the 1/3 radial site.

Treatment of Asymptomatic PHPT

Longitudinal studies of PHPT individuals who have not undergone surgery have documented relative stability in serum calcium, PTH, and creatinine over 10–18 years of follow-up [18–20]. In an observational study with prolonged follow-up of 15 years, approximately 60% of individuals with asymptomatic PHPT experienced more than 10% decrease in BMD at the lumbar spine, proximal femur, or forearm [18]. Unfortunately, this study did not have a control group. Other investigators have documented relative stability in BMD at the lumbar spine and the total body. However, BMD decreases were noted at the femoral neck [20]. Surgical correction of PHPT is associated with reductions in bone turnover and significant improvements in BMD [13, 21–23]. It is, thus, recommended that parathyroidectomy be considered for patients with asymptomatic PHPT. For those in whom surgery is not possible and who have mild disease, monitoring is a safe option [17].

Patients are recommended to be physically active and avoid dehydration. Patients should be advised to avoid the use of thiazide diuretics as well as lithium in order to avoid the possibility of further rises in serum calcium. Additional calcium supplementation is not recommended; however, restriction of dietary calcium is also not advised as this may lead to further rises in PTH. Phosphate supplementation is not recommended due to concerns of extraskeletal calcification.

Medical management includes correction of vitamin D insufficiency. Vitamin D insufficiency may play a role in the severity of PHPT and also in the development of the osteitis fibrosa cystica and further growth of parathyroid tumors [4, 5]. Vitamin D deficiency may result in progressive bone loss and further elevations in

PTH. Vitamin D supplementation has not been associated with increases in serum calcium. Correction of vitamin D insufficiency has, however, been associated with reductions in PTH. Supplementation with cholecalciferol 400 IU daily was not associated with rises in serum calcium or further increases in urinary calcium excretion [24]. Vitamin D_3 in doses of 50,000 IU weekly for 4 weeks followed by once a month for 1 year did not result in elevations in serum calcium in 21 women with PHPT and vitamin D insufficiency [24]. These individuals had vitamin D insufficiency with 25 hydroxy vitamin D levels < 50 nmol/L (20 ng/mL). Serum calcium did not rise; however, PTH decreased by 26% and serum alkaline phosphatase levels also decreased significantly. Following 1 year of supplementation, the mean 25 hydroxy vitamin D levels were 77 nmol/L [24]. It appears that careful vitamin D replacement in individuals with PHPT aiming for a 25-hydroxy vitamin D level of at least 50 nmol/L is well-tolerated and safe and is associated with improvements in serum PTH. Further studies are needed to assess the impact of vitamin D supplementation on bone mineralization and fracture risk in individuals with PHPT.

Aminobisphosphonates, analogs of pyrophosphate, are potent inhibitors of bone resorption and have been evaluated in patients with PHPT. The aminobisphosphonate is preferentially deposited at active remodeling sites in the skeleton, where 50% of the drug is deposited. The remaining 50% is cleared by the kidneys [25]. With bone resorption, the drug is released from the matrix and internalized by osteoclasts, where it inhibits farnesyl pyrophosphate synthase, a key enzyme in the cholesterol synthesis pathway. Inhibiting this enzyme disrupts pathways involved in cytoskeletal organization, cell survival, and proliferation and leads to inhibition of the osteoclast and osteoclast apoptosis [26]. Decreases in bone turnover are associated with enhanced bone mineralization as the resorption phase is shortened.

Aminobisphosphonates have successfully been used in hypercalcemia of malignancy and their effectiveness in lowering serum calcium in PHPT has been evaluated. Early data with etidronate and clodronate demonstrated inconsistent effects on serum calcium in PHPT. The first aminobisphosphonate used in this condition was pamidronate given in 30-mg doses intravenously to ten patients in a randomized crossover study (IV BP from the medical management of PHPT). Transient decreases in serum calcium from 2.72 ± 0.06 to 2.49 ± 0.04 mmol/L (10.88 ± 0.24 to 9.96 ± 0.16 mg/dL) were noted after 1 week [27]. PTH levels were noted to increase during this time period and the effect on serum calcium was only transient [27]. Residronate given in doses of 20 and 40 mg daily for 7 days was evaluated in 19 postmenopausal women and 7 men. This cycle was repeated after 3 weeks. Decreases in serum calcium from 11.04 ± 0.16 to 10.4 ± 0.16 mg/dL (2.76 ± 0.04 to 2.6 ± 0.04 mmol/L) were noted after 1 week. These decreases in serum calcium were accompanied by increases in PTH as well as increases in renal calcium reabsorption [28]. There have been no long-term studies completed evaluating residronate in PHPT. Alendronate has been evaluated in PHPT. Decreases in bone turnover were noted with reductions in alkaline phosphatase and osteocalcin as well as in urinary deoxypyridinoline excretion in 26 elderly women randomized to treatment vs. no treatment over 2 years. BMD increased at the lumbar spine, total hip, and total body with transient decreases in serum calcium phosphate and urinary calcium excretion during the first 3–6 months but returned to baseline following treatment [29]. Alendronate, 10 mg/day, was compared to placebo for 48 weeks followed by treatment withdrawal for 24 weeks in 40 postmenopausal women. BMD was significantly higher with alendronate in comparison to placebo. Serum calcium was reduced with alendronate but not with placebo. Biomarkers were reduced with alendronate treatment. There were no changes in urinary calcium [30]. A multicenter trial evaluated 44 patients with PHPT randomized to placebo or alendronate 10 mg daily after 12 months the placebo group was crossed over to active treatment. All patients were on active treatment in the second year. BMD was evaluated at the lumbar spine, femoral neck, total hip, and distal 1/3 radial sites, every 6 months by DXA. Alendronate over 2 years was associated with increases in the lumbar spine BMD in comparison to baseline ($6.8 \pm 0.94\%$, $p < 0.001$). Total hip BMD increased at 12 months by $4.01 \pm 0.77\%$ ($p < 0.001$) and was stable over the next 12 months of treatment. The distal 1/3 radial site did not show statistically significant changes with the alendronate therapy. Reductions in biomarkers were noted with decreases in urinary N-telopeptide excretion by 66% ($p < 0.001$) at 3 months. Bone-specific alkaline phosphatase decreased by 49% at 6 months ($p < 0.001$). Serum calcium, both total and ionized, PTH, and urinary calcium did not change with alendronate therapy [31]. In this study, 25-hydroxy vitamin D levels were 18.2 ng/mL or 45.5 nmol/L at baseline in the group receiving alendronate for 24 months and 18.6 ng/mL or 46.5 nmol/L in the group receiving placebo. Vitamin D levels were higher than those seen in the study conducted by Chow et al. [30] in whom the mean values of 25-hydroxy vitamin D were 38 nmol/L. The lower vitamin D levels may have contributed to transient decreases in serum calcium in association with elevations in PTH with bisphosphonate therapy. The RCT data with alendronate has demonstrated decreases in bone turnover and increases in BMD at the lumbar spine and the proximal femur. The effect on serum calcium has not been consistent and may have been affected by the baseline vitamin D levels. Unfortunately, Vitamin D levels have not been reported in all the studies conducted to date. Bisphosphonate therapy may lead to improvements in bone strength; however, fracture data is currently not available to confirm this.

Estrogen is an effective treatment for the management of postmenopausal osteoporosis. It may provide skeletal protection by decreasing bone resorption. In a study evaluating 42 postmenopausal women with mild PHPT, conjugated estrogen in doses of 0.625 mg/day and medroxyprogesterone acetate 5 mg/day were compared to placebo. The BMD at the total body and proximal forearm decreased from baseline in the placebo-treated group. In the hormone replacement therapy (HRT) group, BMD increased from baseline. The increases at the total body were $1.3 \pm 0.4\%$ ($p = 0.004$), lumbar spine $5.2 \pm 1.4\%$ ($p = 0.002$), and femoral neck $3.4 \pm 1.5\%$ ($p = 0.05$). In the HRT group, alkaline phosphatase levels decreased by 22% ($p = 0.004$) vs. baseline. Urinary hydroxy proline and urinary cross-linked N-telopeptides (NTX) also decreased by 42 and 54%, respectively. Urinary calcium decreased by 45% ($p = 0.007$). There were no changes noted in ionized calcium or intact PTH [32]. HRT has been shown in limited studies to decrease bone turnover and reduce urinary calcium excretion. Increases in BMD throughout the skeleton have been noted in postmenopausal women with mild PHPT. Estrogen has not been shown to be effective in lowering serum calcium.

Selective estrogen receptor modulators (SERMs) have tissue-specific estrogen agonistic or antagonistic effects. They do provide skeletal protection in postmenopausal women. Raloxifene has been evaluated in postmenopausal women with PHPT. Eighteen postmenopausal women were studied and were randomized to 8 weeks of raloxifene given in 60 mg/day dose vs. placebo followed by a 4-week washout phase. At baseline, the groups were well-matched. Total serum calcium decreased by 8 weeks of raloxifene from 10.8 ± 0.2 to 10.4 ± 0.2 mg/dL ($p < 0.05$). Biomarkers also decreased with decreases in osteocalcin from 11.4 ± 1.6 to 9.9 ± 1.6 nmol/L ($p < 0.05$). Serum NTX decreased from 21.2 ± 3.4 to 17.3 ± 2.8 nmol bce/L ($p < 0.05$). Four weeks following cessation of raloxifene, these values returned to baseline. Raloxifene administration did not affect serum PTH, 125-dihydroxy vitamin D, total alkaline phosphatase, or urinary calcium levels [33]. This study did not evaluate the impact of raloxifene on BMD. There is limited data on the effects of raloxifene on BMD. Raloxifene treatment has been associated with prevention of bone loss at the spine and the hip in three patients with PHPT [34].

Calcimimetic agents increase the sensitivity of calcium-sensing receptor to the serum calcium level. Cinacalcet, a calcimimetic agent, was evaluated in a randomized, double-blind, placebo-controlled trial in patients with PHPT. Seventy-eight patients were randomized to placebo or cinacalcet. In the first 3 months, the dose was titrated from 30 to 50 mg twice a day, followed by a 12th-week maintenance phase and a 28-week follow-up. The primary end point was a predose serum calcium of less than 2.57 mmol/L and a decrease of more than or equal to 0.12 mmol/L. Seventy-three percent of the patients on cinacalcet in comparison to five percent of placebo patients reached the end point. Serum phosphorus values increased significantly in the cinacalcet-treated group from 2.7 ± 0.5 to 3.2 ± 0.5 mg/dL (0.87 ± 0.16 to 1.03 ± 0.16 mmol/L, $p < 0.001$). There were no statistically significant changes in the 24-h urinary calcium/creatinine or 1,25-diydroxyvitamin D levels or the biochemical markers of bone turnover. BMD Z-scores did not change significantly with cinacalcet treatment over the 52-week study [35]. A 4-year open-label extension of this study continued with 45 patients [36]. Eighty percent of patients maintained a normal-range serum calcium during the extension phase. BMD did not improve. Adverse events included nausea and headache; however, the drug was relatively well-tolerated.

In summary, in those unable or unwilling to proceed with surgery medical monitoring is a potential option. It is recommended that patients be closely observed and the guidelines for observation have recently been revised to allow for safe ongoing follow-up. Medical management options include correction of vitamin D insufficiency as well as antiresorptive options, including aminobisphosphonates, and hormone replacement therapy. Data is very limited regarding the effectiveness of raloxifene in the prevention of skeletal complications of PHPT. Cinacalcet has been evaluated in PHPT and is effective in lowering serum calcium and PTH.

HRT and aminobisphosphonates have not been shown to be effective in lowering serum calcium or PTH. Fracture data is not yet available with either bisphosphonates or HRT in those with PHPT. Cinacalcet has not been shown to effect BMD or bone turnover markers. Further study is needed evaluating the effects of these agents on bone strength and fracture risk.

References

1. Khan AA, Hanley DA, O'Brien CJ, Pasieka J, Ste-Marie LG, Rotstein LE, Rosen I, Young JEM, Josse RG, Bilezikian JP. Position paper: asymptomatic primary hyperparathyroidism – standards and guidelines for diagnosis and management in Canada. Endocr Pract. 2003;9(5): 400–5.
2. Rao DS, Agarwal G, Talpos GB, Phillips ER, Bandeira F, Mishra SK, Mithal A. Role of vitamin D and calcium nutrition in disease expression and parathyroid tumor growth in primary hyperparathyroidism: a global perspective. J Bone Miner Res. 2002;17 Suppl 2:N75–80.
3. Moosgaard B, Vestergaard P, Heickendorff L, Melsen F, Christiansen P, Mosekilde L. Vitamin D status, seasonal variations, parathyroid adenoma weight and bone mineral density in primary hyperparathyroidism. Clin Endocrinol (Oxf). 2005;63(5):506–13.
4. Rao DS, Honasoge M, Divine GW, Phillips ER, Lee MW, Ansari MR, Talpos GB, Michael Parfitt A. Effect of vitamin D nutrition on parathyroid adenoma weight: pathogenetic and clinical implications. J Clin Endocrinol Metab. 2000;85:1054–8.
5. Clements MR, Davies M, Fraser DR, Lumb GA, Mawer EB, Adams PH. Metabolic inactivation of vitamin D is enhanced in primary hyperparathyroidism. Clin Sci (Lond). 1987; 73(6):659–64.
6. John MR, Goodman WG, Gao P, Cantor TL, Salusky IB, Jüppner H. A novel immunoradiometric assay detects full-length human PTH but not amino-terminally truncated fragments: implications for PTH measurements in renal failure. J Clin Endocrinol Metab. 1999;84: 4287–90.
7. Freaney R, McBrinn Y, McKenna MJ. Secondary hyperparathyroidism in elderly people: combined effect of renal insufficiency and vitamin D deficiency. Am J Clin Nutr. 1993;58:187–91.
8. Maggio D, Cherubini A, Lauretani F, Russo RC, Bartali B, Pierandrei M, Ruggiero C, Macchiarulo MC, Giorgino R, Minisola S, Ferrucci L. 25(OH)D serum levels decline with age earlier in women than in men and less efficiently prevent compensatory hyperparathyroidism in older adults. J Gerontol. 2005;60A:1414–9.
9. Harris SS, Soteriades E, Coolidge JA, Mudgal S, Dawson-Hughes B. Vitamin D insufficiency and hyperparathyroidism in a low income, multiracial, elderly population. J Clin Endocrinol Metab. 2000;85:4125–30.
10. Steingrimsdottir L, Gunnarsson O, Indridason OS, Franzson L, Sigurdsson G. Relationship between serum parathyroid hormone levels, vitamin D sufficiency, and calcium intake. JAMA. 2005;294:2336–41.
11. Bilezikian JP, Khan AA, Potts Jr JT. Guidelines for the management of asymptomatic primary hyperparathyroidism: summary statement from the third international workshop. J Clin Endocrinol Metab. 2009;94(2):335–9.
12. Khan AA, Syed Z. Bone densitometry in post menopausal women: synthesis and review. J Clin Densitom. 2004;7(1):85–92.
13. Silverberg SJ, Shane E, Jacobs TP, Siris E, Bilezikian JP. A 10 year prospective study of primary hyperparathyroidism with or without parathyroid surgery. N Engl J Med. 1999;341(17): 1249–55.
14. Chen Q, Kaji H, Iu MF, Nomura R, Sowa H, Yamauchi M, Tsukamoto T, Sugimoto T, Chihara K. Effects of an excess and a deficiency of endogenous parathyroid hormone on volumetric bone mineral density and bone geometry determined by peripheral quantitative computed tomography in female subjects. J Clin Endocrinol Metab. 2003;88(10):4655–8.
15. Charopoulos I, Tournis S, Trovas G, Raptou P, Kaldrymides P, Skarandavos G, Katsalira K, Lyritis GP. Effect of primary hyperparathyroidism on volumetric bone mineral density and bone geometry assessed by peripheral quantitative computed tomography in postmenopausal women. J Clin Endocrinol Metab. 2006;91(5):1748–53.
16. Silverberg SJ, Lewiecki EM, Mosekilde L, Peacock M, Rubin MR. Proceedings from the third international workshop on the management of asymptomatic primary hyperparathyroidism: current issues in the presentation of asymptomatic primary hyperparathyroidism. J Clin Endocrinol Metab. 2009;94(2):351–65.

17. Khan AA, Bilezikian JP, Potts Jr JT. The diagnosis and management of asymptomatic primary hyperparathyroidism revisited. J Clin Endocrinol Metab. 2009;94(2):333–4.
18. Rubin MR, Bilezikian JP, McMahon DJ, Jacobs T, Shane E, Siris E, Udesky J, Silverberg SJ. The natural history of primary hyperparathyroidism with or without parathyroid surgery after 15 years. J Clin Endocrinol Metab. 2008;93:3462–70.
19. Iskander J, Rao D. Long term morbidity and mortality in untreated mild primary hyperparathyroidism. J Bone Miner Res. 2007;22:S353.
20. Bolland MJ, Grey AB, Orr-Walker BJ, Horne AM, Evans MC, Clearwater JM, Gamble GD, Reid IR. Prospective 10-year study of postmenopausal women with asymptomatic primary hyperparathyroidism. N Z Med J. 2008;121:18–29.
21. Rao DS, Phillips ER, Divine GW, Talpos GB. Randomized controlled clinical trial of surgery versus no surgery in patients with mild asymptomatic primary hyperparathyroidism. J Clin Endocrinol Metab. 2004;89(11):5415–22.
22. Bollerslev J, Jansson S, Mollerup CL, Nordenstrom J, Lundgren E, Torring O, Varhaug J-E, Baranowski M, Aanderud S, Franco C, Freyschuss B, IsaksenGA UT, Rosen T. Medical observation, compared with parathyroidectomy, for asymptomatic primary hyperparathyroidism: a prospective, randomized trial. J Clin Endocrinol Metab. 2007;92:1687–92.
23. Ambrogini E, Cetani F, Cianferotti L, Vignali E, Banti C, Viccica G, Oppo A, Miccoli P, Berti P, Bilezikian JP, Pinchera A, Marcocci C. Surgery or surveillance of mild asymptomatic primary hyperparathyroidism: a prospective, randomized clinical trial. J Clin Endocrinol Metab. 2007;92:3114–21.
24. Grey A, Lucas J, Horne A, Gamble G, Davidson JS, Reid IR. Vitamin D repletion in patients with primary hyperparathyroidism and coexistent vitamin D insufficiency. J Clin Endocrinol Metab. 2005;90(4):2122–6.
25. Khan SA, Kanis JA, Vasikaran S, Kline WF, Matuszewski BK, McCloskey EV, Beneton MNC, Gertz BJ, Schiberras DG, Holland SD, Orgee J, Coombes GM, Rogers SR, Porras AG. Elimination and biochemical responses to intravenous alendronate in postmenopausal osteoporosis. J Bone Miner Res. 1997;12:1700–7.
26. Meunier PJ, Arlot M, Chavassieux P, Yates AJ. The effects of Alendronate on bone turnover and bone quality. Int J Clin Pract Suppl. 1999;101:14–7.
27. Schmidli RS, Wilson I, Espiner EA, Richards AM, Donald RA. Aminopropylidine diphosphonate (ADP) in mild primary hyperparathyroidism: effects on clinical status. Clin Endocrinol (Oxf). 1990;32:293–300.
28. Reasner CA, Stone MD, Hosking DJ, Ballah A, Mundy GR. Acute changes in calcium homeostasis during treatment of primary hyperparathyroidism with risedronate. J Clin Endocrinol Metab. 1993;77:1067–71.
29. Rossini M, Gatti D, Isaia G, Sartori L, Braga V, Asami S. Effects of oral alendronate in elderly patients with osteoporosis and mild primary hyperparathyroidism. J Bone Miner Res. 2001;16:113–9.
30. Chow CC, Chan WB, Li JK, Chan NW, Chan MHM, Ko GTC, Lo KW, Cockram CS. Oral alendronate increases bone mineral density in postmenopausal women with primary hyperparathyroidism. J Clin Endocrinol Metab. 2003;88:581–7.
31. Khan AA, Bilezikian JP, Kung AW, Ahmed MM, Dubois SJ, Ho AYY, Schussheim D, Rubin MR, Shaikh AM, Silverberg SJ, Standish TI, Syed Z, Syed ZA. Alendronate in primary hyperparathyroidism: a double blind, randomized, placebo controlled trial. J Clin Endocrinol Metab. 2004;89:3319–25.
32. Grey AB, Stapleton JP, Evans MC, Tatnell MA, Reid IR. Effect of hormone replacement therapy on bone mineral density in postmenopausalwomen with mild primary hyperparathyroidism. A randomized, controlled trial. Ann Intern Med. 1996;125:360–8.
33. Rubin MR, Lee KH, McMahon DJ, Silverberg SJ. Raloxifene lowers serum calcium and markers of bone turnover in postmenopausal women with primary hyperparathyroidism. J Clin Endocrinol Metab. 2003;88:1174–8.
34. Zanchetta JR, Bogado CE. Raloxifene reverses bone loss in postmenopausal women with mild asymptomatic primary hyperparathyroidism. J Bone Miner Res. 2001;16:189–90.

35. Peacock M, Bilezikian JP, Bolognese MA, Borofsky M, Scumpia S, Sterling LR, Cheng S, Shoback D. Cinacalcet HCL reduces hypercalcemia in primary hyperparathyroidism across a wide spectrum of disease severity. J Clin Endocrinol Metab. 2011;96(1):E9–18.
36. Peacock M, Scumpia S, Bolognese MA, Borofsky MA, Olson K, McCary LC, Schwanauer LE, Shoback DM. Long term control of primary hyperparathyroidism with cinacalcet HCl. J Bone Miner Res. 2006;21(Suppl1):S38.

Chapter 7
Surgical Management of Asymptomatic Primary Hyperparathyroidism

Rachel Farkas, Jacob Moalem, and Orlo H. Clark

Keywords Asymptomatic pHPT • Bone loss • Neuromuscular symptoms • CV complications • Glucose intolerance • Neuropsychiatric symptoms • NIH treatment criteria • Health status assessment tools • Quality of life • Natural history of PHPT

Introduction

Operative management of primary hyperparathyroidism began in 1925 when Felix Mendl performed the first successful parathyroidectomy for a patient with Von Recklinghousen Disease. This landmark operation initiated the practice of parathyroidectomy for patients with primary hyperparathyroidism and osteitis fibrosa cystica between 1925 and 1932. In 1932, Dr. Fuller Albright noted that 80% of patients treated with parathyroidectomy for primary hyperparathyroidism and osteitis fibrosa cystica also had either nephrolithiasis or nephrocalcinosis. This observation widened the criteria for operative intervention to include patients with hyperparathyroidism and nephrolithiasis and less severe bone disease. Thus, over the subsequent 30 years, the major indication for parathyroidectomy became renal stones without overt bone disease.

Through the 1960s, the clinical manifestations of primary hyperparathyroidism typically involved a classic pentad of symptoms—painful bones, kidney stones, abdominal groans, psychotic moans, and fatigue overtones. In that era, the most common initial symptom among patients diagnosed with primary hyperparathyroidism was the passage of renal stones [1].

R. Farkas, MD • J. Moalem, MD
Department of Surgery, University of Rochester Medical Center, Rochester, NY, USA

O.H. Clark, MD (⊠)
Department of Surgery, University of California, San Francisco, 1600 Divisadero St., Hellman Building Room C-347, Box 1674, San Francisco, CA 94143-1674, USA
e-mail: clarko@surgery.ucsf.edu

A.A. Khan and O.H. Clark (eds.), *Handbook of Parathyroid Diseases:
A Case-Based Practical Guide*, DOI 10.1007/978-1-4614-2164-1_7,
© Springer Science+Business Media, LLC 2012

The advent of the serum channel autoanalyzer in the mid 1960s enabled the routine screening of serum calcium levels. Consequently, the incidence of primary hyperparathyroidism rose precipitously, and a biochemically milder form of the disease became recognized. Currently, most new cases are incidentally discovered by routine blood tests [2]. Although many of these patients have fatigue, weakness, musculoskeletal aches and pains, and osteopenia or osteoporosis, these nonspecific clinical manifestations also occur in patients without hyperparathyroidism [3].

Case: A 59-year-old woman is found to be mildly hypercalcemic (calcium 10.9 mg/dl) on routine testing at her annual physical examination. Upon further questioning, the patient volunteers that she has been fatigued with mild depression and arthralgias for the previous 2 years. Cardiac evaluation reveals that she is hypertensive with a blood pressure of 170/98, mild left ventricular hypertrophy, and hyperlipidemia. She has osteopenia of her lumbar spine. She denies a history of kidney stones, has never had a fracture, and feels relatively "well." The patient has normal renal function and denies any personal or familial history of hypercalcemia or endocrinopathies. Her blood PTH level was 111 pg/ml (normal 16–65 pg/ml) and her 24-h urinary calcium was 257 mg/24 h. How should her case be managed?

Epidemiology

Primary hyperpara thyroidism affects 0.2–0.5% of the general population [4]. There are approximately 100,000 new cases annually in the USA [5]. Hyperparathyroidism is diagnosed in 1 of every 500 women older than 40, and 1 of every 2,000 men [6]. Primary hyperparathyroidism is the third most common endocrine disorder today, after diabetes mellitus and hypothyroidism, and is the most common cause of hypercalcemia in nonhospitalized patients.

The Presentation of Primary Hyperparathyroidism

The manifestations of primary hyperparathyroidism can be divided into two groups, symptoms (which one feels) and associated conditions (which can be measured) [7]. Symptoms of primary hyperparathyroidism include fatigue, musculoskeletal aches and pains, weakness, dyspepsia, polydipsia, constipation, polyuria, nocturia, anorexia, pruritis, nausea, depression, and memory loss. Associated conditions include nephrolithiasis, nephrocalcinosis, hematuria, osteopenia, osteoporosis, proximal muscle weakness as well as weight loss, gout, pancreatitis, left ventricular hypertrophy, hyperlipidemia, and hypertension. While the degree of hypercalcemia does not predict the presence of these symptoms or associated conditions, it correlates, in some investigations, with their severity.

Diagnosis

Primary hyperparathyroidism is characterized by hypersecretion of parathyroid hormone from one or more abnormal parathyroid glands. The diagnosis is confirmed by demonstrating an elevated parathyroid hormone level in a hypercalcemic patient. A normal or increased urinary calcium concentration, in the setting of preserved renal function, excludes benign familial hypocalciuric hypercalcemia (BFHH), which also presents with an elevated parathyroid hormone level and usually mild hypercalcemia but with low urinary calcium (less than 100 mg/24 h). This is an important diagnosis to rule out since it requires no treatment and parathyroidectomy offers no "cure." Patients with BFHH are always hypercalcemic so that documentation of a previously normal blood calcium level also rules out this condition.

Associated laboratory abnormalities that may be detected in patients with primary hyperparathyroidism include decreased serum phosphate level and high-normal or increased serum chloride levels. Some authorities use a chloride:phosphate ratio greater than 33 to differentiate hypercalcemia due to primary hyperparathyroidism from hypercalcemia due to other causes. Recently, the sensitivity of this simple, inexpensive screen was found to be so high (in patients with normal renal function and without emesis) that it was suggested as an adequate replacement for the more expensive parathyroid hormone measurement [8]. Uncommonly, elevated levels of blood urea nitrogen, creatinine, uric acid, and alkaline phosphatase are present in patients with primary hyperparathyroidism. These laboratory tests should, therefore, be evaluated.

Treatment

NIH Consensus Conferences of 1990, 2002, and 2008

The changing presentation and marked increase in the number of patients being treated for primary hyperparathyroidism led to an NIH consensus conference in 1990 to answer the following questions: (1) Are there patients with "asymptomatic" primary hyperparathyroidism who can be followed medically? (2) If these patients are not operated on, how should they be monitored and managed? (3) Are there indications for surgery in patients with asymptomatic primary hyperparathyroidism?

At its conclusion, the panel acknowledged that parathyroidectomy is indicated for all patients who are at risk for progression of their disease, including patients under 50 years of age. Vague symptoms in "asymptomatic" patients with primary hyperparathyroidism were not considered an indication for parathyroidectomy.

Because of the improvements in the understanding of the presentation of primary hyperparathyroidism and the advent of minimally invasive parathyroidectomy, the

Table 7.1 National Institutes of Health Consensus Development Conference

1990	2002	2008
Marked hypercalcemia (1–1.6 mg/dl) above reference range	Marked hypercalcemia *[>0.25 mol/l (1.0 mg/dl)]* above reference range	Unchanged from 2002
History of a life-threatening episode of hypercalcemia	Same	Same
Hypercalciuria [24-h excretion >10 mol (400 mg/dl)]	Same	Eliminated from criteria
Renal insufficiency (creatinine clearance reduced by 30% compared with normal age-matched controls)	Same	Redefined at GFR <60 ml/min
Nephrolithiasis	Same	Same
Age <50	Same	Same
Osteitis fibrosa cystica or marked bone mineral density loss (Z-score density of the spine, hip, or distal radius more than 2 standard deviations below peak bone mass)	Marked bone mineral density loss *(T-score density of the spine, hip, or distal radius more that 2.5 standard deviations below peak bone mass)*	Unchanged from 2002
Neuromuscular symptoms (documented proximal weakness, atrophy, hyperreflexia, gait disturbance)	Same	Same
Patients who request surgery or who do not have consistent follow-up if managed medically	Same	Same
Patients with comorbidities which complicate management	Same	Same

NIH reconvened a workshop in 2002 to refine the indications for parathyroidectomy, particularly for asymptomatic patients [9]:

(1) Marked hypercalcemia [>0.25 mol/l (1.0 mg/dl)] above reference range; (2) history of a life-threatening episode of hypercalcemia; (3) renal insufficiency (creatinine clearance reduced by 30% compared with normal age-matched controls); (4) hypercalciuria [24-h excretion >10 mol (400 mg/dl)]; (5) nephrolithiasis; (6) age <50; (7) osteitis fibrosa cystica or marked bone mineral density loss (*T*-score greater than −2.5 at the spine, hip, or distal radius); (8) neuromuscular symptoms (documented proximal weakness, atrophy, hyperreflexia, gait disturbance); (9) patients who request surgery or who do not have consistent follow-up if managed medically; (10) patients with comorbidities which complicate management.

The proceedings of the most recent conference, in 2008, reaffirmed the majority of the previously published indications for parathyroidectomy in patients with primary hyperparathyroidism. The most notable updates were that hypercalciuria (urinary calcium excretion in excess of 400 mg/day) was removed from the list of indications, and that renal insufficiency was more precisely defined as creatinine clearance less than 60 ml/min [10, 11].

Table 7.1 highlights the differences between the three conferences [5, 9–11].

Table 7.2 Clinical manifestation of primary hyperparathyroidism

Symptoms	Associated conditions
Neuropsychiatric	*Cardiovascular*
Fatigue	Hypertension
Exhaustion	Cardiomegaly
Depression	
Memory loss	
Gastrointestinal	*Gastrointestinal*
Constipation	Peptic ulcer
Anorexia	Pancreatits
Dyspepsia	Weight loss
Nausea	
Musculoskeletal	*Musculoskeletal*
Weakness	Osteopenia
Bone pain	Chondrocalcinois
Joint pain	Osteitis fibrosa cystica
	Fracture
	Gout/pseudogout
Renal	*Renal*
Polydipsia	Nephrolithiasis
Polyuria	Nephrocalcinosis
Nocturia	Hematuria
Renal colic	

Despite three NIH consensus statements, there is still no precise definition for "asymptomatic" primary hyperparathyroidism, and therefore the treatment of these patients remains controversial. It is estimated that only 31% of patients with primary hyperparathyroidism meet one of the above criteria and an additional 20% of patients with hyperparathyroidism meet multiple criteria for parathyroidectomy.

Thus, approximately 50% of patients with primary hyperparathyroidism are excluded from specific NIH criteria for parathyroidectomy, and are managed expectantly [12]. Hence, many patients with associated symptoms that are known to be cured or improved by parathyroidectomy (Table 7.2) are denied treatment. Unfortunately, no investigation to date has been able to predict which patients with "asymptomatic" or mild hyperparathyroidism will develop symptoms, complications, or progressive increase in blood calcium level. Therefore, how do we decide which "asymptomatic" patients with primary hyperparathyroidism should be offered parathyroidectomy? How should our 59-year-old patient with primary hyperparathyroidism be managed?

The "Asymptomatic" Patient

Currently, the diagnosis of primary hyperparathyroidism is most commonly made while patients are asymptomatic or only minimally symptomatic. Fewer than 20% of patients with primary hyperparathyroidism have history of kidney stones, and fewer than 3% demonstrate signs of osteitis fibrosa cystica [13]. Most series [5–7, 12–22] since 1970 demonstrate that at least one-half of patients have a nonrenal, nonosseous presentation. Many patients with primary hyperparathyroidism are affected by vague, nonspecific symptoms, such as fatigue, irritability, and mood swings, which often develop so insidiously that they are misinterpreted as signs of normal aging or stress [21, 23], and are not recognized until these symptoms improve after parathyroidectomy [3, 23].

Prior to the initial consensus meeting, we studied the presence of symptoms and associated conditions in 103 consecutive patients with primary hyperparathyroidism [20]. We demonstrated that (1) truly asymptomatic hyperparathyroidism is exceedingly rare, 98% of patients with primary hyperparathyroidism have symptoms or associated conditions on specific questioning, and that (2) 81% of patients with symptoms improved after parathyroidectomy.

These findings were subsequently confirmed in a review of 250 consecutive patients [24], where 92% of patients were found to be at least mildly symptomatic at presentation. After surgery, symptoms improved in 82% of the older patients and 83% of the younger patients. Older patients (>60) were more likely to have hypertension (47%) than younger patients (28%), whereas younger patients (31%) were more likely to have nephrolithiasis than older patients (12%).

Eigelberger et al. [7] examined the positive effect of parathyroidectomy on 178 consecutive patients, 103 of whom had met the NIH criteria for parathyroidectomy. Twenty-three symptoms and associated conditions were assessed by a questionnaire that was administered pre- and postoperatively. The prevalence of preoperative symptoms did not differ between the patients who met NIH criteria for parathyroidectomy and those who did not, and the extent of improvement was similar in both groups. Similar findings were reported by Perrier et al. [25], and Sosa et al. [1]. Talpos et al. [26] also documented significant improvement in neuropsychiatric status in a prospective trial using SF-36 testing (Table 7.3).

Bone Loss

A well-known complication of primary hyperparathyroidism is progressive demineralization of cortical and trabecular bone, and the accompanying increased fracture risk [27]. The catabolic effect of parathyroid hormone is most pronounced in the distal 1/3 of the radius (cortical bone), but may occur at all skeletal sites [27, 28]. A recent prospective study demonstrated that, on average, bone loss begins to be detectable 9 or 10 years after the diagnosis of primary hyperparathyroidism is made in patients who are managed expectantly [29].

While parathyroidectomy is agreed to induce remineralization in trabecular bone, its effect on cortical bone is more controversial [22, 30]. Nevertheless, the major protective effect of parathyroidectomy is in reducing the risk of spine and hip fractures [22, 30, 31].

Table 7.3 Improvement after parathyroidectomy

	Bone mineral density	Renal function/kidney stones	Myopathy	CV	Glucose	Hyper-lipidemia	Neuro-psychiatric symptoms	Death
Ambrogini [14]	++						++	
Bollerslev [15]	++						0	
Burney [73]							++	
Chan [3]	++		++				++	
Cheung [59]					++			
Chou [41]			++					
Christenson [56]						++		
Cogan [66]							++	
Deaconson [38]		++						
Diamond [51]		++		++				
Eigelberger [7]		++	++					
Hedback [53]				++				++
Hedback [85]								++
Hellstrom [48]				++				
Joborn [42, 68]							++	
Joborn [44]							++	
Lacour [58]						++		
Ljunghal [57]						++		
Mitalek [37]	++	++						
Okamoto [76]							++	
Palmer [45]								++
Paseika [79]							++	
Perrier [25]							++	
Prager [65]					++			
Richards [63]					++			
Ringe [50]				++				
Siverberg [12]	++							
Solomon [74]							++	
Stefenelli [54]				++				
Talpos [26]	++						++	
Uden [24]	++	++		++			++	
Valdemarsson [61]					++			
Vestergaard [31]	++							
Vestergaard [55]				++				++

Vestergaard et al. [31] compared 674 patients who underwent parathyroidectomy to over 2,000 matched controls. In their study, patients with primary hyperparathyroidism had an increased relative risk of fracture (1.8) up to 10 years prior to surgery that returned to normal at 1 year postoperatively. Moreover, the preoperative risk of fracture was independent of serum calcium concentration.

In a recent study of 1,900 premenopausal women in Sweden, 5.1% of the cohort had signs of mild primary hyperparathyroidism. These mild calcium disturbances were associated with lower bone mineral density, significant obesity, and decreased quality of life [32].

Bisphosphonates have been evaluated in patients with asymptomatic primary hyperparathyroidism as a possible alternative to surgery. Two double-blind, randomized clinical trials have been done to compare alendronate to placebo in these patients [33, 34]. Both trials demonstrated an increase in bone density at the lumbar spine (3.8%) and femoral neck (4.2%) in patients receiving alendronate. One of the trials [33] also demonstrated a significant decrease in serum calcium concentration. The value of bisphosphonates following successful parathyroidectomy remains to be elucidated.

In a multicenter, double-blind, placebo-controlled study, Peacock et al. [28] reported that most patients with primary hyperparathyroidism treated with a calcimimetic agent (Cinacalcet) versus placebo achieved stable normocalcemia. Unfortunately, no change occurs in bone mineral density or in blood parathyroid hormone levels.

To date, no medication has been able to mimic the impact of surgery with a sustained decrease in both serum calcium and parathyroid hormone levels and an increase in bone mineral density. More information is needed to determine the effects of bisphosphonates and calcimimetics in patients with "asymptomatic" primary hyperparathyroidism.

Renal Function

Hypercalciuria is a common finding in patients with hyperparathyroidism, and is thought to be the underlying cause of nephrolithiasis and nephrocalcinosis, and ultimately may (rarely) lead to renal failure [35]. Interestingly, urinary calcium excretion has been an uncertain predictor of the risk for kidney stones in patients with untreated primary hyperparathyroidism [9], and renal stones are also commonly seen in normocalcemic hyperparathyroidism [36]. Men, who excrete 20–30% more calcium in their urine than women, are more likely to present with renal stones even with moderate hypercalcemia [21]. Reduction of creatinine clearance and concentrating capacity occurs in over 1/3 of patients with mild hypercalcemia indicating that impairment of glomeruli and tubular function may be silent [37].

Deaconson et al. [38] studied the effect of parathyroidectomy on the future risk of developing renal caliculi. They reported that only 4 of the 71 patients with documented preoperative nephrolithiasis passed stones after parathyroidectomy, resulting in an annual risk reduction from 0.36 to 0.02. Patients with nephrolithiasis should, therefore, be advised that they may continue to pass kidney stones after parathyroidectomy, but should usually stop forming new stones.

Irrespective of nephrocalcinosis or renal calculi, patients with hyperparathyroidism are known to have decreased filtration capacity. In his classic study, Edvall [39] demonstrated that the combination of hypercalcemia and hyperparathyroidism accounts for this finding; patients with hypercalcemia from other causes and patients with nonparathyroid-related renal stones or nephrocalcinosis had preserved concentrating ability.

Mitlak et al. [37] studied 100 patients with primary hyperparathyroidism, 85 of whom had serum calcium less than 12 mg/dl, and denied skeletal, psychiatric, or other signs or symptoms of hyperparathyroidism. Despite this, they discovered premature osteopenia and/or impaired renal function in 29–36% of the patients. They concluded that "silent complications" of primary hyperparathyroidism are common in presumed "asymptomatic" patients.

Hedback et al. [40] reported that parathyroidectomy substantially improves renal concentrating capacity. This improvement often occurred within a week after surgery, and continued over time. Conversely, all patients with primary hyperparathyroidism who did not undergo parathyroidectomy had progressive deterioration of their renal concentrating capacity.

Neuromuscular Symptoms

Severe muscle wasting, which was formerly characteristic of primary hyperparathyroidism, is rarely seen today [41]. The primary neuromuscular symptoms that are currently observed are fatigue and weakness, primarily in the proximal muscles of the lower extremities [42]. Less frequently, patients may also complain of aching muscles, paresthesias, and unsteady gait. The incidence of these symptoms varies from 30 to 80% [43].

Muscle biopsies from patients with primary hyperparathyroidism reveal atrophy of both type I and type II muscle fibers [43]. These findings are attributable to alterations in motor neuron action potentials. Joborn et al. [42] reported that even patients with mild hyperparathyroidism, who denied neuromuscular symptoms, had reduced muscle twitch tension as compared to controls. Chou et al. [41] demonstrated that parathyroidism improved muscle strength and fine motor movement (but not sensation) in supposedly asymptomatic patients. With restoration of normocalcemia, neuromuscular symptoms improved within days to weeks after parathyroidectomy [41, 42, 44].

Cardiovascular Complications

Primary hyperparathyroidism has been reported to be associated with increased mortality from cardiovascular disease [45, 46]. These patients have a high incidence of hypertension, left ventricular hypertrophy, cardiac calcific deposits, and aortic and mitral valve calcifications and carry an increased risk of death. These cardiovascular complications are found in as many as 61% of patients with primary hyperparathyroidism [47].

Hypertension is a common finding in patients with primary hyperparathyroidism. Multiple studies [21, 35, 48] have demonstrated that hypertension is twice as frequent among patients with primary hyperparathyroidism as among the general population. This relationship was recognized over 40 years ago [48] in various series which showed that 30–60% of patients with primary hyperparathyroidism are hypertensive. The severity of hypertension does not parallel the degree of hypercalcemia. While some authors claim that hypertension is unaffected by parathyroidectomy [37, 49], others disagree [48, 50, 51]. Hypertension is agreed to be a risk factor for death [46]. In one study, patients with hypertension had 25–30% increased risk of death in a cohort of over 14,000 patients who were followed for more than 10 years [52].

Hedback and Oden [53] studied the relationship between hyperparathyroidism and cardiovascular disease and survival in a cohort of 845 patients. At a mean follow-up of 10.2 years, patients with hyperparathyroidism who were hypertensive had a 50% higher risk of death as normotensive patients with hyperparathyroidism. Although parathyroidectomy decreased the annual risk of death in all patients, its protective effect was nearly twice as prominent in the hypertensive patients. Younger patients (50–70 years old) with moderate hypercalcemia derived the largest survival benefit from parathyroidectomy.

A high prevalence of left ventricular hypertrophy (LVH) has been reported in both normotensive and hypertensive patients with primary hyperparathyroidism [54]. Although the degree of LVH appears to be unrelated to the degree of hypercalcemia or other hyperparathyroid symptoms [47], hypercalcemia may induce calcifications of heart valves and coronary arteries, and lead to hypertension. While the precise mechanism remains uncertain, the interaction between both hypercalcemia and increased levels of parathyroid hormone is thought to contribute to the development of LVH in these patients [47].

Vestergaard et al. [55] demonstrated that the increased risk from myocardial infarction precedes surgery by 10 years (relative risk 2.5). This higher risk was maintained at 1 year (relative risk 3.6) after parathyroidectomy but subsequently normalized with long-term follow-up.

Steffenelli et al. [54] prospectively studied the impact of parathyroidectomy on cardiac performance of 123 patients with primary hyperparathyroidism. Using echocardiography, they observed stable reversal of LVH and no progression aortic/mitral sclerosis after successful parathyroidectomy. This improvement of LVH is thought to be related to the normalization of PTH levels.

The impact of hyperparathyroidism on patients' lipid profile is controversial. An equal number of reports exist that support or reject the hypothesis that hyperparathyroidism improves serum triglycerides, cholesterol, very-low-density lipoprotiens [56–58].

Glucose Intolerance

The incidence of diabetes among patients with primary hyperparathyroidism is up to five times higher than in the general population (3% versus 16%) [59–61]. Moreover, patients with primary hyperparathyroidism are more likely to develop diabetes in the absence of common risk factors, such as advanced age, obesity, and hypertension [62]. In addition, another 40–80% of patients with primary hyperparathyroidism are found to have glucose intolerance [63]. The underlying mechanism for these findings is multifactorial and includes hyperinsulinism, peripheral insulin insensitivity, and reduced beta cell function [64].

In a recent 20-year retrospective review, Richards et al. [63] identified 61 patients with primary hyperparathyroidism and diabetes. Parathyroidectomy stabilized or improved glucose control in 48/61 (79%) patients. Patients with type II diabetes derived greater benefit, although this improvement could not be predicted by the duration of hyperparathyroidism or diabetes or by the preoperative calcium level.

These findings support earlier reports of improvement in insulin resistance and insulin hypersecretion after parathyroidectomy [59, 61, 65].

Neuropsychiatric Symptoms

A wide spectrum of psychiatric symptoms ranging from mild personality changes to severe depression and psychosis have been attributed to primary hyperparathyroidism. Specifically, easy fatigability, apathy, depression, malaise, mood swings, sleep disorders, irritability, and impaired mental clarity are reported [66–68]. Often, patients do not volunteer these complaints, and in a retrospective review of 441 patients with primary hyperparathyroidism only 23% were reported to have psychiatric complaints [67]. Nevertheless, psychiatric symptoms are found in the majority of patients with primary hyperparathyroidism [44, 69–71], and in a prospective study of 59 consecutive patients over 2/3 were found to have psychiatric complaints [67].

Calcium, which is known to play a central role in neurotransmitter regulation [71, 72], has been implicated in the pathogenesis of neuropsychiatric symptoms in patients with primary hyperparathyroidism [66, 67, 71]. Parathyroid hormone is thought to increase the permeability of the blood–brain barrier [44], and patients with primary hyperparathyroidism were found to have higher cerebrospinal fluid concentrations of total and ionized calcium and lower concentrations of 5-hydroxyindoleacetic acid and homovanillic acid [67]. The severity of patients' psychiatric symptoms correlates well with these abnormalities. Other objective data regarding patients with primary hyperparathyroidism and neuropsychiatric problems are by Cogan et al. [66] who documented changes in 5 and 7 MHz patterns by EEG in these patients that improved after parathyroidectomy.

In a pilot study, Perrier et al. [25] used functional MRI (fMRI) to investigate neurobehavioral dysfunction in patients with primary hyperparathyroidism. They successfully correlated changes in sleep and social behavior with radiographic alterations in the brain, specifically in the medial prefrontal cortex, dorsolateral prefrontal cortex, and parietal cortex. In addition, abnormal electroencephalograms [66], psychological tests [44, 66], and electromyelograms [67] have been reported in patients with primary hyperparathyroidism and often improve after parathyroidectomy.

Burney et al. [73] using the SF-36 survey demonstrated significant 2- and 6-month improvement in mental health status on 110 patients. Talpos et al. [26] used the SF-36 as well, and randomized 53 "asymptomatic" patients with very mild primary hyperparathyroidism to surgery versus observation. They demonstrated a statistically significant improvement in two of the nine domains of the SF-36 survey, social function and emotional role function, in the surgically treated group.

Solomon et al. [74] studied 18 patients with primary hyperparathyroidism and a variety of psychological disturbances (obsession–compulsion, depression, anxiety, hostility, psychosis, sleep disturbance, and lack of concentration). An improvement approaching normal was achieved 1 month after parathyroidectomy, as is seen in most series [17, 20, 67, 75]. Most subsequent studies, but not all, document that the neuropsychiatric improvement lasts for at least several years [76, 77].

Health Status Assessment Tool

Although dramatic improvements in patient's symptoms have been recognized for many years, a specific instrument to measure the effect of parathyroidectomy was only recently developed [78]. In Paseika's study, all 63 patients, including 12 who were considered "asymptomatic" by their referring physician, had symptomatic improvement following parathyroidectomy. This questionnaire uses a visual analog scale to measure quality of life and hyperparathyroid-specific symptoms to determine a patient's parathyroidectomy assessment of symptoms (PAS) score. This instrument has been validated in various subsequent trials [77–79] which demonstrated elevated PAS scores in patients with primary hyperparathyroidism which improved immediately following parathyroidectomy. Prior to this, a standardized health assessment tool, such as the SF-36, as mentioned previously, had been used to demonstrate symptom-specific outcome of parathyroidectomy [26, 73, 80].

Increased Risk of Death

Untreated primary hyperparathyroidism is known to correlate with premature death from cardiovascular disease and malignancy [45, 75, 81, 82]. Data from a large health-screening program in Sweden reveal that even at minimally elevated calcium levels of 9.8–10 mg/dl the risk of premature death was increased by 30% as compared with patients with calcium levels between 9.2 and 9.8. The risk of premature death rose linearly with calcium level, peaking at 120% with calcium levels of 10.4 or higher.

Although three short-term studies suggested that the increased risk of death from primary hyperparathyroidism does not completely disappear after parathyroidectomy, studies with longer follow-up reveal the benefits of parathyroidectomy on life expectancy [75, 83, 84].

A retrospective study of 896 consecutive patients who underwent parathyroidectomy revealed that patients with primary hyperparathyroidism have a higher relative risk of death which decreased after the first postoperative year from 2.6 to 1.6, and normalized by the end of the follow-up period (15 years) [85].

A Swedish study of 3,485 patients who underwent parathyroidectomy for the treatment of multiglandular primary hyperparathyroidism also demonstrated an increased risk of death in these patients as compared to age- and gender-matched controls [86]. Although this increased risk of death persisted for more than 15 years postoperatively, it progressively decreased with follow-up (standardized mortality rate decreased from 2.11 to 1.33 qt with 15-year follow-up). Causes of death included cardiovascular disease, diabetes, malignancy, and genitourinary disease.

A larger study [46] used Sweden's National Patient Registry to study the impact of parathyroidectomy on the risk of death in 4,461 patients who underwent parathyroidectomy between 1987 and 1994. These patients' risk of premature death (as compared to the general population) declined by an average of 17% per year for men and 8% per year for women. In addition to gender, the risk of premature death was related to age, the presence of diabetes mellitus or cardiovascular disease, urine osmolarity [87], the severity of preoperative hypercalcemia, parathyroid hormone level, and adenoma size [46].

Natural History of Untreated Primary Hyperparathyroidism

Scholz et al. [88, 89] reported on 147 patients with asymptomatic primary hyperparathyroidism (serum calcium <11 mg/dl) who were observed for 10 years. Within the first 5 years, 26 patients developed a complication of hyperparathyroidism that warranted parathyroidectomy. By 10 years, 38 patients (26%) had been treated surgically (including one who had a hypercalcemic crisis), 35 patients died, and only 13 patients remained "asymptomatic." Ultimately, 38 of 76 (50%) patients with adequate follow-up developed a complication and required parathyroidectomy [88]. These results support the findings of Silverberg et al. [22], who observed 60 patients who did not meet NIH criteria for surgery. In their series, 27% of patients had progression of disease, and ultimately underwent parathyroidectomy. No one to date has been able to determine who will develop progressive problems and complications of primary hyperparathyroidism.

Recent Randomized-Controlled Studies

Three small, randomized-controlled trials were conducted to compare surgery to observation in patients with asymptomatic primary hyperparathyroidism since the second NIH consensus conference [14, 15, 26]. All three studies demonstrated significant improvements in bone mineral density following parathyroidectomy.

Improvements in quality of life were variably reported, possibly owing to the use of nonparathyroid-specific assessment tools.

Talpos et al. [26] randomized 53 patients with "asymptomatic" primary hyperparathyroidism (serum calcium <10.4 mg/dl and normal parathyroid hormone levels) to surgery versus follow-up. They confirmed statistically significant improvement in 2/9 domains of the SF-36 (social functioning, emotional role functioning) in the surgery group. Rao et al. [80] later reported significant long-term improvements in bone mineral density in the spine, femoral neck, and hip in the group of patients who underwent parathyroidectomy. These patients also enjoyed significant improvements in quality of life and psychological function as compared to the patients who were observed.

Bolerslev et al. [15], on the other hand, failed to demonstrate improvements in psychological symptoms following parathyroidectomy. In their trial of 191 patients, no improvement was conferred in any of the 9 domains of the SF-36, although significant improvement in bone mineral density and hypercalcemia were conferred by parathyroidectomy.

Finally, in 2007, Ambrogini et al. [14] followed 50 patients who did not meet NIH criteria for parathyroidectomy. These "asymptomatic" patients were randomly assigned to surgery or observation and were followed at 6-month intervals for 1 year. The primary focus of this trial was bone mineral density which was found to improve significantly in the lumbar spine and hip in those patients who underwent parathyroidectomy for asymptomatic primary hyperparathyroidism. A modest improvement in quality of life was also seen in patients after parathyroidectomy as compared to the nonsurgical group.

For the reasons outlined in this chapter, we strongly recommend that all patients with asymptomatic hyperparathyroidism and single-gland disease undergo a focused parathyroidectomy, which has a 97% success rate in the hands of an experienced surgeon [90]. Complications, including recurrent laryngeal nerve damage, hematoma, and hypoparathyroidism, are less than 1–2% [91]. Parathyroidectomy has been shown to be more cost-effective than observation or pharmacologic therapy (Cinacalcet) for these patients [92, 93]. Patients who are considered to be poor surgical candidates should be referred to a high-volume center for appropriate management.

Conclusion

Parathyroidectomy offers the only cure for primary hyperparathyroidism and should be recommended to all patients with classical symptoms or complications of the disease [3, 5–7, 16–20]. Although two consensus conferences have defined indications for parathyroidectomy, these exclude half of the patients with hyperparathyroidism [9], who we believe still benefit from parathyroidectomy.

Beyond the NIH criteria, it is clear that the majority of patients with primary hyperparathyroidism are symptomatic, and that most benefit symptomatically and metabolically following parathyroidectomy [20, 23]. In addition to improvement in the classic parameters used by the NIH (bone disease, renal function, and neuromuscular disorders), parathyroidectomy has been convincingly shown to improve neuropsychiatric symptoms [2, 3], LVH [47], and hypertension [48, 50, 51]. Most importantly, parathyroidectomy has been demonstrated to normalize the increased risk of death that patients with primary hyperparathyroidism have as compared with controls. Therefore, we believe that the patient described, and many patients like her, who are "asymptomatic" and fall short of fulfilling the current NIH criteria for parathyroidectomy, would benefit from parathyroidectomy [2, 7].

References

1. Sosa JA, Udelsman R. New directions in the treatment of patients with primary hyperparathyroidism. Curr Probl Surg. 2003;40(12):812–49.
2. AACE/AAES Task Force on Primary Hyperparathyroidism. The American Association of Clinical Endocrinologists and the American Association of Endocrine Surgeons position statement on the diagnosis and management of primary hyperparathyroidism. Endocr Pract. 2005;11(1):49–54.
3. Chan AK, Duh QY, Katz MH, et al. Clinical manifestations of primary hyperparathyroidism before and after parathyroidectomy. A case–control study. Ann Surg. 1995;222(3):402–12. discussion 412–4.
4. Christensson T, Hellstrom K, Wengle B, et al. Prevalence of hypercalcaemia in a health screening in Stockholm. Acta Med Scand. 1976;200(1–2):131–7.
5. Diagnosis and management of asymptomatic primary hyperparathyroidism. National Institutes of Health Consensus Development Conference, October 29–31, 1990. Consens Statement 1990;8(7):1–18.
6. Clark OH, Duh QY. Primary hyperparathyroidism. A surgical perspective. Endocrinol Metab Clin North Am. 1989;18(3):701–14.
7. Eigelberger MS, Cheah WK, Ituarte PH, et al. The NIH criteria for parathyroidectomy in asymptomatic primary hyperparathyroidism: are they too limited? Ann Surg. 2004;239(4): 528–35.
8. Boughey JC, Ewart CJ, Yost MJ, et al. Chloride/phosphate ratio in primary hyperparathyroidism. Am Surg. 2004;70(1):25–8.
9. Bilezikian JP, Potts Jr JT, Fuleihan Gel H, et al. Summary statement from a workshop on asymptomatic primary hyperparathyroidism: a perspective for the 21st century. J Clin Endocrinol Metab. 2002;87(12):5353–61.
10. Bilezikian JP, Khan AA, Potts Jr JT. Guidelines for the management of asymptomatic primary hyperparathyroidism: summary statement from the third international workshop. J Clin Endocrinol Metab. 2009;94(2):335–9.
11. Udelsman R, Pasieka JL, Sturgeon C, et al. Surgery for asymptomatic primary hyperparathyroidism: proceedings of the third international workshop. J Clin Endocrinol Metab. 2009;94(2):366–72.
12. Silverberg SJ, Bilezikian JP. Evaluation and management of primary hyperparathyroidism. J Clin Endocrinol Metab. 1996;81(6):2036–40.
13. Mack LA, Pasieka JL. Asymptomatic primary hyperparathyroidism: a surgical perspective. Surg Clin North Am. 2004;84(3):803–16.
14. Ambrogini E, Cetani F, Cianferotti L, et al. Surgery or surveillance for mild asymptomatic primary hyperparathyroidism: a prospective, randomized clinical trial. J Clin Endocrinol Metab. 2007;92(8):3114–21.

15. Bollerslev J, Jansson S, Mollerup CL, et al. Medical observation, compared with parathyroidectomy, for asymptomatic primary hyperparathyroidism: a prospective, randomized trial. J Clin Endocrinol Metab. 2007;92(5):1687–92.
16. Clark OH. "Asymptomatic" primary hyperparathyroidism: is parathyroidectomy indicated? Surgery. 1994;116(6):947–53.
17. Clark OH. Surgical treatment of primary hyperparathyroidism. Adv Endocrinol Metab. 1995; 6:1–16.
18. Clark OH. Current management of patients with hyperparathyroidism. Adv Surg. 1996; 30:179–87.
19. Clark OH. How should patients with primary hyperparathyroidism be treated? J Clin Endocrinol Metab. 2003;88(7):3011–4.
20. Clark OH, Wilkes W, Siperstein AE, Duh QY. Diagnosis and management of asymptomatic hyperparathyroidism: safety, efficacy, and deficiencies in our knowledge. J Bone Miner Res. 1991;6 Suppl 2:S135–42. discussion 151–2.
21. Lafferty FW, Hubay CA. Primary hyperparathyroidism. A review of the long-term surgical and nonsurgical morbidities as a basis for a rational approach to treatment. Arch Intern Med. 1989;149(4):789–96.
22. Silverberg SJ, Shane E, Jacobs TP, et al. A 10-year prospective study of primary hyperparathyroidism with or without parathyroid surgery. N Engl J Med. 1999;341(17):1249–55.
23. Hasse C, Sitter H, Bachmann S, et al. How asymptomatic is asymptomatic primary hyperparathyroidism? Exp Clin Endocrinol Diabetes. 2000;108(4):265–74.
24. Uden P, Chan A, Duh QY, et al. Primary hyperparathyroidism in younger and older patients: symptoms and outcome of surgery. World J Surg. 1992;16(4):791–7. discussion 798.
25. Perrier ND, Coker LH, Rorie KD, et al. Preliminary report: functional MRI of the brain may be the ideal tool for evaluating neuropsychologic and sleep complaints of patients with primary hyperparathyroidism. World J Surg. 2006;30(5):686–96.
26. Talpos GB, Bone III HG, Kleerekoper M, et al. Randomized trial of parathyroidectomy in mild asymptomatic primary hyperparathyroidism: patient description and effects on the SF-36 health survey. Surgery. 2000;128(6):1013–20. discussion 1020–1.
27. Larsson K, Ljunghall S, Krusemo UB, et al. The risk of hip fractures in patients with primary hyperparathyroidism: a population-based cohort study with a follow-up of 19 years. J Intern Med. 1993;234(6):585–93.
28. Peacock M, Bilezikian JP, Klassen PS, et al. Cinacalcet hydrochloride maintains long-term normocalcemia in patients with primary hyperparathyroidism. J Clin Endocrinol Metab. 2005;90(1):135–41.
29. Silverberg SJ, Lewiecki EM, Mosekilde L, et al. Presentation of asymptomatic primary hyperparathyroidism: proceedings of the third international workshop. J Clin Endocrinol Metab. 2009;94(2):351–65.
30. Nomura R, Sugimoto T, Tsukamoto T, et al. Marked and sustained increase in bone mineral density after parathyroidectomy in patients with primary hyperparathyroidism; a six-year longitudinal study with or without parathyroidectomy in a Japanese population. Clin Endocrinol (Oxf). 2004;60(3):335–42.
31. Vestergaard P, Mollerup CL, Frokjaer VG, et al. Cohort study of risk of fracture before and after surgery for primary hyperparathyroidism. BMJ. 2000;321(7261):598–602.
32. Siilin H, Rastad J, Ljunggren O, Lundgren E. Disturbances of calcium homeostasis consistent with mild primary hyperparathyroidism in premenopausal women and associated morbidity. J Clin Endocrinol Metab. 2008;93(1):47–53.
33. Chow CC, Chan WB, Li JK, et al. Oral alendronate increases bone mineral density in postmenopausal women with primary hyperparathyroidism. J Clin Endocrinol Metab. 2003;88(2): 581–7.
34. Khan AA, Bilezikian JP, Kung AW, et al. Alendronate in primary hyperparathyroidism: a double-blind, randomized, placebo-controlled trial. J Clin Endocrinol Metab. 2004;89(7): 3319–25.

35. Nikkila MT, Saaristo JJ, Koivula TA. Clinical and biochemical features in primary hyperparathyroidism. Surgery. 1989;105(2 Pt 1):148–53.
36. Yang AH, Hsu CW, Chen JY, et al. Normocalcemic primary hyperparathyroidism in patients with recurrent kidney stones: pathological analysis of parathyroid glands. Virchows Arch. 2006;449(1):62–8.
37. Mitlak BH, Daly M, Potts Jr JT, et al. Asymptomatic primary hyperparathyroidism. J Bone Miner Res. 1991;6 Suppl 2:S103–10. discussion S121–4.
38. Deaconson TF, Wilson SD, Lemann Jr J. The effect of parathyroidectomy on the recurrence of nephrolithiasis. Surgery. 1987;102(6):910–3.
39. Edvall CA. Renal function in hyperparathyroidism; a clinical study of 30 cases with special reference to selective renal clearance and renal vein catheterization. Acta Chir Scand Suppl. 1958;114 Suppl 229:1–56.
40. Hedback G, Abrahamsson K, Oden A. The improvement of renal concentration capacity after surgery for primary hyperparathyroidism. Eur J Clin Invest. 2001;31(12):1048–53.
41. Chou FF, Sheen-Chen SM, Leong CP. Neuromuscular recovery after parathyroidectomy in primary hyperparathyroidism. Surgery. 1995;117(1):18–25.
42. Joborn C, Rastad J, Stalberg E, et al. Muscle function in patients with primary hyperparathyroidism. Muscle Nerve. 1989;12(2):87–94.
43. Patten BM, Bilezikian JP, Mallette LE, et al. Neuromuscular disease in primary hyperparathyroidism. Ann Intern Med. 1974;80(2):182–93.
44. Joborn C, Hetta J, Niklasson F, et al. Cerebrospinal fluid calcium, parathyroid hormone, and monoamine and purine metabolites and the blood–brain barrier function in primary hyperparathyroidism. Psychoneuroendocrinology. 1991;16(4):311–22.
45. Palmer M, Adami HO, Bergstrom R, et al. Survival and renal function in untreated hypercalcaemia. Population-based cohort study with 14 years of follow-up. Lancet. 1987;1(8524): 59–62.
46. Hedback G, Oden A. Increased risk of death from primary hyperparathyroidism–an update. Eur J Clin Invest. 1998;28(4):271–6.
47. Piovesan A, Molineri N, Casasso F, et al. Left ventricular hypertrophy in primary hyperparathyroidism. Effects of successful parathyroidectomy. Clin Endocrinol (Oxf). 1999;50(3): 321–8.
48. Hellstrom J, Birke G, Edvall CA. Hypertension in hyperparathyroidism. Br J Urol. 1958;30(1): 13–24.
49. Heath III H. Clinical spectrum of primary hyperparathyroidism: evolution with changes in medical practice and technology. J Bone Miner Res. 1991;6 Suppl 2:S63–70. discussion S83–4.
50. Ringe JD. Reversible hypertension in primary hyperparathyroidism–pre- and posteroperative blood pressure in 75 cases. Klin Wochenschr. 1984;62(10):465–9.
51. Diamond TW, Botha JR, Wing J, et al. Parathyroid hypertension. A reversible disorder. Arch Intern Med. 1986;146(9):1709–12.
52. Havlik RJ, LaCroix AZ, Kleinman JC, et al. Antihypertensive drug therapy and survival by treatment status in a national survey. Hypertension. 1989;13(5 Suppl):I28–32.
53. Hedback GM, Oden AS. Cardiovascular disease, hypertension and renal function in primary hyperparathyroidism. J Intern Med. 2002;251(6):476–83.
54. Stefenelli T, Abela C, Frank H, et al. Cardiac abnormalities in patients with primary hyperparathyroidism: implications for follow-up. J Clin Endocrinol Metab. 1997;82(1):106–12.
55. Vestergaard P, Mollerup CL, Frokjaer VG, et al. Cardiovascular events before and after surgery for primary hyperparathyroidism. World J Surg. 2003;27(2):216–22.
56. Christensson T, Einarsson K. Serum lipids before and after parathyroidectomy in patients with primary hyperparathyroidism. Clin Chim Acta. 1977;78(3):411–5.
57. Ljunghall S, Lithell H, Vessby B, Wide L. Glucose and lipoprotein metabolism in primary hyperparathyroidism. Effects of parathyroidectomy. Acta Endocrinol (Copenh). 1978;89(3): 580–9.

58. Lacour B, Roullet JB, Liagre AM, et al. Serum lipoprotein disturbances in primary and secondary hyperparathyroidism and effects of parathyroidectomy. Am J Kidney Dis. 1986;8(6):422–9.
59. Cheung PS, Thompson NW, Brothers TE, Vinik AI. Effect of hyperparathyroidism on the control of diabetes mellitus. Surgery. 1986;100(6):1039–47.
60. Ljunghall S, Palmer M, Akerstrom G, Wide L. Diabetes mellitus, glucose tolerance and insulin response to glucose in patients with primary hyperparathyroidism before and after parathyroidectomy. Eur J Clin Invest. 1983;13(5):373–7.
61. Valdemarsson S, Lindblom P, Bergenfelz A. Metabolic abnormalities related to cardiovascular risk in primary hyperparathyroidism: effects of surgical treatment. J Intern Med. 1998;244(3):241–9.
62. Kumar S, Olukoga AO, Gordon C, et al. Impaired glucose tolerance and insulin insensitivity in primary hyperparathyroidism. Clin Endocrinol (Oxf). 1994;40(1):47–53.
63. Richards ML, Thompson NW. Diabetes mellitus with hyperparathyroidism: another indication for parathyroidectomy? Surgery. 1999;126(6):1160–6.
64. Fadda GZ, Akmal M, Lipson LG, Massry SG. Direct effect of parathyroid hormone on insulin secretion from pancreatic islets. Am J Physiol. 1990;258(6 Pt 1):E975–84.
65. Prager R, Schernthaner G, Niederle B, Roka R. Evaluation of glucose tolerance, insulin secretion, and insulin action in patients with primary hyperparathyroidism before and after surgery. Calcif Tissue Int. 1990;46(1):1–4.
66. Cogan MG, Covey CM, Arieff AI, et al. Central nervous system manifestations of hyperparathyroidism. Am J Med. 1978;65(6):963–70.
67. Joborn C, Hetta J, Johansson H, et al. Psychiatric morbidity in primary hyperparathyroidism. World J Surg. 1988;12(4):476–81.
68. Joborn C, Hetta J, Lind L, et al. Self-rated psychiatric symptoms in patients operated on because of primary hyperparathyroidism and in patients with long-standing mild hypercalcemia. Surgery. 1989;105(1):72–8.
69. Karpati G, Frame B. Neuropsychiatric disorders in primary hyperparathyroidism. Clinical analysis with review of the literature. Arch Neurol. 1964;10:387–97.
70. Mallette LE, Bilezikian JP, Heath DA, Aurbach GD. Primary hyperparathyroidism: clinical and biochemical features. Medicine (Baltimore). 1974;53(2):127–46.
71. Joborn C, Hetta J, Rastad J, et al. Psychiatric symptoms and cerebrospinal fluid monoamine metabolites in primary hyperparathyroidism. Biol Psychiatry. 1988;23(2):149–58.
72. Dubovsky SL, Franks RD. Intracellular calcium ions in affective disorders: a review and an hypothesis. Biol Psychiatry. 1983;18(7):781–97.
73. Burney RE, Jones KR, Peterson M, et al. Surgical correction of primary hyperparathyroidism improves quality of life. Surgery. 1998;124(6):987–91. discussion 991–2.
74. Solomon BL, Schaaf M, Smallridge RC. Psychologic symptoms before and after parathyroid surgery. Am J Med. 1994;96(2):101–6.
75. Sivula A, Ronni-Sivula H. The changing picture of primary hyperparathyroidism in the years 1956–1979. Ann Chir Gynaecol. 1984;73(6):319–24.
76. Okamoto T, Gerstein HC, Obara T. Psychiatric symptoms, bone density and non-specific symptoms in patients with mild hypercalcemia due to primary hyperparathyroidism: a systematic overview of the literature. Endocr J. 1997;44(3):367–74.
77. Pasieka JL, Parsons LL, Demeure MJ, et al. Patient-based surgical outcome tool demonstrating alleviation of symptoms following parathyroidectomy in patients with primary hyperparathyroidism. World J Surg. 2002;26(8):942–9.
78. Pasieka JL, Parsons LL. Prospective surgical outcome study of relief of symptoms following surgery in patients with primary hyperparathyroidism. World J Surg. 1998;22(6):513–8. discussion 518–9.
79. Pasieka JL, Parsons LL. A prospective surgical outcome study assessing the impact of parathyroidectomy on symptoms in patients with secondary and tertiary hyperparathyroidism. Surgery. 2000;128(4):531–9.
80. Rao DS, Phillips ER, Divine GW, Talpos GB. Randomized controlled clinical trial of surgery versus no surgery in patients with mild asymptomatic primary hyperparathyroidism. J Clin Endocrinol Metab. 2004;89(11):5415–22.

81. Hedback G, Oden A. Survival of patients operated on for primary hyperparathyroidism. Surgery. 1999;125(2):240–1.
82. Posen S, Clifton-Bligh P, Reeve TS, et al. Is parathyroidectomy of benefit in primary hyperparathyroidism? Q J Med. 1985;54(215):241–51.
83. Palmer M, Ljunghall S, Akerstrom G, et al. Patients with primary hyperparathyroidism operated on over a 24-year period: temporal trends of clinical and laboratory findings. J Chronic Dis. 1987;40(2):121–30.
84. Hedback G, Tisell LE, Bengtsson BA, et al. Premature death in patients operated on for primary hyperparathyroidism. World J Surg. 1990;14(6):829–35. discussion 836.
85. Hedback G, Oden A, Tisell LE. The influence of surgery on the risk of death in patients with primary hyperparathyroidism. World J Surg. 1991;15(3):399–405. discussion 406–7.
86. Nilsson IL, Wadsten C, Brandt L, et al. Mortality in sporadic primary hyperparathyroidism: nationwide cohort study of multiple parathyroid gland disease. Surgery. 2004;136(5):981–7.
87. Hedback G, Oden A. Death risk factor analysis in primary hyperparathyroidism. Eur J Clin Invest. 1998;28(12):1011–8.
88. Scholz DA, Purnell DC. Asymptomatic primary hyperparathyroidism. 10-year prospective study. Mayo Clin Proc. 1981;56(8):473–8.
89. Purnell DC, Smith LH, Scholz DA, et al. Primary hyperparathyroidism: a prospective clinical study. Am J Med. 1971;50(5):670–8.
90. Kebebew E, Hwang J, Reiff E, et al. Predictors of single-gland vs. multigland parathyroid disease in primary hyperparathyroidism: a simple and accurate scoring model. Arch Surg. 2006;141(8):777–82. discussion 782.
91. Clark OH, Duh Q-Y, Kebebew E. Textbook of endocrine surgery. 2nd ed. Philadelphia: W.B. Saunders; 2005.
92. Zanocco K, Angelos P, Sturgeon C. Cost-effectiveness analysis of parathyroidectomy for asymptomatic primary hyperparathyroidism. Surgery. 2006;140(6):874–81. discussion 881–2.
93. Sejean K, Calmus S, Durand-Zaleski I, et al. Surgery versus medical follow-up in patients with asymptomatic primary hyperparathyroidism: a decision analysis. Eur J Endocrinol. 2005;153(6):915–27.

Chapter 8
Nonclassic, Extraskeletal Manifestations of Primary Hyperparathyroidism

Associated Symptoms and Possible Mechanisms

Nancy D. Perrier, Storm Weaver, Swaroop Gantela, and D. Sudhaker Rao

Keywords Nonclassic manifestations • Sleep disturbance • Psychiatric complications • Psychological symptoms • Neurocognitive issues • Pathophysiology of disease complications • Cardiovascular disease • Endothelial dysfunction • Arrhythmias • Hypertension • Mortality • Muscular function • PTH receptors • Cerebral blood flow

Introduction

Historically, patients with PHPT presented with manifestations of hypercalcemia, such as kidney stones, overt bone disease, and neuromuscular dysfunction. Today, patients are often diagnosed with PHPT in the course of routine biochemical screening and frequently have vague, nonspecific symptoms. Recognizing the changing presentation of PHPT, the NIH convened two consensus conferences to determine which subset of patients with PHPT might be safely observed and have their disease medically managed and which patients would benefit from operative intervention.

The classic manifestations of bone disease and nephrolithiasis with PHPT have been well described in the medical literature, owing in part to the facility with which they can be objectively documented. Since 1929 [1], however, there have been numerous reports [2–10] of constellations of other signs and symptoms that

N.D. Perrier, MD, FACS (✉) • S. Weaver
Department of Surgical Oncology, Unit 1484, The University of Texas
M. D. Anderson Cancer Center, 1400 Pressler Street Boulevard, Houston, TX 77030, USA
e-mail: nperrier@mdanderson.org

S. Gantela, MD
Human Neuroimaging Laboratory, Baylor College of Medicine, Houston, TX, USA

D.S. Rao, MBBS, FACP, FACE
Bone & Mineral Metabolism, Bone & Mineral Research Laboratory, Henry Ford Medical Center,
New Center One, Henry Ford Hospital, Suite 800, 3031 W. Grand Blvd., Detroit, MI 48202, USA

A.A. Khan and O.H. Clark (eds.), *Handbook of Parathyroid Diseases:*
A Case-Based Practical Guide, DOI 10.1007/978-1-4614-2164-1_8,
© Springer Science+Business Media, LLC 2012

appear to be associated with PHPT but that have no clearly established connection with the disease nor can easily be measured objectively. Subjective neurobehavioral symptoms have been described with PHPT since the 1940s [11, 12]. Lethargy, drowsiness, depressed mood, neurasthenia, paranoia, hallucinations, disorientation, confusion, and cognitive (mostly memory) complaints have been documented in a number of early case reports [13–18]. More recent studies have described biochemically confirmed PHPT to be characterized by a number of symptoms previously thought to be atypical of the condition. These include low energy and/or fatigue [6, 19, 20], weakness [19], bone and joint pain [19–21], cognitive dysfunction [4, 19, 22], sleep disorders [6], psychological and psychiatric symptoms that range from depression and anxiety to psychosis and coma [6, 19, 21, 23–25], decreased ability to complete daily tasks at home [20] or work [26], and decreased social interaction [6, 20, 21]. Some patients with mild hypercalcemia report either no symptoms or only neurobehavioral complaints [27]. Presumably, these signs and symptoms of "nonclassic" PHPT have a negative impact on health-related quality of life (HRQL). Despite the number and frequency of these findings, recommendations for their management are not addressed in the current NIH guidelines for surgical intervention. Despite a large number of published reports on these symptoms over the past 75 years, the pathophysiologic mechanisms by which they occur remain lacking. The purpose of this chapter is to review the recent literature on the nonclassic symptoms of PHPT and possible causes of these manifestations.

Nonclassic Manifestations

Psychiatric Manifestations

Case studies and series have reported a wide range of psychiatric manifestations thought to be associated with PHPT, including depression, anxiety, agitation, irascibility, delusions, auditory and visual hallucinations, and paranoid ideations [6–10, 21, 28–34]. Case studies have also demonstrated dramatic clearing of the symptoms after curative parathyroidectomy [27–29, 32, 33]. The series [6–10, 21, 27, 34–36] report on groups of PHPT patients with psychiatric symptoms, with some providing data on the prevalence of these symptoms, which ranged from 32 to 66% [6, 9, 27]. However, the response of psychiatric symptoms to parathyroidectomy has been inconsistent: some series showed general improvement [6, 7, 35], others showed no improvement [10, 27], while still others showed mixed results [8, 9, 21, 34, 36]. This may be related in part to the different methods used to assess symptoms, including systematic psychiatric interviews, self-reported responses to questionnaires, and observer rating scales. The psychiatric symptoms may, in fact, be the most difficult nonclassic PHPT manifestations to quantify objectively.

Neurocognitive Manifestations

Neurocognitive symptoms that have been associated with PHPT include impairments in concentration, memory, processing speed, and executive functioning [6–10, 33, 37, 38]. As with the psychiatric symptoms, a variety of neurocognitive impairments have been reported in patients with PHPT; however, data on the prevalence of these symptoms is sparse. Similar to the psychiatric symptoms, the response to parathyroidectomy has been mixed: improvement in some series [6, 37, 38], varied response in some [8, 9, 21, 36], and no improvement in others [10, 39]. Coker et al. [40], and Roman and Sosa [41] reviewed some of the recent studies, and both underscored the need for larger, longitudinal studies evaluating neurocognitive function. Future studies should employ the currently available robust battery of objective tests to better characterize the neurocognitive impairments in patients with PHPT and their response to parathyroidectomy.

Several examples of such studies are cited in detail. Studies that used a battery of neuropsychiatric tests pre- and post-surgery to assess multiple cognitive domains include Numann et al. [4], who compared ten patients with PHPT who were scheduled for parathyroidectomy to ten normocalcemic orthopedic patients using seven cognitive tests: the Wechsler Memory Scale, Form I (WMS) [42]; the Information, Vocabulary, Similarities, and Block Design subtests of the Wechsler Adult Intelligence Scale (WAIS) [43]; the Facial Recognition Test [44]; the Benton Revised Visual Retention Test [45]; Forms A and B of the Trail Making Test [46]; and the Finger Tapping Test [47]. Several tests were clustered to measure-specific cognitive domains: the Information and Orientation subtests of the WMS were combined to measure orientation; the Logical Memory and Associate Learning subtests of the WMS were grouped to measure short-term verbal memory; both forms of the Trail Making Test were scored together as measures of visuomotor tracking and planning. Analyses of the data indicated improvement across trials for the hyperparathyroid group on the combined scores of the Logical Memory and Associate Learning subtests of the WMS (measures of short-term verbal memory); improvement in scores of the Digit Span subtest of the WMS (a measure of verbal attention); and improvement on the Similarities subtests of the WAIS (a measure of logical, categorical reasoning). Significant improvements by both groups on the Block Design subtest of the WAIS and the Facial Recognition subtest of the WMS were attributed to practice effects. The results of the Trail Making Test indicated that the hyperparathyroid group had faster times than the orthopedic group both pre- and postsurgery. There were no significant differences between conditions or across trials for the remaining measures. Collectively, these results indicated that PHPT patients demonstrated improved NP functioning across several cognitive skills, including attention, memory, and reasoning following parathyroidectomy.

Chiang et al. [39] administered four NP tests, including the Stroop Color Word Test [48] (executive functioning); the Digit Symbol Subtest of the WAIS-R [49] (attention, perceptuo-motor coordination); the Royal Melbourne Memory for Prose Test [50] (verbal memory); and the Unusual Shapes Test [51] (visual recognition) to 20 patients with PHPT and 20 patients scheduled for orthopedic surgery as control subjects matched for age, gender, and intellectual function based on the National Adult Reading Test. A battery of tests was also administered to assess symptoms of anxiety and depression. All tests were administered preoperatively and at a single follow-up interval that varied widely from 30 to 380 days (mean, 125 days) for PHPT patients and 14 to 162 days (mean, 82 days) for the orthopedic patients. No significant changes were found between groups on the NP tests or measures of mood from preoperative to postoperative follow-up periods.

In the 2005 study by Sosa, patients with PHPT were preoperatively evaluated with validated psychometric and neurocognitive instruments, such as the Beck and Stait test to assess if learning, memory or concentration improved after parathyroidectomy. The group was compared to patients undergoing thyroidectomy. Greater depression was noted in the PHPT group compared to the thyroidectomy patients. Patients with PHPT showed deficits in spatial learning and those with the greatest change in PTH had the greatest improvement in learning efficiency following parathyroidectomy.

Similarly, the M. D. Anderson Cancer Center study of 55 patients with PHTP who underwent parathyroidectomy with both pre- and postoperative neurocognitive evaluations has been reported [38]. The study of 43 women and 12 men with an average age of 63 years consisted of pre- and postoperative evaluations utilizing the Stroop Color and Word Test. The Stroop Color and Word Test measures cognitive processing speed (Word and Color subtests) and executive function (Color-Word subtest). The Stroop Color subset measures selective attention and the ability to inhibit a preferred response. Impairment, defined as a greater than 1.5 standard deviation from the normal, below the mean was identified in 13% of patients all of whom experienced improvement after surgery. Impaired cognitive processing speed was identified in 26% of the 47 patients; 75% of whom improved after parathyroidectomy. In total, 15 (32%) of 47 patients had neurocognitive impairment preoperatively. Twelve of 15 patients (80%) improved after parathyroidectomy. There was no difference between the impaired and nonimpaired groups with respect to age, or serum calcium or intact PTH levels.

Sleep Disturbance

PHPT has been associated with disturbances in sleep and has been shown to disrupt the circadian rhythms of both parathyroid hormone (PTH) secretion [52] and autonomic function related to heart rate variability [53]. These changes may be indicative of a deeper connection between sleep and PHPT. Interestingly, the neurocognitive complaints in patients with PHPT are similar to the patients with sleep inefficiency, but few authors have reported sleep disturbance with PHPT [7, 14, 37, 54, 55]. Bridging this data suggests that disruption of sleep itself is associated with mood disturbance [56], impaired executive functioning [57], and declines in memory [57]. However, the response of sleep symptoms to parathyroidectomy have been mixed, though the outcomes data may have been weakened by the use of self-report questionnaires [7, 37, 54] and there are only a few reports using polysomnography as an objective sleep measure in patients with PHPT [55, 58].

A prospective, randomized, controlled trial to measure sleep-related outcomes following parathyroidectomy was designed by our group at MDACC using actigraphy. Twenty-one patients were randomly assigned to either parathyroidectomy (treatment group) or control group. Wrist actigraphy was used to estimate total sleep time and sleep efficiency, and the Epworth Sleepiness Scale (ESS) to quantify daytime hypersomnolence. Measurements were made at baseline, 6 weeks and 6 months after parathyroidectomy. There was a significant improvement in ESS in the surgery group versus control (−8 versus −2, $p=0.017$) at 6 weeks, and although the difference between the groups persisted as a trend at 6 months, it did not reach statistical significance. However, there was no significant difference in total sleep time or efficiency either at 6 weeks or at 6 months. This suggests that despite the lack of significant change in sleep architecture following parathyroidectomy, there is improvement in the perception of daytime sleepiness. Further studies correlating with serum PTH and calcium levels may elucidate underlying pathophysiology.

Cardiovascular Disease

The impact of PHPT on overall mortality, mainly due to increases in cardiovascular disease, may be as high as 20–58%, as shown in the study by Leifsson et al. In this study of 33,346 patients, each patient was followed after a single serum calcium measurement for 11 years. Those with elevated serum calcium levels had 20–58% higher mortality, often due to cardiovascular disease, than the age-matched counterparts who were normocalcemic [59].

Cardiac Structural Abnormalities

Among the cardiovascular abnormalities in patients with PHPT, cardiac structural changes, such as coronary artery disease (CAD) [60, 61] valvular and myocardial calcifications, and increased left ventricular (LV) hypertrophy are the most common. In addition, there is increased vascular and aortic stiffness [61, 62] increased carotid artery intima media thickness (IMT) with subsequent reduced distensibility [63], and reduced diastolic function. These changes, either singly or together, appear to contribute to the increased cardiovascular morbidity and mortality in patients with PHPT.

Recently, Walker et al. conducted a case controlled study evaluating the cardiac structure and diastolic function in patients with PHPT [64]. Patients with biochemically mild PHPT did not have evidence of increased left ventricular mass, diastolic dysfunction, or increased valvular calcifications. However, there was an association between low 25-hydroxyvitamin D levels and the development of left ventricular hypertrophy in PHPT. In addition, the higher serum calcium and PTH levels in those with diastolic dysfunction suggested that severity of PHPT may determine the presence of cardiac manifestations. On the contrary, recent data has suggested that PHPT is associated with a significant dysfunction of the coronary microcirculation. It was hypothesized that this might contribute to the high cardiovascular risk seen in conditions characterized by chronic elevation in serum PTH levels [65]. Although the study was small it suggested that the duration of the disease reasonably correlated with the degree of coronary blood vessel flow impairment ($p < 0.02$).

The effect of parathyroidectomy on cardiac structural parameters has not been uniform. Faranak et al. performed a prospective case controlled study of 51 PHPT patients without cardiovascular risk factors and compared the findings to 51 healthy matched controls. Echocardiography, Doppler tissue imaging, blood pressure, and heart rate were measured. No significant differences in systolic, or diastolic function, or cardiac morpholology was noted between the cases or controls. However, systolic blood pressure at baseline was higher in patients compared to controls ($p < 0.05$). After parathyroidectomy regional peak systolic myocardial velocities measured with Doppler decreased at tricuspid and mitral annulus and septal and lateral sites. In addition, both systolic and diastolic blood pressures decreased ($p < 0.05$) after parathyroidectomy approximating the values in the control group. This change in blood pressures warrants further investigation.

In another study, Bakyan et al. determined that endothelial dysfunction, which reflects an early stage of atherosclerosis, can be aggravated due to increased PTH levels, even in early PHPT. Using high-resolution ultrasonography to measure postischemic flow-mediated dilation of the brachial artery, and independent of other confounding factors, the study found that elevated PTH levels can induce endothelial dysfunction and reduce arterial dilatory capacity. Additionally, it was noted that attempts to manage endothelial dysfunction in PHPT patients without parathyroidectomy could result in increased morbidity and mortality [60].

The relationship of carotid arterial intima-media thickening to PHPT was examined by Nuzzo et al. in 20 patients with PHPT and 20 matched asymptomatic, nonhypertensive controls. Although the carotid artery IMT was increased in PHPT patients compared to normotensive healthy controls in this study [66], other studies, also examining the impact of PHPT on carotid IMT, found no such relationship [67, 68].

Cardiac Functional Abnormalities

Although the mechanistic explanation for the negative impact of PHPT on overall survival among PHPT patients, most agree that cardiac functional abnormalities are relevant to the development of cardiovascular disease in PHPT [69–71]. Earlier studies on direct impact of PTH and serum calcium levels on cardiovascular structures have been inconclusive [63, 67, 68, 71], but more recent studies suggest potential links between PHPT and cardiovascular risk factors, such as altered serum glucose levels, insulin resistance, dyslipidemia, and the presence of abnormal and increased coagulation factors. Such changes in PHPT patients may explain the cardiac functional and structural abnormalities [72]. In addition, the relationship between metabolic syndrome, cardiovascular disease, and PHPT have been explored in greater detail. Functional changes in cardiovascular system, including hormone-exacerbated cardiovascular symptomotology and subsequent structural damage are becoming an area of great interest.

Heart Rate Changes

Since electro-mechanical cardiac function and heart rate is highly regulated, in part, by a careful balance of electrolytes, including calcium, hypercalcemia associated with PHPT may affect cardiac electrical conductivity. Increased serum calcium levels, found even in nominally asymptomatic PHPT patients, contributes to arrhythmias and increased risk of cardiac death—even in patients without prior history or risk factors for cardiovascular disease [73].

Hypertension and Increased Left Ventricular Pressure

Hypertension and/or increased left ventricular pressure are the best predictors of increased risk of cardiovascular morbidity and mortality. The renin-angiotensin-aldosterone system is fundamental in the management of blood pressure, and interference in the system due to increased PTH levels has been examined to determine the impact of PHPT on hypertensive cardiovascular disease [74]. Other aspects of the relationship between hypertension and PHPT, including evidence that increased calcium levels may contribute to increased risk of developing hypertension in PHPT and the possibility that fragments of PTH can instigate hypertension, have also been evaluated [69, 75].

Work by Lehmann et al. may shed light on the prevalence of hypertension in PHPT patients. In their 2008 study, Lehmann et al. showed that two fragments PTH induce hypertension in rats. Both PTH (25–34) and the acetylated amide analogue of PTH(25–30), (Ac-PTH(25–30)-NH(2))-induced hypertension in physiologic doses, suggesting that in patients with increased PTH levels, excessive levels of these fragments could contribute to hypertension.

There is some evidence that curative parathyroidectomy in PHPT does have an overall impact on long-term mortality even in nonclassical, mild, or near-asymptomatic PHPT [76]. Mihai et al., emphasize the need for further study of the potential links between subclinical PHPT and cardiovascular abnormalities, as this relationship is poorly understood in patients with "asymptomatic" PHPT. There is growing evidence that life expectancy may be reduced in asymptomatic PHPT patients, even beyond that of patients with similar cardiovascular disease but without PHPT [77].

Muscular Function

Much has been written about symptoms of muscle function, myalgias and arthralgias in patients with PHPT. Most studies, albeit small, suggest improvement after surgery. Similar to other endocrine myopathies, proximal muscle weakness is typical and is more common in the lower than in the upper extremities. Muscle weakness also occurs in other forms of hyperparathyroidism (renal or nonrenal) and thus is more likely related to serum PTH rather than calcium levels. In 2005, Giles, Tezelman et al. reviewed the involvement of respiratory muscle group in patients with PHPT. This work and that of the others show improvement following parathyroidectomy. All of the 15 patients had generalized fatigue and muscle weakness at baseline, and 11 of the 15 patients also had impaired functional vital capacity (FVC) and 9 of the 15 had reduced functional expiratory volume (FEV1) at baseline. There was a significant improvement in the PHPT group who underwent parathyroidectomy, but no change in the control group of thyroidectomy patients [78, 79]. In addition, using a hand dynamometer Chou and Leong demonstrated improved muscle strength following parathyroidectomy [80].

Possible Mechanisms of Nonclassic Manifestations

Calcium

That calcium can have central nervous system (CNS) effects is reasonably clear; in fact, severe hypercalcemia often presents with somnolence or coma [81]. However, it is unclear whether hypercalcemia has graded CNS effects. An early study reported close relationship between hypercalcemia and the severity of psychiatric and neurocognitive symptoms [3], which was corroborated in a more recent study [27]. However, other recent studies have failed to find such an association [6, 10, 38]. These apparent discrepancies may reflect patients' varying susceptibility to changes in serum calcium levels.

Other evidence that calcium may play a role in the nonclassic manifestations of PHPT can be found in early case studies that reported on psychiatric symptoms in patients who had hypercalcemia but normal PTH levels, as is seen in hypervitaminosis D [82]. The psychiatric symptoms in these unusual cases resolved as the serum calcium levels normalized.

More evidence comes from studies on cerebrospinal fluid (CSF) calcium levels. It is generally regarded that CSF calcium is tightly and independently regulated and that there is no correlation between plasma and CSF calcium levels [83]. However, one study found significantly increased CSF calcium levels in patients with PHPT, a finding that may have been due to compromises in blood–brain barrier integrity in these patients [84].

Parathyroid Hormone

The role of PTH in the nonclassic symptoms of PHPT remains undetermined. It has been conjectured that elevated levels of PTH may have primary and/or secondary

Table 8.1 Characteristics of PTH receptors

Characteristic	PTH1R	PTH2R	C-PTHR
First cloned	1991	1995	Has not been cloned
Tissue distribution	Wide, most prevalent in bone and kidney	Limited, most prevalent in the cardiovascular and central nervous systems	Unknown
Function	Regulating calcium homeostasis	Unknown	Unknown
Ligands	PTH, PTHrP	TIP39, PTH (partial agonist)	PTH, C-terminal PTH fragments
Sequence identity	–	Overall sequence homology with PTHR1 is 70%, amino-terminal homology 50% [89]	Unknown

PTHrP parathyroid hormone-related protein; *TIP39* tuberoinfundibular protein 39

Table 8.2 Regional distribution of PTH receptors in CNS and potential role

Region	Pertinent roles
Basal forebrain [86]	Memory, information processing [117]
Midline thalamus [86]	Memory, emotion, cognition [118]
Hypothalamus [119] suprachiasmatic nucleus [90]	Circadian rhythm [120]
Septum [90]	Limbic system [90]

effects on the CNS, yet serum levels of PTH do not correlate with the severity of nonclassic symptoms [10, 38]. It has been hypothesized that the nonclassic symptoms of PHPT are mediated by PTH receptors in the CNS. The elucidation of the role of PTH receptors in the CNS may have significant clinical impact toward understanding the variable penetrance of the nonclassic symptoms and their variable degree of resolution after surgical cure.

CNS Distribution of PTH Receptors

PTH receptors belong to the family of G protein-coupled receptors and at least three different receptors exist: PTH type 1 receptor (PTH1R) [85]; PTH type 2 receptor (PTH2R) [86]; and the putative carboxy-PTH receptor (C-PTHR) [87]. To date, the PTH type 3 receptor has only been cloned from zebrafish [88]. Some characteristics of the PTH receptors are summarized in Table 8.1. There has been a growing body of recent work on the distribution of PTH receptors in the CNS. Studies have demonstrated the expression of PTH1R and PTH2R mRNA in human CNS tissue [89]. To date, no CNS localization studies have been performed for PTH1R, but detailed studies in rat have shown extensive distribution of PTH2R [90] in the CNS. Some distinct areas of interest are shown in Table 8.2.

Primary Effects

There is preclinical evidence of primary effects of PTH on the CNS. In animal studies, PTH administered intracerebrally has been reported to increase dopamine turnover [91] and neurotransmitter release, thereby affecting learning and memory [92, 93]. Such effects may be mediated by PTH1 and PTH2 receptors that have been demonstrated in the rat brain [89, 91, 94, 95]. The function of PTH receptors in the CNS has not been made clear, but animal studies have implicated PTH2 receptors in affecting behavior and anxiety [96]. PTH receptors have also been found to be expressed in the human brain [89].

Critical toward clarifying the role of PTH in mediating CNS effects is the elucidation of the interaction between PTH and the blood–brain barrier. As yet, studies on PTH and the blood–brain barrier are sparse and conflicting. The interaction between the blood–brain barrier and the various circulating fragments of PTH (carboxy-terminal PTH, N-truncated PTH, short N-terminal forms, PTH with midregion modifications) [97, 98] also has not yet been clarified.

Secondary Effects

Elevated levels of PTH may induce other pathophysiologic perturbations that could cause the nonclassic symptoms of PHPT. It has been conjectured that PTH may affect the permeability of blood–brain barrier, thereby affecting CSF constituents [84, 99]. Interleukin-6, which is influenced by PTH, has also been considered as having secondary effects on the CNS. In one study, patients with PHPT were shown to have higher levels of IL-6 than healthy controls and a significant decrease in IL-6 after parathyroidectomy [100]. However, another similar study found contradictory results [101]. Elevations in PTH and one of its fragments have been shown to increase hepatic production of IL-6 [102]. With respect to the nonclassic symptoms of PHPT, IL-6 levels were found to be significantly higher in patients with depression, and these patients also had significantly decreased total sleep time and longer sleep latency [103]. Other studies have provided further evidence of an association between elevations in IL-6 and altered sleep [104, 105]. In healthy men, administration of IL-6 increased fatigue and altered sleep architecture [106]. Associations have also been made between IL-6 and cognitive impairment [107].

Vitamin D: Vitamin D is another factor implicated in the etiology of the nonclassic symptoms of PHPT. The relationship between PHPT and vitamin D deficiency is not completely clear. Since PTH stimulates conversion of 25-hydroxyvitamin D (25-OHD) to its active metabolite 1,25-dihydroxyvitamin D (1,25-OH$_2$D), it has been proposed that the excess PTH of PHPT causes excessive conversion, leading to "conditional" 25-OHD deficiency [108, 109]. However, it is unlikely that significant depletion could occur by this mechanism alone considering the large molar ratio of 25-OHD to 1,25-OH$_2$D (1,000/1) [110, 111]. Others have suggested that PHPT may cause increased hepatic inactivation of 25-OHD [110]. Vitamin D deficiency, which is more common in PHPT patients, itself has been implicated in myopathy, most likely mediated by vitamin D receptors in the myocytes, independent of high PTH levels. In addition, vitamin D deficiency itself has been reported to be associated with impaired cognitive function and low moods [112].

Cerebral Blood Flow

Recent studies using single-photon emission computed tomography have shown decreases in regional cerebral blood flow in patients with PHPT [113, 114]. Similar decreases in regional cerebral blood flow have been seen in patients with depression, anxiety disorders, and chronic fatigue [113, 114]. In one study, 13 of the 14 patients with PHPT had normalization of regional cerebral flow after parathyroidectomy [113]. The authors proposed that elevated calcium levels due to high PTH were affecting cerebral blood flow. Using a different imaging modality, a recent study also demonstrated the feasibility of using functional magnetic resonance imaging to document changes in regional blood oxygenation levels [37].

Conclusions

Elucidation of the mechanisms by which the vast array of nonclassic symptoms of PHPT occur could improve patient management, and thereby improve the quality of life for the affected patients, prevent downstream potential disability, and preserve patient independence. A key component to uncovering these mechanisms lies in outcomes-based research [19, 115, 116]. The importance of such research increases with the projected growth of the geriatric population, the group who is at increased risk for developing PHPT in the upcoming decades.

References

1. Boyd JD, Milgram JE, Stearns G. Clinical hyperparathyroidism. J Am Med Assoc. 1929;93:684–8.
2. Karpati G, Frame B. Neuropsychiatric disorders in primary hyperparathyroidism. Clinical analysis with review of the literature. Arch Neurol. 1964;10:387–97.
3. Petersen P. Psychiatric disorders in primary hyperparathyroidism. J Clin Endocrinol Metab. 1968;28:1491–5.
4. Numann PJ, Torppa AJ, Blumetti AE. Neuropsychologic deficits associated with primary hyperparathyroidism. Surgery. 1984;96(6):1119–23.
5. Joborn C, Hetta J, Palmer M, Akerstrom G, Ljunghall S. Psychiatric symptomatology in patients with primary hyperparathyroidism. Ups J Med Sci. 1986;91(1):77–87.
6. Joborn C, Hetta J, Johansson H, et al. Psychiatric morbidity in primary hyperparathyroidism. World J Surg. 1988;12(4):476–81.
7. McAllion SJ, Paterson CR. Psychiatric morbidity in primary hyperparathyroidism. Postgrad Med J. 1989;65(767):628–31.

8. Goyal A, Chumber S, Tandon N, Lal R, Srivastava A, Gupta S. Neuropsychiatric manifestations in patients of primary hyperparathyroidism and outcome following surgery. Indian J Med Sci. 2001;55(12):677–86.

9. Roman SA, Sosa JA, Mayes L, et al. Parathyroidectomy improves neurocognitive deficits in patients with primary hyperparathyroidism. Surgery. 2005;138(6):1121–8. discussion 8–9.

10. Dotzenrath CM, Kaetsch AK, Pfingsten H, et al. Neuropsychiatric and cognitive changes after surgery for primary hyperparathyroidism. World J Surg. 2006;30(5):680–5.

11. Nielsen HE, Steffensen K. Geographic distribution and surgical therapy of hyperparathyroidism in connection with 2 cases. Nord Med. 1941;9:115–21.

12. Nielson H. Familial occurrence, gastrointestinal symptoms and mental disturbances in hyperparathyroidism. Acta Med Scand. 1955;151:359–66.

13. Fitz TE, Hallman BL. Mental changes associated with hyperparathyroidism; report of two cases. AMA Arch Intern Med. 1952;89(4):547–51.

14. Reinfrank RF. Primary hyperparathyroidism with depression. Arch Intern Med. 1961;108:606–10.

15. Agras S, Oliveau DC. Primary hyperparathyroidism and psychosis. Can Med Assoc J. 1964;91:1366–7.

16. Flanagan TA, Goodwin DW, Alderson P. Psychiatric illness in a large family with familial hyperparathyroidism. Br J Psychiatry. 1970;117(541):693–8.

17. Gatewood JW, Organ Jr CH, Mead BT. Mental changes associated with hyperparathyroidism. Am J Psychiatry. 1975;132(2):129–32.

18. Rosenblatt S, Faillace LA. Psychiatric manifestations of hyperparathyroidism. Tex Med. 1977;73(2):59–60.

19. Pasieka JL, Parsons LL. Prospective surgical outcome study of relief of symptoms following surgery in patients with primary hyperparathyroidism. World J Surg. 1998;22(6):513–8. discussion 8–9.

20. Sheldon DG, Lee FT, Neil NJ, Ryan Jr JA. Surgical treatment of hyperparathyroidism improves health-related quality of life. Arch Surg. 2002;137(9):1022–6. discussion 6–8.

21. Okamoto T, Kamo T, Obara T. Outcome study of psychological distress and nonspecific symptoms in patients with mild primary hyperparathyroidism. Arch Surg. 2002;137(7):779–83. discussion 84.

22. Prager G, Kalaschek A, Kaczirek K, et al. Parathyroidectomy improves concentration and retentiveness in patients with primary hyperparathyroidism. Surgery. 2002;132(6):930–5. discussion 5–6.

23. Rastad J, Joborn C, Akerstrom G, Ljunghall S. Incidence, type and severity of psychic symptoms in patients with sporadic primary hyperparathyroidism. J Endocrinol Invest. 1992;15(9 Suppl 6):149–56.

24. Joborn C, Hetta J, Lind L, Rastad J, Akerstrom G, Ljunghall S. Self-rated psychiatric symptoms in patients operated on because of primary hyperparathyroidism and in patients with long-standing mild hypercalcemia. Surgery. 1989;105(1):72–8.

25. Doherty GM. Parathyroid glands. In: Greenfield LJ, Mulholland MW, Oldham KT, Zelenock GB, Lillemoe KD, editors. Surgery – scientific principles and practice. Philadelphia: Lippincott Williams & Wilkins; 2001. p. 1284–306.

26. Lundgren E, Szabo E, Ljunghall S, Bergstrom R, Holmberg L, Rastad J. Population based case–control study of sick leave in postmenopausal women before diagnosis of hyperparathyroidism. BMJ. 1998;317(7162):848–51.

27. Brown GG, Preisman RC, Kleerekoper M. Neurobehavioral symptoms in mild primary hyperparathyroidism: related to hypercalcemia but not improved by parathyroidectomy. Henry Ford Hosp Med J. 1987;35(4):211–5.

28. Kleinfeld M, Peter S, Gilbert GM. Delirium as the predominant manifestation of hyperparathyroidism: reversal after parathyroidectomy. J Am Geriatr Soc. 1984;32(9):689–90.

29. Alarcon RD, Franceschini JA. Hyperparathyroidism and paranoid psychosis. Case report and review of the literature. Br J Psychiatry. 1984;145:477–86.

30. Borer MS, Bhanot VK. Hyperparathyroidism: neuropsychiatric manifestations. Psychosomatics. 1985;26(7):597–601.
31. Brown Jr RS, Fischman A, Showalter CR. Primary hyperparathyroidism, hypercalcemia, paranoid delusions, homicide, and attempted murder. J Forensic Sci. 1987;32(5):1460–3.
32. Hayabara T, Hashimoto K, Izumi H, Morioka E, Hosokawa K. Neuropsychiatric disorders in primary hyperparathyroidism. Jpn J Psychiatry Neurol. 1987;41(1):33–40.
33. Spivak B, Radvan M, Ohring R, Weizman A. Primary hyperparathyroidism, psychiatric manifestations, diagnosis and management. Psychother Psychosom. 1989;51(1):38–44.
34. Solomon BL, Schaaf M, Smallridge RC. Psychologic symptoms before and after parathyroid surgery. Am J Med. 1994;96(2):101–6.
35. Linder J, Brimar K, Granberg PO, Wetterberg L, Werner S. Characteristic changes in psychiatric symptoms, cortisol and melatonin but not prolactin in primary hyperparathyroidism. Acta Psychiatr Scand. 1988;78(1):32–40.
36. Bollerslev J, Jansson S, Mollerup CL, et al. Medical observation, compared with parathyroidectomy, for asymptomatic primary hyperparathyroidism: a prospective, randomized trial. J Clin Endocrinol Metab. 2007;92(5):1687–92.
37. Perrier ND, Coker LH, Rorie KD, et al. Preliminary report: functional MRI of the brain may be the ideal tool for evaluating neuropsychologic and sleep complaints of patients with primary hyperparathyroidism. World J Surg. 2006;30(5):686–96.
38. Mittendorf EA, Wefel JS, Meyers CA, et al. Improvement of sleep disturbance and neurocognitive function after parathyroidectomy in patients with primary hyperparathyroidism. Endocr Pract. 2007;13(4):338–44.
39. Chiang CY, Andrewes DG, Anderson D, Devere M, Schweitzer I, Zajac JD. A controlled, prospective study of neuropsychological outcomes post parathyroidectomy in primary hyperparathyroid patients. Clin Endocrinol (Oxf). 2005;62(1):99–104.
40. Coker LH, Rorie K, Cantley L, et al. Primary hyperparathyroidism, cognition, and health-related quality of life. Ann Surg. 2005;242(5):642–50.
41. Roman S, Sosa JA. Psychiatric and cognitive aspects of primary hyperparathyroidism. Curr Opin Oncol. 2007;19(1):1–5.
42. Wechsler D. A standardized memory scale for clinical use. J Psychol. 1945;19:87–95.
43. Wechsler D. Wechsler adult intelligence scale manual. New York: Psychological Corporation; 1949.
44. Milner B. Visual recognition and recall after right temporal-lobe excision in a man. Neuropsychologia. 1968;6:191–209.
45. Benton AL. The revised visual retention test. New York: Psychological Corporation; 1963.
46. Reitan RM. Validity of the trail making test as an indicator of organic brain damage. Percept Mot Skills. 1958;8:271–6.
47. Reitan RM. Manual for administration of neuropsychological test batteries for adults and children. Indianapolis: Reitan; 1969.
48. Golden CJ. The stroop color and word test: a manual for clinical and experimental uses. Chicago: Stoelting; 1960.
49. Matarazzo JD. Wechler's measurement and appraisal of adult intelligence. Baltimore: Williams & Wilkins; 1972.
50. Andrewes DG, Puce A, Bladin PF. Post-ictal recognition memory predicts laterality of temporal lobe seizure focus: comparison with post-operative data. Neuropsychologia. 1990;28(9): 957–67.
51. Puce A, Andrewes DG, Berkovic SF, Bladin PF. Visual recognition memory. Neurophysiological evidence for the role of temporal white matter in man. Brain. 1991;114(Pt 4):1647–66.
52. Logue FC, Fraser WD, Gallacher SJ, et al. The loss of circadian rhythm for intact parathyroid hormone and nephrogenous cyclic AMP in patients with primary hyperparathyroidism. Clin Endocrinol (Oxf). 1990;32(4):475–83.

53. Nilsson IL, Aberg J, Rastad J, Lind L. Circadian cardiac autonomic nerve dysfunction in primary hyperparathyroidism improves after parathyroidectomy. Surgery. 2003;134(6): 1013–9. discussion 9.
54. Walker RP, Paloyan E, Gopalsami C. Symptoms in patients with primary hyperparathyroidism: muscle weakness or sleepiness. Endocr Pract. 2004;10(5):404–8.
55. Lim LL, Dinner D, Tham KW, Siraj E, Shields Jr R. Restless legs syndrome associated with primary hyperparathyroidism. Sleep Med. 2005;6(3):283–5.
56. Dinges DF, Pack F, Williams K, et al. Cumulative sleepiness, mood disturbance, and psychomotor vigilance performance decrements during a week of sleep restricted to 4–5 hours per night. Sleep. 1997;20(4):267–77.
57. Durmer JS, Dinges DF. Neurocognitive consequences of sleep deprivation. Semin Neurol. 2005;25(1):117–29.
58. Kripke DF, Lavie P, Parker D, Huey L, Deftos LJ. Plasma parathyroid hormone and calcium are related to sleep stage cycles. J Clin Endocrinol Metab. 1978;47(5):1021–7.
59. Leifsson BG, Ahren B. Serum calcium and survival in a large health screening program. J Clin Endocrinol Metab. 1996;81(6):2149–53.
60. Baykan M, Erem C, Erdogan T, et al. Impairment of flow mediated vasodilatation of brachial artery in patients with primary hyperparathyroidism. Int J Cardiovasc Imaging. 2007;23(3): 323–8.
61. Neunteufl T, Katzenschlager R, Abela C, et al. Impairment of endothelium-independent vasodilation in patients with hypercalcemia. Cardiovasc Res. 1998;40(2):396–401.
62. Rubin MR, Maurer MS, McMahon DJ, Bilezikian JP, Silverberg SJ. Arterial stiffness in mild primary hyperparathyroidism. J Clin Endocrinol Metab. 2005;90(6):3326–30.
63. Streeten EA, Munir K, Hines S, et al. Coronary artery calcification in patients with primary hyperparathyroidism in comparison with control subjects from the multi-ethnic study of atherosclerosis. Endocr Pract. 2008;14(2):155–61.
64. Walker MD, Fleischer JB, Di Tullio MR, et al. Cardiac structure and diastolic function in mild primary hyperparathyroidism. J Clin Endocrinol Metab. 2010;95(5):2172–9.
65. Marini C, Giusti M, Armonino R, et al. Reduced coronary flow reserve in patients with primary hyperparathyroidism: a study by G-SPECT myocardial perfusion imaging. Eur J Nucl Med Mol Imaging. 2010;37(12):2256–63.
66. Nuzzo V, Tauchmanova L, Fonderico F, et al. Increased intima-media thickness of the carotid artery wall, normal blood pressure profile and normal left ventricular mass in subjects with primary hyperparathyroidism. Eur J Endocrinol. 2002;147(4):453–9.
67. Lumachi F, Ermani M, Frego M, et al. Intima-media thickness measurement of the carotid artery in patients with primary hyperparathyroidism. A prospective case–control study and long-term follow-up. In Vivo. 2006;20(6B):887–90.
68. Fallo F, Camporese G, Capitelli E, Andreozzi GM, Mantero F, Lumachi F. Ultrasound evaluation of carotid artery in primary hyperparathyroidism. J Clin Endocrinol Metab. 2003;88(5): 2096–9.
69. Ybarra J, Donate T, Jurado J, Pou JM. Primary hyperparathyroidism, insulin resistance, and cardiovascular disease: a review. Nurs Clin North Am. 2007;42(1):79–85. vii.
70. Kiernan TJ, O'Flynn AM, McDermott JH, Kearney P. Primary hyperparathyroidism and the cardiovascular system. Int J Cardiol. 2006;113(3):E89–92.
71. Kamycheva E, Sundsfjord J, Jorde R. Serum parathyroid hormone levels predict coronary heart disease: the Tromso study. Eur J Cardiovasc Prev Rehabil. 2004;11(1):69–74.
72. Erem C, Kocak M, Hacihasanoglu A, Yilmaz M, Saglam F, Ersoz HO. Blood coagulation, fibrinolysis and lipid profile in patients with primary hyperparathyroidism: increased plasma factor VII and X activities and D-dimer levels. Exp Clin Endocrinol Diabetes. 2008;116(10): 619–24.
73. Curione M, Letizia C, Amato S, et al. Increased risk of cardiac death in primary hyperparathyroidism: what is a role of electrical instability? Int J Cardiol. 2007;121(2):200–2.
74. Bernini G, Moretti A, Lonzi S, Bendinelli C, Miccoli P, Salvetti A. Renin-angiotensin-aldosterone system in primary hyperparathyroidism before and after surgery. Metabolism. 1999;48(3):298–300.

75. Letizia C, Ferrari P, Cotesta D, et al. Ambulatory monitoring of blood pressure (AMBP) in patients with primary hyperparathyroidism. J Hum Hypertens. 2005;19(11):901–6.
76. Wermers RA, Khosla S, Atkinson EJ, et al. Survival after the diagnosis of hyperparathyroidism: a population-based study. Am J Med. 1998;104(2):115–22.
77. Mihai R, Wass JA, Sadler GP. Asymptomatic hyperparathyroidism – need for multicentre studies. Clin Endocrinol (Oxf). 2008;68(2):155–64.
78. Giles Y, Baspinar I, Tunca F, Terzioglu T, Tezelman S. Impact of surgical treatment on respiratory muscle dysfunction in symptomatic hyperparathyroidism. Arch Surg. 2005;140(12): 1167–71.
79. Kristoffersson A, Bostrom A, Soderberg T. Muscle strength is improved after parathyroidectomy in patients with primary hyperparathyroidism. Br J Surg. 1992;79(2):165–8.
80. Chou FF, Sheen-Chen SM, Leong CP. Neuromuscular recovery after parathyroidectomy in primary hyperparathyroidism. Surgery. 1995;117(1):18–25.
81. Ziegler R. Hypercalcemic crisis. J Am Soc Nephrol. 2001;12 Suppl 17:S3–9.
82. Lehrer GM, Levitt MF. Neuropsychiatric presentation of hypercalcemia. J Mt Sinai Hosp NY. 1960;27:10–8.
83. Keep RF, Ulanski II LJ, Xiang J, Ennis SR, Lorris Betz A. Blood–brain barrier mechanisms involved in brain calcium and potassium homeostasis. Brain Res. 1999;815(2):200–5.
84. Joborn C, Hetta J, Niklasson F, et al. Cerebrospinal fluid calcium, parathyroid hormone, and monoamine and purine metabolites and the blood–brain barrier function in primary hyperparathyroidism. Psychoneuroendocrinology. 1991;16(4):311–22.
85. Chorev M. Parathyroid hormone 1 receptor: insights into structure and function. Receptors Channels. 2002;8(3–4):219–42.
86. Usdin TB, Bonner TI, Hoare SR. The parathyroid hormone 2 (PTH2) receptor. Receptors Channels. 2002;8(3–4):211–8.
87. Murray TM, Rao LG, Divieti P, Bringhurst FR. Parathyroid hormone secretion and action: evidence for discrete receptors for the carboxyl-terminal region and related biological actions of carboxyl-terminal ligands. Endocr Rev. 2005;26(1):78–113.
88. Hoare SR, Rubin DA, Juppner H, Usdin TB. Evaluating the ligand specificity of zebrafish parathyroid hormone (PTH) receptors: comparison of PTH, PTH-related protein, and tuberoinfundibular peptide of 39 residues. Endocrinology. 2000;141(9):3080–6.
89. Usdin TB, Gruber C, Bonner TI. Identification and functional expression of a receptor selectively recognizing parathyroid hormone, the PTH2 receptor. J Biol Chem. 1995;270(26): 15455–8.
90. Wang T, Palkovits M, Rusnak M, Mezey E, Usdin TB. Distribution of parathyroid hormone-2 receptor-like immunoreactivity and messenger RNA in the rat nervous system. Neuroscience. 2000;100(3):629–49.
91. Harvey S, Hayer S, Sloley BD. Parathyroid hormone-induced dopamine turnover in the rat medial basal hypothalamus. Peptides. 1993;14(2):269–74.
92. Clementi G, Drago F, Prato A, et al. Effects of calcitonin, parathyroid hormone and its related fragments on acquisition of active avoidance behavior. Physiol Behav. 1984;33(6):913–6.
93. Harvey S, Hayer S. Parathyroid hormone binding sites in the brain. Peptides. 1993;14(6): 1187–91.
94. Hoare SR, Bonner TI, Usdin TB. Comparison of rat and human parathyroid hormone 2 (PTH2) receptor activation: PTH is a low potency partial agonist at the rat PTH2 receptor. Endocrinology. 1999;140(10):4419–25.
95. Weaver DR, Deeds JD, Lee K, Segre GV. Localization of parathyroid hormone-related peptide (PTHrP) and PTH/PTHrP receptor mRNAs in rat brain. Brain Res Mol Brain Res. 1995;28(2):296–310.
96. LaBuda CJ, Usdin TB. Tuberoinfundibular peptide of 39 residues decreases pain-related affective behavior. Neuroreport. 2004;15(11):1779–82.
97. D'Amour P. Circulating PTH, molecular forms: what we know and what we don't. Kidney Int Suppl. 2006;102:S29–33.
98. Souberbielle JC, Friedlander G, Cormier C. Practical considerations in PTH testing. Clin Chim Acta. 2006;366(1–2):81–9.

99. Akmal M, Tuma S, Goldstein DA, Pattabhiraman R, Bernstein L, Massry SG. Intact and carboxyterminal PTH do not cross the blood-cerebrospinal fluid barrier. Proc Soc Exp Biol Med. 1984;176(4):434–7.

100. Grey A, Mitnick MA, Shapses S, Ellison A, Gundberg C, Insogna K. Circulating levels of interleukin-6 and tumor necrosis factor-alpha are elevated in primary hyperparathyroidism and correlate with markers of bone resorption – a clinical research center study. J Clin Endocrinol Metab. 1996;81(10):3450–4.

101. Ogard CG, Engelmann MD, Kistorp C, Nielsen SL, Vestergaard H. Increased plasma N-terminal pro-B-type natriuretic peptide and markers of inflammation related to atherosclerosis in patients with primary hyperparathyroidism. Clin Endocrinol (Oxf). 2005;63(5): 493–8.

102. Mitnick MA, Grey A, Masiukiewicz U, et al. Parathyroid hormone induces hepatic production of bioactive interleukin-6 and its soluble receptor. Am J Physiol Endocrinol Metab. 2001;280(3):E405–12.

103. Motivala SJ, Sarfatti A, Olmos L, Irwin MR. Inflammatory markers and sleep disturbance in major depression. Psychosom Med. 2005;67(2):187–94.

104. Vgontzas AN, Papanicolaou DA, Bixler EO, Kales A, Tyson K, Chrousos GP. Elevation of plasma cytokines in disorders of excessive daytime sleepiness: role of sleep disturbance and obesity. J Clin Endocrinol Metab. 1997;82(5):1313–6.

105. Vgontzas AN, Papanicolaou DA, Bixler EO, et al. Circadian interleukin-6 secretion and quantity and depth of sleep. J Clin Endocrinol Metab. 1999;84(8):2603–7.

106. Spath-Schwalbe E, Hansen K, Schmidt F, et al. Acute effects of recombinant human interleukin-6 on endocrine and central nervous sleep functions in healthy men. J Clin Endocrinol Metab. 1998;83(5):1573–9.

107. Meyers CA, Albitar M, Estey E. Cognitive impairment, fatigue, and cytokine levels in patients with acute myelogenous leukemia or myelodysplastic syndrome. Cancer. 2005;104(4):788–93.

108. Boudou P, Ibrahim F, Cormier C, Sarfati E, Souberbielle JC. A very high incidence of low 25 hydroxy-vitamin D serum concentration in a French population of patients with primary hyperparathyroidism. J Endocrinol Invest. 2006;29(6):511–5.

109. Silverberg SJ, Shane E, Dempster DW, Bilezikian JP. The effects of vitamin D insufficiency in patients with primary hyperparathyroidism. Am J Med. 1999;107(6):561–7.

110. Clements MR, Davies M, Fraser DR, Lumb GA, Mawer EB, Adams PH. Metabolic inactivation of vitamin D is enhanced in primary hyperparathyroidism. Clin Sci (Lond). 1987;73(6):659–64.

111. Moosgaard B, Vestergaard P, Heickendorff L, Melsen F, Christiansen P, Mosekilde L. Vitamin D status, seasonal variations, parathyroid adenoma weight and bone mineral density in primary hyperparathyroidism. Clin Endocrinol (Oxf). 2005;63(5):506–13.

112. Wilkins CH, Sheline YI, Roe CM, Birge SJ, Morris JC. Vitamin D deficiency is associated with low mood and worse cognitive performance in older adults. Am J Geriatr Psychiatry. 2006;14(12):1032–40.

113. Mjaland O, Normann E, Halvorsen E, Rynning S, Egeland T. Regional cerebral blood flow in patients with primary hyperparathyroidism before and after successful parathyroidectomy. Br J Surg. 2003;90(6):732–7.

114. Cermik TF, Kaya M, Ugur-Altun B, Bedel D, Berkarda S, Yigitbasi ON. Regional cerebral blood flow abnormalities in patients with primary hyperparathyroidism. Neuroradiology. 2007;49(4):379–85.

115. Chan AK, Duh QY, Katz MH, Siperstein AE, Clark OH. Clinical manifestations of primary hyperparathyroidism before and after parathyroidectomy. A case–control study. Ann Surg. 1995;222(3):402–12. discussion 12–4.

116. Burney RE, Jones KR, Christy B, Thompson NW. Health status improvement after surgical correction of primary hyperparathyroidism in patients with high and low preoperative calcium levels. Surgery. 1999;125(6):608–14.

117. Baxter MG, Chiba AA. Cognitive functions of the basal forebrain. Curr Opin Neurobiol. 1999;9(2):178–83.
118. Vertes RP. Interactions among the medial prefrontal cortex, hippocampus and midline thalamus in emotional and cognitive processing in the rat. Neuroscience. 2006;142(1):1–20.
119. Dobolyi A, Irwin S, Wang J, Usdin TB. The distribution and neurochemistry of the parathyroid hormone 2 receptor in the rat hypothalamus. Neurochem Res. 2006;31(2):227–36.
120. Mistlberger RE. Circadian regulation of sleep in mammals: role of the suprachiasmatic nucleus. Brain Res Brain Res Rev. 2005;49(3):429–54.

Chapter 9
Secondary Hyperparathyroidism

Naifa Lamki Busaidy*, Amit Lahoti*, and David A. Hanley

Keywords Secondary hyperparathyroidism • Vitamin D homeostasis • Vitamin D inadequacy and manifestations • Secondary hyperparathyroidism in CKD • Diagnosis and management of sHPT • Phosphate binders • Vitamin D therapy and derivatives • Calcimimetics • Parathyroid hyperplasia • Low phosphate diet • Osteomalacia • Vascular calcification • Diagnosis • Calcitriol • Phosphate binders

Introduction

Parathyroid hormone (PTH) is an 84 amino acid polypeptide produced by the chief cells of the parathyroid gland, and its primary role in human physiology is the maintenance of normal extracellular fluid-ionized calcium (Ca^{2+}) concentration. PTH secretion rises in response to a low Ca^{2+}. Under high Ca^{2+} conditions, PTH secretion is reduced, and intracellular degradation of PTH increases, with resultant increased proportional secretion of biologically inactive fragments of PTH. The influence of secreted fragments of PTH on the measurement of serum PTH is discussed in Chap. 3.

*Naifa Lamki Busaidy and Amit Lahoti contributed equally to this work

N.L. Busaidy, MD, FACP (✉)
Department of Endocrine Neoplasia & Hormonal Disorders, University of Texas
M. D. Anderson Cancer Center, 1515 Holcombe Blvd, Unit 1461, Houston 77031, TX, USA
email: naifa99gmail.com

A. Lahoti, MD (✉)
Section of Nephrology, Department of General Internal Medicine, University of Texas
M. D. Anderson Cancer Center, Houston, TX, USA

D.A. Hanley, MD, FRCPC
Department of Medicine, University of Calgary, Calgary, AB, Canada

A.A. Khan and O.H. Clark (eds.), *Handbook of Parathyroid Diseases:
A Case-Based Practical Guide*, DOI 10.1007/978-1-4614-2164-1_9,
© Springer Science+Business Media, LLC 2012

Table 9.1 Causes of secondary hyperparathyroidism

Chronic kidney disease	Multiple mechanisms (Fig. 9.2)
Lack of intake or production of vitamin D	Insufficient oral intake, insufficient sunshine exposure
	Malabsorption syndromes: Celiac disease, chronic pancreatitis, small bowel disease, bariatric surgery
Lack of conversion of vitamin D	Impaired 25-hydroxylation (late stage liver disease)
	Impaired 1α-hydroxylation: inherited 1α-hydroxylase deficiency, ketoconazole
Decreased 1,25(OH)$_2$ vitamin D	Increased vitamin D catabolism: accelerated loss (medications), overexpression of 24-hydroxylase
True resistance to 1,25 (OH)$_2$D	Vitamin D receptor deficiency
Calcium deficiency	Deficient intake, malnutrition
	Hypercalciuria
	Impaired 1α-hydroxylation and complexing of ionized calcium
Other conditions causing hypocalcemia	Osteoblastic metastases
	Hungry bone syndrome
	Medications (chemotherapy, EDTA, citrate)
	Hyperphosphatemia (e.g., rhabdomyolysis)
	Pseudohypoparathyroidism (PTH resistance)

A number of stimuli of PTH secretion have been identified, but clinically, the most important regulators are calcium, vitamin D, and, directly or indirectly, phosphate metabolism. The regulation of parathyroid function is discussed in Dr. Brown's chapter (Chap. 1) on calcium homeostasis, and he calls attention to the sequential nature of the parathyroid's response to stimulation by low Ca^{2+}: increased secretion of PTH, followed by decreased intracellular degradation. Then, after the stimulus becomes more chronic (hours), increased PTH gene expression occurs. Chronic stimulation of PTH secretion by low Ca^{2+} or by vitamin D deficiency eventually results in parathyroid chief cell proliferation and hyperplasia. Therefore, while primary hyperparathyroidism may be defined as excessive PTH secretion that is inappropriate for the serum Ca^{2+}, secondary hyperparathyroidism (sHPT) is an appropriate increase in synthesis and secretion of PTH in response to an excess of a normal stimulus, such as low serum Ca^{2+}. Although there are many causes of sHPT (Table 9.1), this chapter concentrates on the most common causes, vitamin D deficiency (which causes calcium deficiency, an additional stimulus for sHPT) and chronic kidney disease (CKD). Recent research has provided insight into the pathogenesis and treatment of sHPT.

Vitamin D

Vitamin D metabolism is outlined in Fig. 9.1a, b. Humans synthesize vitamin D$_3$ (cholecalciferol) from 7-dehydrocholesterol via ultraviolet B irradiation of the skin. A smaller amount of vitamin D is absorbed from dietary sources, predominantly

a

Vitamin D Metabolism

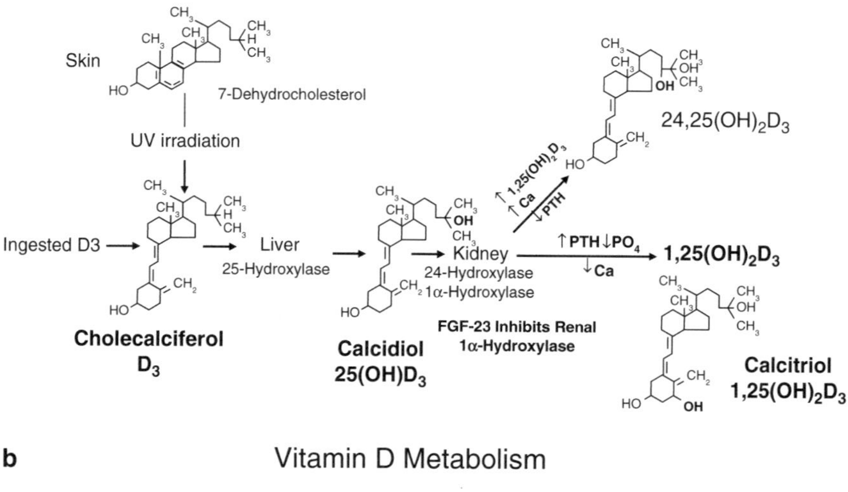

b

Vitamin D Metabolism

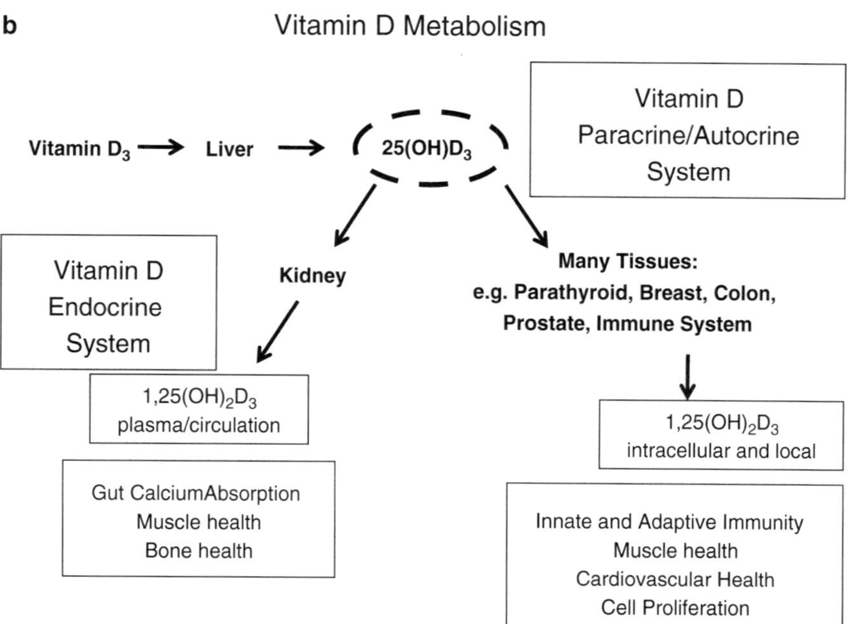

Fig. 9.1 (**a**) Vitamin D metabolism. The two sources of vitamin D are skin synthesis and diet. The hydroxyl groups added by the respective enzymes are *bolded* and *enlarged* in each step. Vitamin D_2 (ergocalciferol) follows the same pathway as vitamin D_3 and is probably 1/3–1/2 as active as D_3. Vitamin D_2 differs from vitamin D_3 by having a double bond at C_{22}–C_{23} and a methyl group at C_{24}. (**b**) Vitamin D metabolism: Vitamin D endocrine system is responsible for the traditional actions of vitamin D on the skeleton and calcium metabolism. The paracrine/autocrine system is important in the nontraditional actions of vitamin D but this may also involve regulation of parathyroid function

fatty fish and fortified food. In the USA, prescription vitamin D supplements are ergocalciferol (vitamin D_2), as are most over-the-counter preparations. Vitamin D_3 is the usual supplement in most other countries in the world. Vitamin D_2 follows the same metabolic pathways as native vitamin D_3, and is very similar in its biological activity. In this chapter, "vitamin D" is used to refer to either form, except where specific reference to ergocalciferol is made. Cholecalciferol is further metabolized by the liver via 25-hydroxylase to 25(OH)D or calcidiol. Serum measurement of 25(OH)D is the best functional indicator of vitamin D nutritional status and most methods measure both $25(OH)D_2$ and $25(OH)D_3$. The most active form of vitamin D is the vitamin D hormone, $1,25(OH)_2D$ or calcitriol, which is converted from 25(OH)D by the enzyme 1-alpha-hydroxylase in the kidney and released into the circulation. Circulating calcitriol increases calcium and phosphate absorption from the gut, increases bone turnover facilitates bone mineralization, and provides feedback inhibition of PTH synthesis and secretion. More recently, 1-alpha hydroxylase has been identified in most tissues of the body, including the parathyroid gland itself. It is therefore postulated that vitamin D may play an important regulatory role in many physiological pathways via local tissue conversion of circulating 25(OH)D, rather than responding to circulating calcitriol, which is primarily involved in regulation of calcium and phosphate metabolism. The more recent concept of endocrine and paracrine/autocrine metabolism of vitamin D is depicted in Fig. 9.1b.

Deficiency of vitamin D results in reduced gut calcium absorption, which, in turn, results in calcium deficiency and elevated PTH. Low circulating levels of calcitriol in CKD, secondary to decreased 1-alpha-hydroxylase activity in the kidney, lead to increased PTH secretion and parathyroid hyperplasia. However, in keeping with the model of vitamin D metabolism outlined in Fig. 9.1b, it has been shown that the parathyroid gland itself can convert 25(OH)D to calcitriol [1]. This may explain the observation that serum PTH levels are more strongly associated with serum 25(OH)D than serum calcitriol, which are often within the normal laboratory range in the setting of severe nutritional vitamin D deficiency [2].

Patients with CKD commonly have hypocalcemia, hyperphosphatemia, and calcitriol deficiency, all of which are stimuli for excessive PTH secretion and sHPT. If left untreated, sHPT leads to severe bone disease (osteitis fibrosa cystica) and soft tissue and vascular calcifications, all of which contribute to the increased morbidity and mortality seen in patients with CKD. The term, chronic kidney disease–mineral and bone disorder (CKD-MBD), has been recently coined to describe the effects of hyperphosphatemia, hypocalcemia, and sHPT in the setting of CKD [3].

Pathophysiology

sHPT is a result of dysregulation and imbalance of calcium, phosphate, and vitamin D metabolism. Parathyroid gland function is dependent on the G-protein-coupled calcium-sensing receptor (CaSR), the vitamin D receptor, and the putative extracellular

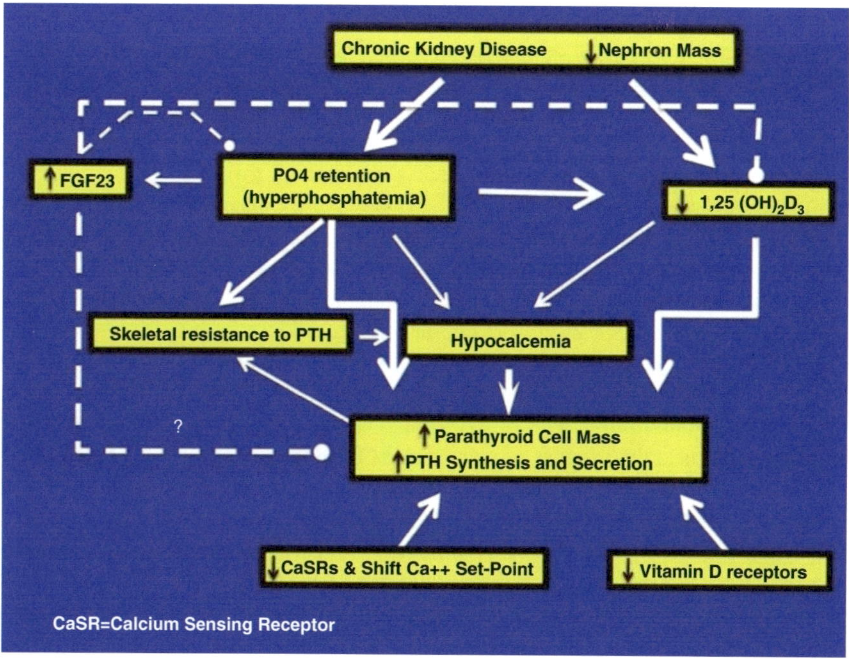

Fig. 9.2 Pathophysiology of secondary hyperparathyroidism in chronic kidney disease. *Dashed line* indicates inhibition

phosphate sensor. Parathyroid gland hyperfunction in vitamin D deficiency results from negative calcium balance and probably deficient parathyroid conversion of 25(OH)D to calcitriol.

Parathyroid gland hyperfunction in individuals with CKD results from a combination of hypocalcemia, decreased 1,25 dihydroxyvitamin D levels, and hyperphosphatemia (Fig. 9.2). Disordered calcium and phosphate metabolism occurs early in CKD prior to any obvious biochemical abnormalities. When the glomerular filtration rate decreases below 90 mL/min, fibroblast growth factor-23 (FGF-23) is released from osteocytes and osteoblasts prior to detectable elevations in PTH or serum phosphate. FGF-23 levels increase with progressive CKD and maintain phosphate homeostasis by (1) inhibition of phosphate reabsorption in the proximal tubule of the nephron (2) inhibition of renal 1-alpha hydroxylase activity, thereby reducing circulating calcitriol, and (3) inhibition of PTH secretion. The increased levels of FGF-23 in renal failure may therefore have a moderating effect on the development of sHPT. Interestingly, FGF-23 has been shown to increase parathyroid 1-alpha hydroxylase, which would tend to further contribute to its suppression of PTH secretion [4]. However, the progressive loss of nephron mass results in decreased ability to excrete phosphate. The parathyroid gland eventually develops resistance to FGF-23 inhibition [5]. This is a result of decreased expression of the receptor for FGF-23 (a co-receptor complex of Klotho and FGF receptor 1-c) in renal failure [5].

Both hyperphosphatemia and FGF-23 inhibit renal 1-alpha hydroxylase, and the decreased calcitriol contributes to increased PTH synthesis directly and indirectly through the reduced vitamin D-mediated gut Ca^{2+} absorption.

The high content of phosphate in a normal diet contributes to hyperphosphatemia and the development of sHPT. Canine studies have shown that a phosphate restricted diet in the setting of reduced nephron mass can prevent the development of sHPT until the late stages of CKD [6]. As CKD progresses, the kidneys are unable to maintain sufficient phosphate excretion in the urine despite high levels of FGF-23, and hyperphosphatemia ensues. High serum phosphate binds to Ca^{2+} causing hypocalcemia, and but also has a direct stimulatory effect on PTH synthesis, and perhaps also stimulates parathyroid cell proliferation [7].

Finally, there is downregulation of the calcium-sensing receptor, vitamin D receptor, and FGF-23 receptor and its co-receptor, Klotho, in the parathyroid gland. There is loss of inhibition of PTH secretion in an attempt to increase serum calcium to normal levels at the expense of calcium loss from the bones (sHPT). The chronic overstimulation of PTH results in parathyroid gland hyperplasia. When sHPT is untreated, parathyroid cell proliferation continues and in many patients the increased parathyroid mass results in the development of chronic hypercalcemia. This is termed "tertiary hyperparathyroidism," and is a result of two factors: a shift in the set-point for Ca^{2+} suppression of PTH secretion [8]; and the normal basal, nonsuppressible, Ca^{2+} independent component of PTH secretion that is "autonomous" in the setting of markedly increased chief cell mass [9, 10]. Tertiary hyperparathyroidism was initially described as the development of a parathyroid adenoma in the setting of sHPT—either vitamin D deficiency or CKD [11], and is the subject of another chapter in this volume.

Clinical Features

Vitamin D Deficiency

Vitamin D deficiency causes rickets in children and osteomalacia in adults. It may be a significant contributor to osteopenia and osteoporosis as suboptimal levels of vitamin D have been noted in a large minority of the population. As vitamin D is necessary for intestinal calcium absorption, vitamin D deficiency can result in hypocalcemia with its resultant symptoms: spasms, cramps, and weakness. Epidemiologic studies have shown that vitamin D deficiency may also be associated with several chronic illnesses [2].

There is some controversy regarding what constitutes vitamin D adequacy. Although most clinical laboratories have been reporting optimal levels for serum 25(OH)D to be above 30 ng/mL (75 nmol/L), the Institute of Medicine (IOM) Committee on Dietary Reference Intakes for Calcium and Vitamin D defined serum levels of 25(OH)D of 20 ng/mL (50 nmol/L) as adequate for bone health [12]. There have been studies and commentaries by experts in the field suggesting higher levels of vitamin D may be beneficial for many health issues outside the bone field and many have, therefore, advocated attaining higher levels of serum 25(OH)D [2]. The IOM report is a recommendation for vitamin D intake for the general (healthy) population, and of necessity, must be a cautious interpretation of the literature. The report concluded the literature describing nonskeletal effects of vitamin D was not consistent enough to be used for making recommendations regarding intake or optimal blood levels. There is reasonable agreement, however, that 25(OH)D levels below 10 ng/mL (25 nmol/L) would place a patient at very high risk for sHPT and the bone disease of vitamin D deficiency [2].

The relationship between PTH and vitamin D is complex, given that serum PTH is also dependent on dietary calcium and calcium balance [13, 14]. Several studies have shown that while there is a general inverse trend between serum vitamin D 25(OH) and PTH levels, a direct inverse relationship between vitamin D and PTH levels has not been demonstrated [13, 15]. This relationship is even less clear in renal failure patients [16–19]. Nevertheless, the relationship between serum 25(OH) D and PTH is stronger than that between calcitriol and PTH [2]. In an autopsy series, when serum 25(OH)D was below 30 ng/mL (75 nmol/L), bone histology changes consistent with vitamin D deficiency (early osteomalacia and signs of sHPT) began to be seen, and were more consistently seen when serum 25(OH)D levels fell below 20 ng/mL (50 nmol/L) [20].

Chronic Kidney Disease

sHPT in the setting of CKD leads to an array of bone abnormalities involving bone mineralization and turnover. Patients generally present with varying degrees of skeletal pain, deformities, and fractures. The most common skeletal abnormality is osteitis fibrosa cystica, which is characterized by subperiosteal bone resorption, commonly in the fingers, clavicles, and tibia. This is a high-turnover bone disease characterized by marked increased osteoclastic and osteoblastic activity, which results in mechanically weak bones. Histologically, there is marrow fibrosis, excess osteoid (unmineralized matrix) and woven bone. In patients with CKD impaired mineralization (osteomalacia), with marked increase in osteoid volume may rarely result from vitamin D deficiency, or severe phosphate depletion by excessive use of phosphate-binding agents. Patients who are aggressively treated with active vitamin D metabolites to suppress sHPT may develop adynamic bone disease, which presents clinically as fractures and chronic pain. Bone biopsies show relatively normal looking bone, but extremely low bone turnover and virtually no evidence of new bone formation, which is in sharp contrast to bone disease in untreated sHPT. This problem was seen more commonly in the past when aluminum was used as a phosphate binder, which would subsequently deposit in bone. Although aluminum-related bone disease is now rarely seen, it has not disappeared. Desferoxamine mesylate is used as a chelating agent to help remove aluminum from affected patients. More commonly, adynamic bone disease is now thought to be a reflection of aggressive suppression of PTH with vitamin D metabolites, and other bone toxins that accumulate in the higher stages of CKD. Affected patients have little capacity to buffer exogenous calcium, and frequently develop hypercalcemia. This is commonly seen in patients receiving large doses of vitamin D or treated with high calcium containing dialysate. Mixed lesions combining high and low bone turnover diseases may also be present.

Vascular calcification contributes to the high morbidity and mortality seen in patients with CKD. Recent evidence has demonstrated an association between elevated FGF-23 levels and increased arterial stiffness, endothelial dysfunction, progression of CKD, and increased mortality in dialysis patients [21, 22]. In addition to atherosclerosis, which involves intimal thickening and plaque formation, patients with CKD also have arteriosclerosis, which is characterized by concentric thickening of the blood vessels and deposition of hydroxyapatite crystals through the media. This is a highly regulated process that involves the transformation of vascular smooth muscle cells into osteoblastic vascular cells, and is stimulated by hyperphosphatemia [23, 24]. This process leads to arterial stiffness, increased pulse pressure, left ventricular hypertrophy, and cardiac ischemia [25]. Valvular calcifications in the heart are also common in patients on dialysis. In extreme cases of soft tissue calcification, some patients develop ischemic necrosis of the distal extremities (calciphylaxis).

Diagnosis

sHPT is mainly a diagnosis based on a combination of clinical and laboratory findings, namely: calcium, phosphate, creatinine, PTH, and 25-(OH)D levels. Serum PTH rises in response to vitamin D deficiency, and many clinicians use an elevated serum PTH as an indicator of vitamin D deficiency in the setting of normal serum calcium and renal function. Unfortunately, as noted above, other factors regulate PTH secretion, which may mitigate against the detection of a high serum PTH in the setting of vitamin D deficiency. An increase in PTH in response to vitamin D deficiency may be blunted by magnesium deficiency [26] which is commonly found in cases of malabsorption syndrome.

Vitamin D Deficiency

Although calcitriol is the active vitamin D metabolite, in vitamin D deficiency states, serum calcitriol levels are usually normal because of the high serum PTH and low serum phosphate increase renal 1-alpha hydroxylase activity. Vitamin D deficiency is therefore best diagnosed by measuring serum 25(OH)D levels. Reference ranges for 25(OH)D were 10–55 ng/mL (25–137 nmol/L), and as noted above, within that range, levels between 10 and 20–30 ng/mL considered to be inadequate.

As noted above, the relationship between 25(OH)D and PTH is not generally agreed upon, but serum PTH is elevated in vitamin D deficiency, and declines as the deficiency is corrected. In one study, PTH levels came down nicely when vitamin D was replaced to achieve a 25(OH)D level of approximately 20 ng/mL and they plateau when vitamin D levels reach 20–25 ng/mL (50–63 nmol/L) [27]. Because calcium absorption increased in postmenopausal women with levels vitamin D levels up to 30–32 ng/mL (75–80 nmol/L), it was suggested that perhaps vitamin D insufficiency is present at 20–30 ng/mL or 50–75 nmol/L [2, 28]. The recent IOM report called into question the validity of calcium absorption studies and the need to aim for 25(OH)D levels above 20 ng/mL [12].

The relationship between PTH and vitamin D is complex and dependent on calcium in one's diet [13, 14]. Several studies have shown that while there is a general inverse trend between serum vitamin D 25(OH) and PTH levels, there is no direct inverse relationship between vitamin D and PTH levels [15]. This relationship is even less clear in renal failure patients [16–19]. Nevertheless, the relationship between serum 25(OH)D and PTH is stronger than that between calcitriol and PTH.

Not only is the definition of vitamin D sufficiency controversial, it is also unclear as to who should be screened for vitamin D deficiency. Several studies have shown an association of vitamin D deficiency with numerous chronic diseases including, but not limited to: cancers, wheezing, metabolic syndrome, glucose intolerance, hypertension, etc. [29–32]. As a result of this, many have advocated screening of the entire population for vitamin D. Although some advocate vitamin D supplementation to achieve a target level of 25(OH)D of >40 ng/mL (100 nmol/L) as a preventive measure, there are no adequately powered randomized controlled trials showing that therapeutic replacement decreases the risk of these illnesses.

Those at highest risk of developing vitamin D deficiency include: those with darker skin, obese patients, increased winter time, those with illnesses that can cause a malabsorption of vitamin D or increased clearance [31, 33, 34]. Hence, measuring vitamin D levels is most needed in patients with conditions that put them at higher risk for vitamin D deficiency, such as: osteoporosis/penia, inflammatory bowel diseases, liver and kidney disease, cystic fibrosis, malabsorption syndromes (e.g., celiac disease), gastric or intestinal bypass surgery, patients on medications, such as glucocorticoids, antiseizure medications or therapy for AIDS.

There is controversy regarding what level of serum 25(OH)D constitutes vitamin D deficiency. The Institute of Medicine (IOM) Committee on Vitamin D and Calcium defined serum levels of 25(OH)D of 20 ng/mL (50 nmol/L) as a safe and appropriate target for adequate bone health for the majority of the population. After careful review of the available literature, they further concluded a level above 50 ng/mL (125 nmol/L) might have the potential for adverse health effects. There have been other studies, meta-analyses and commentaries by experts in the field suggesting higher intakes of vitamin D may be necessary. Many have, therefore, advocated doses of vitamin D aimed at attaining levels of serum 25(OH)D higher than 20 ng/mL, but the evidence is not consistent. There is no clear-cut evidence that higher levels of vitamin D are necessary and there may even be potential for harm.

Clinically, patients with sHPT due to vitamin D deficiency may complain of musculoskeletal pain, and muscle weakness. Muscle weakness is a prominent feature of severe vitamin D deficiency, and is made worse by the hypophosphatemia that accompanies nutritional deficiency resulting form malabsorption syndromes, and the phosphaturia stimulated by the sHPT. Severe bone disease due to sHPT in renal failure features pain and increased fracture risk.

Chronic Kidney Disease

The PTH assays have evolved over the years and aid in the diagnosis and management of sHPT due to renal failure [35]. Early radioimmunoassays (RIA) were poor predictors of CKD-MBD. The development of immunoradiometric assays (IRMA) in the 1990s made it possible to correlate elevated intact PTH levels and bone disease in patients with CKD. However, it was later determined that these first-generation assays not only detected "intact" PTH(1–84), but also fragments such as PTH(7–84). In an effort to improve the diagnostic accuracy of intact PTH, second generation assays have been developed, which have better discrimination between intact PTH and fragments. The values for these second generation assays are 40–50% lower than the first generation assays, but have similar diagnostic accuracy. Unfortunately, there are now many different commercial assays available with significant interassay variability. Therefore, it is generally felt that trends in serial values for intact PTH using the same assay are more clinically meaningful than single isolated values.

Management

Vitamin D and Calcium Deficiency as a Cause of sHPT

Due to increased risk of aging and skin cancer effects of ultraviolet exposure, recommendations to treat and prevent vitamin D deficiency focus on nutrition and/or supplements. For prevention of vitamin D deficient bone disease in the general population and to maintain a healthy 25(OH)D level above 20 ng/mL (50 nmol/L), the recent Institute of Medicine (IOM) report recommended a daily intake of 600 international units (IU) vitamin D for people aged 1–70 years and 800 IU/day for those over 70 years.

However, the IOM recommendations for vitamin D are not relevant to the treatment of vitamin D deficiency causing bone disease (rickets or osteomalacia). This would always feature sHPT, and much larger doses of vitamin D are indicated to correct the abnormal physiology. The vitamin D preparation used should be vitamin D_3 or D_2 (not calcitriol), and the article by Holick provides a reasonable outline of doses recommended for the treatment of established vitamin D deficiency [2]. Obviously, the cause of the vitamin D deficiency has to be identified and addressed (e.g., celiac disease treated with a gluten-free diet), but for the correction of the deficiency, Holick recommends 50,000 IU vitamin D_2 once weekly for at least 8 weeks. His target serum 25-(OH)D is 30 ng/mL (75 nmol/L), but even if one prefers the IOM recommendations, the patient should be treated for another 8 weeks to build up body stores if 20 ng/mL (50 nmol/L) is not achieved with the initial therapy. Patients with sHPT due to vitamin D deficiency associated with a short gut syndrome may best be treated with phototherapy (ultraviolet B irradiation via a tanning bed or portable UVB lamp) [2].

Recently, a greater degree of caution has been advised regarding the use of calcium supplements, and the 2011 report of the IOM report reflects this concern. Their recommended total calcium intake from all sources (diet and supplements) for people over age 9 years varied with age and sex, but was generally in the range of 1,000–1,300 mg daily. The tolerable upper intake level for safety was 3,000 mg from ages 9–18, 2,500 mg/day for ages 19–50 years, and 2,000 mg/day for men and women over the age of 50 [12]. A recent meta-analysis suggested an increased risk of cardiovascular disease in clinical trials of calcium supplements [36], and this has particular relevance for patients with CKD, who are known to be at high risk for vascular calcification and cardiovascular mortality and high doses of calcium supplements have been used as phosphate binders to reduce hyperphosphatemia. However, in the initial treatment of osteomalacia and rickets, replacement of vitamin D may be associated with a form of "hungry bone syndrome" with a rise in alkaline phosphatase and even a drop in serum calcium and phosphate below the normal range as the skeleton remineralizes. Attention to the serum calcium response to high-dose vitamin D supplementation is important, and there is also potential for later vitamin D toxicity.

Chronic Kidney Disease

Assessment and treatment of sHPT should begin at CKD stage III (estimated GFR <60 mL/min). The treatment at this stage includes: low phosphate diet, vitamin D derivatives, phosphate binders, calcimimetics, and parathyroidectomy if necessary. Target ranges for PTH, calcium, and phosphorus are recommended to be in the normal range for those with CKD stages III–V not yet on dialysis [37]. For patients on dialysis, the earlier guidelines recommended pith levels (second-generation assay) remain between 150 and 300 pg/mL in patients with a GFR <15 mL/min to minimize risk of bone disease progression, vascular calcification, and mortality [38]; however, because the PTH assay on which the original guidelines were based is no longer available, and with recent refinements to PTH assays, the latest KDIGO guidelines (based mainly on bone and mineral effects) simply suggest PTH levels should be maintained between two and nine times the upper normal limit of the assay in patients on dialysis [37]. Calcium levels should be maintained in the normal range and phosphorus should be lowered toward the normal range in dialysis patients.

Phosphate Binders

With mounting evidence that hyperphosphatemia is associated with increased mortality in CKD patients, prevention and treatment of hyperphosphatemia is the initial treatment of secondary hyperparathyroidism. Dietary restriction of protein, dairy, and processed foods may be recommended. Unfortunately, foods that are high in phosphate may also be rich sources of calcium and vitamin D. When the GFR falls below 30 mL/min, hyperphosphatemia develops despite dietary restriction, and phosphate binders are generally necessary to prevent absorption of phosphate from the gut. Until the mid-1980s, aluminum was the main phosphate binder available. Although effective, its use was associated with aluminum toxicity manifested by encephalopathy, osteomalacia, and anemia. Therefore, the use of aluminum has largely been abandoned except in limited circumstances for short periods of time. The main drugs used as phosphate binders currently include calcium, sevelamer, and lanthanum carbonate. Several studies and meta-analyses have compared calcium-based binders (calcium acetate and calcium carbonate) with sevelamer (sevelamer hydrochloride and sevelamer carbonate) [39–42]. There is no conclusive evidence that either binder is superior in terms of mortality, vascular calcification, or safety. Sevelamer does have a lower incidence of hypercalcemia, but is also more expensive and has a higher incidence of adverse GI side effects. Lanthanum carbonate is a nonaluminum, noncalcium phosphate binder, but there have not been good-quality studies examining its effects on mortality or vascular calcification. Moreover, the potential adverse effects of lanthanum accumulation in soft tissues over the time are not known.

Vitamin D Therapy in CKD

Vitamin D Deficiency

There is some controversy as to whether nutritional stores of vitamin D should be repleted to provide substrate for the production of calcitriol in patients on hemodialysis, but it may be beneficial in patients with stages III–V predialysis.

Data in favor of repleting cholecalciferol in deficient patients include animal data suggesting beneficial bone effects of 25(OH)D separate from 1,25-dihydroxyvitamin D. There may also be a biologic effect on reduction of inflammation [43]. Low vitamin D levels have also been associated with increased mortality in dialysis patients. However, it is unknown whether repletion with vitamin D or 25-(OH)D is beneficial or necessary. Studies that evaluated therapy with a vitamin D supplement to treat vitamin D insufficiency in patients with stages 3 to 4 CKD have shown significant increases in serum vitamin D 25(OH), but only minimal decreases in PTH [44]. However, the potential nonskeletal benefits of attaining normal serum 25(OH)D levels [2] are likely still relevant in the setting of CKD.

Repletion with 50,000 IU of vitamin D_2 monthly in hemodialysis patients does appear safe and increases 25-(OH)D levels, with no significant increase in the $Ca \times P$ product [45]. Other dosage recommendations include 8–10,000 IU weekly.

The K/DOQI guidelines recommend in stages III and IV CKD, serum 25-(OH)D levels should be maintained around 30 ng/mL and replaced with nutritional vitamin D (ergocalciferol or cholecalciferol) if levels are <30 ng/mL [38]. The data are inadequate to make this recommendation for patients on dialysis (stage V), but there is no evidence of harm. As with any vitamin D therapy, calcium and phosphorus levels should be monitored.

Vitamin D Derivatives

The deficiency of calcitriol in CKD patients forms the rationale for the use of calcitriol in these patients. In predialysis patients, the administration of active vitamin D analogs is not routine. Vitamin D analogs are used if PTH levels are not suppressed, despite correction of nutritional vitamin D deficiency, calcium administration and control of phosphorus with diet and phosphate binders. Placebo controlled randomized trials have documented benefit from therapy with calcitriol or active vitamin D analogs, in terms of reduction of PTH and improvement in bone disease [46–49]. All of the available active vitamin D metabolites and analogs seem effective. One must be careful, however, as all these agents have been shown to increase calcium and phosphorus levels.

In patients on dialysis with increased PTH levels, the use of calcitriol or vitamin D analogs is advocated to lower PTH levels (<300 pg/mL). Retrospective studies have suggested a survival advantage with the use of vitamin D analogs [50–53]. In a meta-analysis of 76 trials, however, (albeit most were small studies with short-term follow-up) while vitamin D analogs lower PTH and do not tend to increase phosphate, calcium levels were increased and no clear benefit in endpoints, such as death, hospitalization, fracture, or cardiovascular events, were seen [54].

Because of the ability of active vitamin D analogs to increase GI absorption of calcium and phosphate and, hence, worsen hyperphosphatemia and hypercalcemia, the dose of vitamin D analog should be judiciously monitored and adjusted. Therapy with these agents is contraindicated in patients with hyperphosphatemia or low PTH levels (<150 pg/mL) due to the potential for metastatic calcification and adynamic bone disease, respectively. More selective vitamin D analogs have been developed, but all vitamin D analogs have the potential to increase serum calcium and phosphate at high doses.

The recommendations for initiation of vitamin D analog therapy in dialysis patients include: PTH above goal, serum calcium <9.5 mg/dL (<2.38 mmol/L) and serum phosphate <5.5 mg/dL (<1.78 mmol/L). The agent chosen is the clinician's choice and dose should be titrated to suppress PTH, but often this goal can be achieved with lower doses if vitamin D analogs are combined with calcimimetics (see below).

Calcimimetics

Calcimimetics are a class of drugs that increase the sensitivity of the calcium sensing receptor (CaSR) on the parathyroid. These drugs either mimic the effects of calcium or change the conformation of the CaSR and increase its sensitivity to calcium. This results in decreases in PTH secretion and in parathyroid cell growth. Cinacalcet has been one of the best studied in this class and is approved by the US Food and Drug Administration and the European Medicines Agency for the treatment of sHPT in dialysis patients. In patients on dialysis, the target intact PTH level is between 150 and 300 pg/mL (15.9–31.8 pmol/L). The serum calcium (corrected for albumin) goal is >8.4 mg/dL (2.10 mmol/L).

Phase III studies investigating cinacalcet at 20–180 mg/day have shown reduction in PTH levels by 33 and 65% after 18 weeks and 3 years of treatment, respectively [55–57]. Serum calcium–phosphorus product decreased by 6–15%. Calcium, phosphorus, and PTH National Kidney Foundation-Kidney Disease Outcomes and Quality Initiative (NKF-K/DOQI) goals were met more often on the treatment arm. Compared with placebo cinacalcet-treated patients had a significant increase in the likelihood of achieving target serum PTH levels <300 pg/mL and obtaining goals for calcium, phosphorus, and the calcium x phosphate product [58]. A post-hoc analysis of four studies suggests decreases in fractures, risk for parathyroidectomy and hospitalization for cardiovascular complications [59].

The most frequent side effects of cinacalcet were gastrointestinal related, including vomiting and nausea. Hypocalcemia was also seen at an increased rate, but was easily manageable in most patients. Cinacalcet is indicated in dialysis patients with PTH levels >300 pg/mL with serum calcium levels >8.4 mg/dL (>2.1 mmol/L). Unlike vitamin D analogs, cinacalcet can be initiated in the setting of hyperphosphatemia. Calcium levels need to be maintained at 8.4 mg/dL (≥2.1 mmol/L) or above to avoid the development of hypocalcemia. Frequent monitoring of calcium and PTH levels is advised to avoid QT prolongation and seizures.

At this time, it is unclear which combination of the above therapies is ideal. Cinacalcet is more costly than the other therapies mentioned above. More studies are needed to determine the ideal treatment regimen in combination with cinacalcet in order to improve clinically relevant endpoints.

Cinacalcet is not approved in predialysis patients in the USA, but has been evaluated in patients with CKD. Cinacalcet did suppress PTH and calcium, but it also has the potential to raise serum phosphorus in predialysis patients [60, 61]. The hypocalcemia and hyperphosphatemia seen with cinacalcet was managed with titrating vitamin D supplements, calcium supplements, or other phosphate binders, however, some patients did have to discontinue cinacalcet due to hypocalcemia seen with the lowest dose of cinacalcet.

Regression of Parathyroid Hyperplasia

Chronic sHPT results in parathyroid cell proliferation and hyperplastic glands. When the cause of the sHPT is corrected, or when suppression of PTH secretion is achieved with active vitamin D metabolites and/or calcimimetic therapy in CKD, the enlarged parathyroids may regress [62, 63]. But if the hyperplasia is longstanding, the regression may not be complete, particularly if nodular hyperplasia is present. Parathyroid cells have not been documented to be highly susceptible to apoptosis, but more recent studies have vitamin D metabolites and/or calcimimetic therapy induce apoptosis of chief cells (the major PTH secreting cells) in hyperplastic glands, resulting in an increased ratio of oxyphil cell to chief cells and perhaps an increased residual nodular hyperplasia [64]. Despite the suppression of PTH secretion and potential for regression of parathyroid hyperplasia associated with these drugs, some patients will still require surgical reduction of parathyroid mass.

Conclusion

The major causes of sHPT are CKD and vitamin D deficiency. The correction of vitamin D deficiency with the appropriate vitamin D metabolite (vitamin D for nutritional deficiency, calcitriol for disorders of calcitriol synthesis), and the cause of the deficiency (e.g., celiac disease) will usually result in regression of symptoms and PTH hypersecretion. The management of sHPT in CKD is usually more complex, requiring control of calcium and phosphate intake, and a combination of vitamin D metabolites. Although calcitriol is widely used in CKD to control sHPT, there is increasing evidence of the importance of maintaining an adequate intake of vitamin D itself (as reflected by serum 25(OH)D), in order to gain potential benefits of the nonskeletal functions of vitamin D. Control of hyperphosphatemia is extremely important in the management of sHPT in CKD and cinacalcet is a promising addition to the therapeutic armamentarium for suppression of sHPT.

References

1. Ritter CS, Armbrecht HJ, Slatopolsky E, et al. 25-Hydroxyvitamin D(3) suppresses PTH synthesis and secretion by bovine parathyroid cells. Kidney Int. 2006;70:654–9.
2. Holick MF. Vitamin D deficiency. N Engl J Med. 2007;357:266–81.
3. Moe S, Drueke T, Cunningham J, et al. Definition, evaluation, and classification of renal osteodystrophy: a position statement from Kidney Disease: Improving Global Outcomes (KDIGO). Kidney Int. 2006;69:1945–53.
4. Krajisnik T, Bjorklund P, Marsell R, et al. Fibroblast growth factor-23 regulates parathyroid hormone and 1alpha-hydroxylase expression in cultured bovine parathyroid cells. J Endocrinol. 2007;195:125–31.
5. Silver J, Naveh-Many T. FGF23 and the parathyroid glands. Pediatr Nephrol. 2010;25: 2241–5.

6. Slatopolsky E, Caglar S, Pennell JP, et al. On the pathogenesis of hyperparathyroidism in chronic experimental renal insufficiency in the dog. J Clin Invest. 1971;50:492–9.
7. Silver J, Naveh-Many T. Phosphate and the parathyroid. Kidney Int. 2009;75:898–905.
8. Brown EM, Wilson RE, Eastman RC, et al. Abnormal regulation of parathyroid hormone release by calcium in secondary hyperparathyroidism due to chronic renal failure. J Clin Endocrinol Metab. 1982;54:172–9.
9. Mayer GP, Habener JF, Potts Jr JT. Parathyroid hormone secretion in vivo. Demonstration of a calcium-independent nonsuppressible component of secretion. J Clin Invest. 1976;57:678–83.
10. Gittes RF, Radde IC. Experimental model for hyperparathyroidism: effect of excessive numbers of transplanted isologous parathyroid glands. J Urol. 1966;95:595–603.
11. Davies DR, Dent CE, Watson L. Tertiary hyperparathyroidism. Br Med J. 1968;3:395–9.
12. IOM (Institute of Medicine). Dietary reference intakes for calcium and vitamin D. Washington, DC: The National Academies Press; 2011.
13. Steingrimsdottir L, Gunnarsson O, Indridason OS, et al. Relationship between serum parathyroid hormone levels, vitamin D sufficiency, and calcium intake. JAMA. 2005;294:2336–41.
14. Adami S, Viapiana O, Gatti D, et al. Relationship between serum parathyroid hormone, vitamin D sufficiency, age, and calcium intake. Bone. 2008;42:267–70.
15. Rucker D, Allan JA, Fick GH, et al. Vitamin D insufficiency in a population of healthy western Canadians. CMAJ. 2002;166:1517–24.
16. Gonzalez EA, Sachdeva A, Oliver DA, et al. Vitamin D insufficiency and deficiency in chronic kidney disease. A single center observational study. Am J Nephrol. 2004;24:503–10.
17. Taskapan H, Ersoy FF, Passadakis PS, et al. Severe vitamin D deficiency in chronic renal failure patients on peritoneal dialysis. Clin Nephrol. 2006;66:247–55.
18. Mucsi I, Almasi C, Deak G, et al. Serum 25(OH)-vitamin D levels and bone metabolism in patients on maintenance hemodialysis. Clin Nephrol. 2005;64:288–94.
19. Zehnder D, Landray MJ, Wheeler DC, et al. Cross-sectional analysis of abnormalities of mineral homeostasis, vitamin D and parathyroid hormone in a cohort of pre-dialysis patients. The chronic renal impairment in Birmingham (CRIB) study. Nephron Clin Pract. 2007;107:c109–16.
20. Priemel M, von Domarus C, Klatte TO, et al. Bone mineralization defects and vitamin D deficiency: histomorphometric analysis of iliac crest bone biopsies and circulating 25-hydroxyvitamin D in 675 patients. J Bone Miner Res. 2010;25:305–12.
21. Gutierrez OM, Mannstadt M, Isakova T, et al. Fibroblast growth factor 23 and mortality among patients undergoing hemodialysis. N Engl J Med. 2008;359:584–92.
22. Gutierrez OM, Januzzi JL, Isakova T, et al. Fibroblast growth factor 23 and left ventricular hypertrophy in chronic kidney disease. Circulation. 2009;119:2545–52.
23. Mizobuchi M, Towler D, Slatopolsky E. Vascular calcification: the killer of patients with chronic kidney disease. J Am Soc Nephrol. 2009;20:1453–64.
24. Mathew S, Tustison KS, Sugatani T, et al. The mechanism of phosphorus as a cardiovascular risk factor in CKD. J Am Soc Nephrol. 2008;19:1092–105.
25. Raggi P, Kleerekoper M. Contribution of bone and mineral abnormalities to cardiovascular disease in patients with chronic kidney disease. Clin J Am Soc Nephrol. 2008;3:836–43.
26. Sahota O, Mundey MK, San P, et al. Vitamin D insufficiency and the blunted PTH response in established osteoporosis: the role of magnesium deficiency. Osteoporos Int. 2006;17:1013–21.
27. Malabanan A, Veronikis IE, Holick MF. Redefining vitamin D insufficiency. Lancet. 1998;351:805–6.
28. Heaney RP, Dowell MS, Hale CA, et al. Calcium absorption varies within the reference range for serum 25-hydroxyvitamin D. J Am Coll Nutr. 2003;22:142–6.
29. Lappe JM, Travers-Gustafson D, Davies KM, et al. Vitamin D and calcium supplementation reduces cancer risk: results of a randomized trial. Am J Clin Nutr. 2007;85:1586–91.
30. Bischoff-Ferrari HA, Giovannucci E, Willett WC, et al. Estimation of optimal serum concentrations of 25-hydroxyvitamin D for multiple health outcomes. Am J Clin Nutr. 2006;84:18–28.
31. Looker AC, Pfeiffer CM, Lacher DA, et al. Serum 25-hydroxyvitamin D status of the US population: 1988–1994 compared with 2000–2004. Am J Clin Nutr. 2008;88:1519–27.

32. Wang TJ, Pencina MJ, Booth SL, et al. Vitamin D deficiency and risk of cardiovascular disease. Circulation. 2008;117:503–11.
33. Holick MF, Biancuzzo RM, Chen TC, et al. Vitamin D2 is as effective as vitamin D3 in maintaining circulating concentrations of 25-hydroxyvitamin D. J Clin Endocrinol Metab. 2008;93: 677–81.
34. Kumar J, Muntner P, Kaskel FJ, et al. Prevalence and associations of 25-hydroxyvitamin D deficiency in US children: NHANES 2001–2004. Pediatrics. 2009;124:e362–70.
35. Gao P, D'Amour P. Evolution of the parathyroid hormone (PTH) assay – importance of circulating PTH immunoheterogeneity and of its regulation. Clin Lab. 2005;51:21–9.
36. Bolland MJ, Avenell A, Baron JA, et al. Effect of calcium supplements on risk of myocardial infarction and cardiovascular events: meta-analysis. BMJ. 2010;341:c3691.
37. Kidney Disease: Improving Global Outcomes (KDIGO) CKD-MBD Work Group. KDIGO clinical practice guideline for the diagnosis, evaluation, prevention, and treatment of Chronic Kidney Disease-Mineral and Bone Disorder (CKD-MBD). Kidney Int Suppl. 2009;113:S1–130.
38. National Kidney Foundation. K/DOQI clinical practice guidelines for bone metabolism and disease in chronic kidney disease. Am J Kidney Dis. 2003;42:S1–201.
39. Jamal SA, Fitchett D, Lok CE, et al. The effects of calcium-based versus non-calcium-based phosphate binders on mortality among patients with chronic kidney disease: a meta-analysis. Nephrol Dial Transplant. 2009;24:3168–74.
40. Chertow GM, Burke SK, Raggi P. Sevelamer attenuates the progression of coronary and aortic calcification in hemodialysis patients. Kidney Int. 2002;62:245–52.
41. Block GA, Raggi P, Bellasi A, et al. Mortality effect of coronary calcification and phosphate binder choice in incident hemodialysis patients. Kidney Int. 2007;71:438–41.
42. Qunibi W, Moustafa M, Muenz LR, et al. A 1-year randomized trial of calcium acetate versus sevelamer on progression of coronary artery calcification in hemodialysis patients with comparable lipid control: the Calcium Acetate Renagel Evaluation-2 (CARE-2) study. Am J Kidney Dis. 2008;51:952–65.
43. Stubbs JR, Idiculla A, Slusser J, et al. Cholecalciferol supplementation alters calcitriol-responsive monocyte proteins and decreases inflammatory cytokines in ESRD. J Am Soc Nephrol. 2010;21:353–61.
44. Al-Aly Z, Qazi RA, Gonzalez EA, et al. Changes in serum 25-hydroxyvitamin D and plasma intact PTH levels following treatment with ergocalciferol in patients with CKD. Am J Kidney Dis. 2007;50:59–68.
45. Saab G, Young DO, Gincherman Y, et al. Prevalence of vitamin D deficiency and the safety and effectiveness of monthly ergocalciferol in hemodialysis patients. Nephron Clin Pract. 2007;105:c132–8.
46. Hamdy NA, Kanis JA, Beneton MN, et al. Effect of alfacalcidol on natural course of renal bone disease in mild to moderate renal failure. BMJ. 1995;310:358–63.
47. Slatopolsky E, Berkoben M, Kelber J, et al. Effects of calcitriol and non-calcemic vitamin D analogs on secondary hyperparathyroidism. Kidney Int Suppl. 1992;38:S43–9.
48. Rix M, Eskildsen P, Olgaard K. Effect of 18 months of treatment with alfacalcidol on bone in patients with mild to moderate chronic renal failure. Nephrol Dial Transplant. 2004;19:870–6.
49. Coyne D, Acharya M, Qiu P, et al. Paricalcitol capsule for the treatment of secondary hyperparathyroidism in stages 3 and 4 CKD. Am J Kidney Dis. 2006;47:263–76.
50. Wolf M, Shah A, Gutierrez O, et al. Vitamin D levels and early mortality among incident hemodialysis patients. Kidney Int. 2007;72:1004–13.
51. Teng M, Wolf M, Ofsthun MN, et al. Activated injectable vitamin D and hemodialysis survival: a historical cohort study. J Am Soc Nephrol. 2005;16:1115–25.
52. Teng M, Wolf M, Lowrie E, et al. Survival of patients undergoing hemodialysis with paricalcitol or calcitriol therapy. N Engl J Med. 2003;349:446–56.
53. Shoji T, Shinohara K, Kimoto E, et al. Lower risk for cardiovascular mortality in oral 1alpha-hydroxy vitamin D3 users in a haemodialysis population. Nephrol Dial Transplant. 2004;19: 179–84.

54. Palmer SC, McGregor DO, Macaskill P, et al. Meta-analysis: vitamin D compounds in chronic kidney disease. Ann Intern Med. 2007;147:840–53.
55. Block GA, Martin KJ, de Francisco AL, et al. Cinacalcet for secondary hyperparathyroidism in patients receiving hemodialysis. N Engl J Med. 2004;350:1516–25.
56. Quarles LD, Sherrard DJ, Adler S, et al. The calcimimetic AMG 073 as a potential treatment for secondary hyperparathyroidism of end-stage renal disease. J Am Soc Nephrol. 2003;14: 575–83.
57. Lindberg JS, Moe SM, Goodman WG, et al. The calcimimetic AMG 073 reduces parathyroid hormone and calcium×phosphorus in secondary hyperparathyroidism. Kidney Int. 2003;63: 248–54.
58. Moe SM, Chertow GM, Coburn JW, et al. Achieving NKF-K/DOQI bone metabolism and disease treatment goals with cinacalcet HCl. Kidney Int. 2005;67:760–71.
59. Cunningham J, Danese M, Olson K, et al. Effects of the calcimimetic cinacalcet HCl on cardiovascular disease, fracture, and health-related quality of life in secondary hyperparathyroidism. Kidney Int. 2005;68:1793–800.
60. Chonchol M, Locatelli F, Abboud HE, et al. A randomized, double-blind, placebo-controlled study to assess the efficacy and safety of cinacalcet HCl in participants with CKD not receiving dialysis. Am J Kidney Dis. 2009;53:197–207.
61. Charytan C, Coburn JW, Chonchol M, et al. Cinacalcet hydrochloride is an effective treatment for secondary hyperparathyroidism in patients with CKD not receiving dialysis. Am J Kidney Dis. 2005;46:58–67.
62. Olgaard K, Lewin E. Can hyperparathyroid bone disease be arrested or reversed? Clin J Am Soc Nephrol. 2006;1:367–73.
63. Komaba H, Fukagawa M. Regression of parathyroid hyperplasia by calcimimetics – fact or illusion? Nephrol Dial Transplant. 2009;24:707–9.
64. Lomonte C, Vernaglione L, Chimienti D, et al. Does vitamin D receptor and calcium receptor activation therapy play a role in the histopathologic alterations of parathyroid glands in refractory uremic hyperparathyroidism? Clin J Am Soc Nephrol. 2008;3:794–9.

Chapter 10
Secondary Hyperparathyroidism: Surgical

John Yoo and J.E.M. Young

Keywords Refractory secondary HPT • Total and subtotal parathyroidectomy • Parathyroid autotransplantation • Transcervical thymectomy • Parathyroid cryo-preservation • Intraoperative PTH • Preoperative imaging

Surgical Management of Refractory Secondary Hyperparathyroidism

The most common cause of refractory secondary hyperparathyroidism (2HPT) requiring surgical intervention is end-stage renal disease (ESRD) requiring dialysis. Renal insufficiency gradually results in low serum calcium and high phosphate levels. These factors in association with vitamin D deficiency stimulate parathyroid hormone (PTH) production in an attempt to keep the serum calcium within the normal range. However, in rare instances excessive PTH production leads to progressive hypercalcemia. Medical management, such as Vitamin D therapy, has improved 2HPT for patients with ESRD and most patients do not require parathyroid surgery [1–5]. However, it is estimated that currently almost 1% of patients on dialysis per year and up to 15% of dialysis patients at 10 years will require parathyroidectomy [6–8] due to rising levels of PTH as the parathyroid glands become hyperplasic and eventually autonomous (Fig. 10.1) [9]. Other causes of 2HPT include malabsorption or rarer conditions, such as congenital hypophosphatemic osteomalacia, but these rarely cause hypercalcemia requiring surgery.

J. Yoo, MD, FRCS(C), FACS (✉)
Department of Otolaryngology-Head and Neck Surgery, University of Western Ontario, London, ON, Canada
e-mail: john.yoo@lhsc.on.ca

J.E.M. Young, BSc, MD, FRCS, FACS
Department of Surgery, McMaster University, Hamilton, ON, Canada

A.A. Khan and O.H. Clark (eds.), *Handbook of Parathyroid Diseases: A Case-Based Practical Guide*, DOI 10.1007/978-1-4614-2164-1_10, © Springer Science+Business Media, LLC 2012

Although the strict definition of refractory 2HPT remains elusive, it is a condition of markedly elevated PTH levels that cannot be corrected with the appropriate doses of calcium and vatamin D. Thus, the standard indication for surgery is hyperphosphatemia and/or hypercalcemia that are refractory to medical management in the presence of advanced hyperparathyroidism [10]. In particular, hyperparathyroidism leads to significant health consequences, including cardiovascular disease, calciphylaxis, skeletal and neuromuscular weakness, physiological tiredness, and increased mortality (Figs. 10.2–10.4) [11–15].

Parathyroidectomy is highly effective in correcting biochemical abnormalities and mitigating the physiologic consequences of refractory 2HPT. The initial success rates with parathyroidectomy approaches 95% [10, 16, 17]. However, recurrent and persistent diseases remain significant problems with rates up to 30% even by experienced surgeons [18–21]. Although there is universal agreement that parathyroidectomy is the optimal treatment for refractory 2HPT, there is considerable controversy regarding the type of surgical approach. Three different operations have been described: subtotal parathyroidectomy (SPTX), total parathyroidectomy with autotransplantation (TPTX + AT), and total parathyroidectomy without autotransplantation (TPTX without AT). The predominant debate concerns recurrence and the increased difficulty of reoperation. There are strong proponents of each surgical approach who highlight specific advantages and disadvantages. Unfortunately, a definitive prospective randomized clinical trial has not been conducted and surgeons often select the type of procedure based on personal experience and opinion [10].

The objective of this chapter is to describe and review the three surgical approaches that are most commonly employed for the management of refractory 2HPT.

1. Subtotal parathyroidectomy
   The technique of SPTX for renal 2HPT was described in 1960 by Stanbury [22]. The technique requires the identification of all parathyroid glands (usually four), complete removal of three parathyroid glands, and partial removal from the most normal appearing fourth gland. The remaining gland remnant (approximately 50 mg) is left in-situ in the neck keeping the blood supply to it intact. The advantage of this approach is its potential to retain functioning parathyroid tissue in the neck immediately following surgery. The main disadvantages of this technique are that persistent hyperparathyroidism can result if the remnant is too large or conversely, significant persistent hypoparathyroidism if the remnant is too small or undergoes infarction. Recurrence caused by regrowth of the remnant hyperplasia may require re-exploration of the neck, and consequently a higher risk of surgical complications [23, 44]. This technique may be best used for patients with refractory 2HPT who are candidates for renal transplantation.

2. Total parathyroidectomy with autotransplantation
   TPTX + AT was first reported by Alveryd in 1969 [24]. This technique requires the identification of all parathyroid gland but unlike SPTX, all identified parathyroid glands are completely removed. Autotransplantation of parathyroid tissue is then carried out by sectioning small pieces of one hyperplastic parathyroid gland and implanting them into a heterotopic site that is readily accessible for subsequent removal should the need arise. As popularized by Wells [25], the forearm

brachioradialis muscle has traditionally been the most common recipient site. Other parathyroid surgeons have used the sternocleidomastoid (SCM) for its convenience and ease of access under local anesthesia should a subsequent operation become necessary. Over time, the transplanted nests of parathyroid tissue recruit blood supply from its host bed and regain function. High success rates and the ease of access of the forearm in patients with recurrent hyperparathyroidism are proposed as the main advantages of this technique [26].

3. Total parathyroidectomy without autotransplantation
   Identical to the TPTX + AT, this technique requires the removal of all parathyroid tissue from the neck. However, parathyroid tissue is not re-implanted. This approach was first proposed by Ogg in 1967 because of the concern of recurrent disease [27]. Proponents of this technique suggest significantly lower recurrence rates and that even without autotransplantation; some parathyroid function is retained in most cases likely due to residual parathyroid nests [28–30]. However, this approach is generally considered to be appropriate only for patients who are not candidates for reoperation or kidney transplantations because of the difficulty in managing hypoparathyroidism following successful renal transplantation.

Subtotal Parathyroidectomy Versus Total Parathyroidectomy with Autotransplantation

SPTX and TPTX + AT have the longest history and remain the two most widely accepted surgical approaches. There is considerable debate between these two techniques in the management of renal 2HPT. Proponents of SPTX argue that the advantages include earlier normalization of PTH following surgery, similar recurrence rates to TPTX + AT, and lower risk of permanent hypoparathyroidism. Advocates for TPTX + AT claim reduced recurrence rates and safer reoperation when failures do occur. Both approaches are highly effective, with initial success rates of up to 95% in normalizing PTH levels and improving symptoms, such as bone pain and pruritis [10, 17, 26, 31]. With both approaches, understanding the anatomy and embryology of normal, abnormal, and ectopic parathyroid glands are essential to success [32, 33]. The objective of both operations is to identify all parathyroid glands. The failure to identify at least four glands necessitates a concurrent transcervical thymectomy and/or partial thyroidectomy [34–36]. Furthermore, some experts believe that finding fewer than four parathyroid glands obviates the need for either autotransplantation or keeping a remnant and all identified glands should be completely removed [32–37].

The likelihood of maintaining adequate parathyroid function is considered an important advantage with both SPTX and TPTX + AT over TPTX without AT. Particularly, for patients who are candidates for renal transplantation, it is important to maintain normal parathyroid function following renal transplantation [12]. However, some investigators have shown similar success rates with all three techniques [28, 38]. Even when at least four glands were removed, two-thirds of patients had either normal or increased PTH levels following renal transplantation [28, 38].

Some studies have directly compared SPTX and TPTX + AT, with most evaluating the short-term outcomes of both approaches. Overall, both have similar rates of early success, persistence of disease, and recurrence of hyperparathyroidism [31, 39–44]. One retrospective comparison did evaluate both short-term and long-term outcomes of the two techniques [45]. As expected, they found excellent early results with both techniques but two-thirds of all patients experienced suboptimal long-term outcomes of either persistent hypoparathyroidism or development of recurrent disease. There was no significant difference between surgical approaches.

Important differences between SPTX and TPTX + AT have been noted in some studies. A randomized trial of 40 patients comparing the two techniques was conducted by Rothmund et al. [20]. A significant difference favoring TPTX + AT in normalizing serum calcium and alkaline phosphatase was found. Furthermore, the study noted the difficulty in re-exploration for recurrence after SPTX over the relatively simpler reoperation of the forearm. For these reasons, TPTX + AT was their recommended surgical technique. However, the interpretation of this study should be done with caution. This study was severely limited by a small sample size with only 17 patients remaining for long-term analysis. Melck et al. conducted a 32-year retrospective review and reported higher failure rates requiring reoperation in patients who underwent TPTX + AT versus SPTX (26% vs. 6%) [46]. Unfortunately, in Melck's study the cohorts were disproportional with only 19 patients undergoing TPTX + AT while 193 patients underwent SPTX.

Recurrent 2PHT is an expected outcome in a proportion of patients and will occasionally necessitate reoperation. Richards et al. conducted a meta-analysis of reoperations for recurrent or persistent 2HPT, and looked for important clinical differences in outcome between first-operation SPTX and TPTX + AT [32]. Overall the most common cause of failure was autograft hyperplasia, with 49% of the cases they reviewed. Inadequate initial cervical exploration was deemed in 42% and 34% of the SPTX and TPTX + AT revision, respectively. The two surgical approaches appeared to be similar in causes of failure (most commonly due to inadequate initial exploration) and perioperative complications when reoperation is carried out. They did find a higher recurrence rate with TPTX + AT versus SPTX (49% vs. 17%), but these findings were difficult to interpret since the number of total original operations was not ascertained for either group.

The potential advantage of exploring the forearm versus the neck may seem self-evident but actual results from studies have contradicted this belief [33, 44]. Cattan and colleagues reviewed success rates of revision surgery for 2HPT and found that the likelihood of successful reoperation was significantly higher in patients who originally underwent SPTX versus TPTX + AT [33]. The main reason for the higher failure rate in TPTX + AT was the difficulty in eradicating the hyperplastic glands at the autografted site. In contrast, when recurrence was due to remnant hypertrophy, identification and removal were easier and with acceptable morbidity. They recommended SPTX as the preferred approach for renal 2HPT. As expected, the success of treating persistent disease was similar in both groups, as the cause was due to missed glands in the neck or mediastinum. Several other studies have found that autograft proliferation within the forearm and parathyromatosis were formidable problems and required extensive removal of the forearm muscle [46–48], and sometimes with unsuccessful results [46, 48]. A strong recommendation was made in favor of SPTX for refractory renal 2HPT [46].

Various modifications of the standard techniques have since been described. Authors have reported sophisticated techniques of selecting areas of the gland with lower proliferative potential for autotransplantation [47, 49]. Several other anatomic sites for reimplantation have also been recommended. These included subcutaneous tissue of the abdomen, forearm, neck, or the SCM muscle [50–55]. Implantation into the inner aspect of the SCM muscle marked with metal clips may have several advantages [50]. Reoperation under local anesthetic of the SCM muscle is manageable with minimal risk to the recurrently laryngeal and vagus nerves. Sestamibi scanning to exclude residual parathyroid tissue in the neck or mediastinum can identify tissue in the SCM without the need for forearm imaging. Endoscopic-assisted parathyroidectomy for 2HPT is an emerging technology. These procedures may have limited short-lived advantages, such as less pain and smaller incision but is more expensive and there is no evidence of improved overall outcome in the management of 2HPT [56–59].

SPTX and TPTX+AT are both safe operations that offer excellent short-term success rates. However, both approaches require good medical management because there are significant rates of recurrent HPT with long-term dialysis. When recurrence does arise, the likelihood of successful reoperation may be better in patients who initially underwent SPTX. The risk of parathyromatosis after SPTX appears to be lower than after TPTX+AT.

Total Parathyroidectomy Without Autotransplantation

Recent studies have suggested that TPTX without AT is a viable alternative to SPTX and TPTX+AT for refractory 2HPT [29, 30, 60–67]. Supporters of this approach argue higher success rates and lower recurrence rates over the other two options. In addition, when patients experience severe acute life threatening complications, such as calciphylaxis TPTX without AT may be a better option [1, 11]. Especially for dialysis patients who are unlikely to receive kidney transplantation, some investigators have recommended TPTX without AT over SPTX or TPTX+AT as the treatment of choice [28, 60]. However, there is controversy whether TPTX without AT should be considered in patients awaiting kidney transplantation because of the potential of permanent hypoparathyroidism. In 2003, the National Kidney Foundation recommended that TPTX without AT be contraindicated in this cohort of patients [12]. However, compelling counter-arguments have been made by other investigators. Stracke and colleagues have advocated TPTX without AT in all patients based on their comprehensive long-term evaluation of 46 patients [28]. A prospective clinical trial is currently underway that compares TPX without AT versus TPTX+AT [68]. As more data becomes available with this technique, its value is sure to be revisited.

Several studies have compared TPTX without AT versus the other two traditional surgical approaches. A prospective nonrandomized trial was conducted by Shih et al. looking at long-term recurrence rates [63]. Group A patients were not expected to undergo kidney transplantation, and TPTX without AT was performed. Group B patients were considered candidates for renal transplantation and underwent either SPTX or TPTX + AT. After 60 months, the TPTX without AT experience significantly lower recurrence rates (4.5% vs. 18.0%). The weakness of this study is that the authors did not report the rate of persistent hypoparathyroidism in either group.

A retrospective comparison of three surgical techniques was conducted by Nicholson et al. [41]. Although there were only a few patients in the study they found reduced recurrence rates in the TPTX without AT over SPTX and TPTX + AT (0/24, 3/11, 2/13). They also noted that residual PTH function was seen in 14/16 patients who underwent TPTX without AT. Coulston retrospectively reviewed 115 patients who underwent TPTX without AT over a 10 year period, with a median follow-up period of 31 months [61]. They reported a recurrence rate of 12% and a reoperation rate of 3.5%, which was significantly lower than seen with SPTX or TPTX + AT. However, they also reported that 28.7% of patients had undetectable PTH. Interestingly, many studies have demonstrated that even when at least four hyperplastic parathyroid glands were removed, most patients had persistent measureable PTH levels. The explanation for this was either uncontrolled parathyroid nests of cells or a supernumerary gland [28–30].

In summary, TPTX without AT has been reported to have lower rate of recurrent 2HPT as compared to SPTX or TPTX + AT. Patients undergoing TPTX however, clearly have a higher risk of hypoparathyroidism or undetectable levels of PTH creating difficulties with calcium homeostasis following renal transplantation.

Success rates with parathyroidectomy in refractory secondary HPT

	Rates	Subtotal parathyroidectomy	Total parathyroidectomy with AT	Total parathyroidectomy without AT
Post-op success	90–95%	+++	+++	+++
Persistent hypoparathyroidism	10–30%	+	+	+++
Persistent hyperparathyroidism	5–10%	+	+	+
Recurrence	10–30%	++	+++	+

Transcervical Thymectomy

The thymus is the most common site of ectopic and supernumerary parathyroid glands. Both autopsy and surgical studies have demonstrated that intrathymic parathyroid glands occur in up to 40% of cases [34, 37]. Schneider et al. analyzed 461 consecutive patients who underwent bilateral thymectomies as part of their routine surgical approach [34]. They reported the rate of intrathymic parathyroid glands to be over 40% of patients, and the incidence of thymic supernumerary glands was 7.4%. However, the incidence of clinically significant supernumerary intrathymic glands in patients with 2HPT appeared to be about 15% [28, 34].

Initial identification of fewer than four glands at the time of surgery requires the deliberate search for additional glands. In these situations, there is agreement that thymectomy is indicated [28, 33–37]. Several authors recommend routine bilateral thymectomies to be included for all parathyroidectomies conducted for 2HPT [19, 34, 35, 69, 70]. Although there may be theoretical advantages to this approach, the routine practice of thymectomy remains controversial. Most series reporting surgical outcomes describe routine exploration of the upper thymus as opposed to bilateral thymectomy. Furthermore, numerous clinical series, especially those who advocate TPTX without AT have reported comparable success and recurrence rates when thymectomy was not performed routinely [29, 30, 60–66].

Parathyroid Cryopreservation

Cryopreservation is the practice of storing an individual's excised parathyroid tissue in the event that future reimplantation becomes necessary due to persistent hypoparathyroidism. The technique was first described by Wells in 1972 [25, 71] and has subsequently been advocated by other authors [72, 73]. There are numerous theoretical advantages to this approach, but recent studies have demonstrated some practical limitations [74–77]. A multicenter retrospective study by Borot and colleagues reported that of 1,376 samples cryopreserved, only 22 were eventually autografted into 20 patients. Of the 22 autografts 80% were nonfunctional. No patient was autografted after 1 year from their original surgery [74]. Guerrero and colleagues found that parathyroid glands preserved for longer than 24 months were no longer viable [75]. A cryopreservation program is unlikely to be successful except in selected institutions with considerable experience in parathyroid surgery. In addition, the likelihood of requiring autotransplantation is small and diminishes over time from the initial operation. Nevertheless, in rare occasions when cryopreserved parathyroid tissue can be successfully reimplanted, it may prevent permanent hypoparathyroidism.

Imaging

Preoperative imaging to localize multiple hyperplastic parathyroid glands in patients with 2HPT is not necessary [78–83]. Ultrasound and sestamibi scintigraphy are the two most commonly used imaging studies but inconsistently identify hyperplastic glands. Regardless of whether some abnormal parathyroid glands can be identified preoperatively, a targeted surgical approach is not indicated for patients with 2HPT. These patients require a comprehensive bilateral neck and upper mediastinal

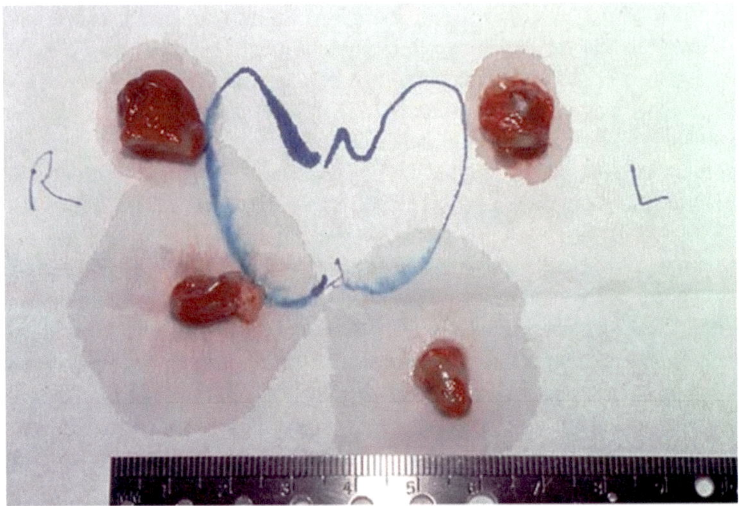

Fig. 10.1 Appearance and position of usual hyperplastic glands in secondary hyperparathyroidism

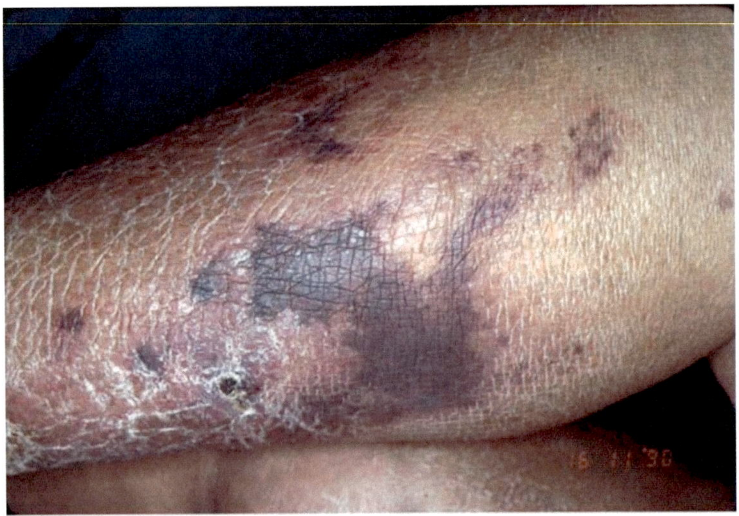

Fig. 10.2 Advanced secondary hyperparathyroidism with massive calcium deposits in soft tissue of the upper arm

exploration in an attempt to identify at least four parathyroid glands. Imaging modalities that consistently identify mediastinal or ectopic parathyroid glands would be useful. There is emerging data that suggests CT scanning may be valuable for this application but further clinical experience will be necessary before this practice can be broadly recommended [84].

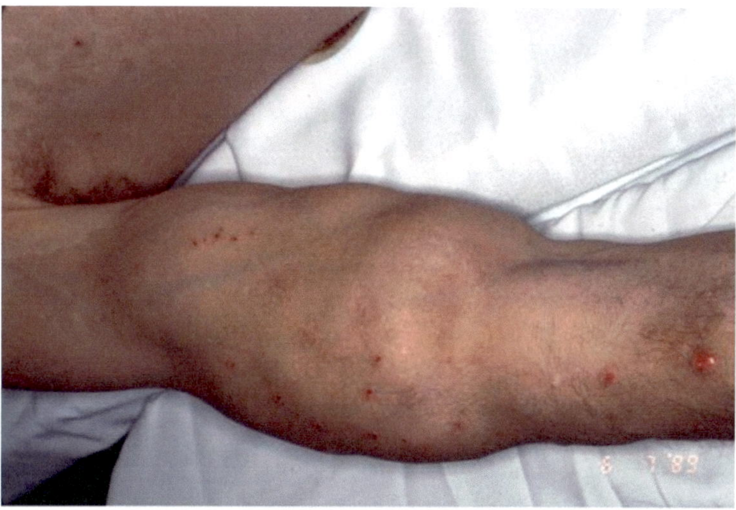

Fig. 10.3 Advanced secondary hyperparathyroidism with plaques of calcium deposited in skin and dermis

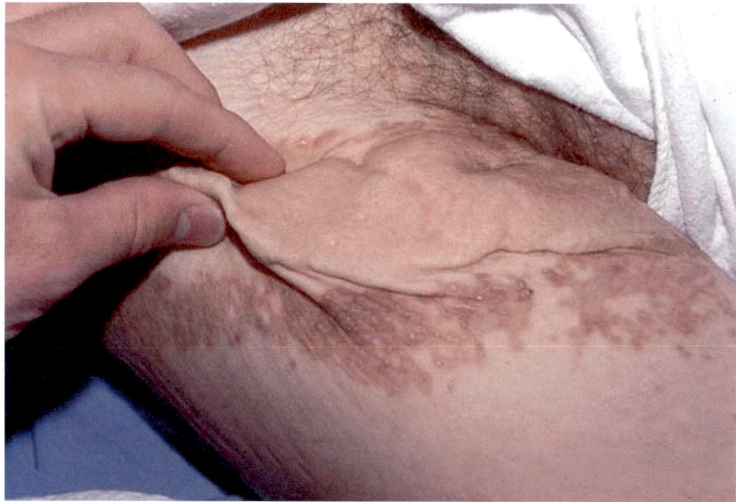

Fig. 10.4 Calciphylaxis with developing skin hemorrhage and necrosis with calcium deposits in skin ulcers

In contrast to patients undergoing initial surgery for 2HPT, there is strong evidence that preoperative imaging is helpful for patients with recurrent or persistent hyperparathyroidism [85, 86]. A study by Hindie utilized SPECT or SPECT/CT and reported positive findings in 20 of 21 recurrent or persistent cases [85]. Reoperation was carried out in 13 patients with no false positives. In over half of all revision operations the neck required exploration [32, 86]. Reoperation may be challenging and a targeted approach aided by appropriate imaging is preferred and can improve rates of success [86].

Ultrasound is helpful in identifying parathyroid glands adjacent to and within the thyroid gland but overall is inferior to sestamibi scanning. Ultrasound fails to detect mediastinal and retroesophageal abnormalities [23]. The ability to accurately evaluate the thyroid gland is an advantage of ultrasonography. Concurrent thyroid and parathyroid disorders occur and surgical management of both at the same time is ideal [87].

Intraoperative PTH

It is well established that monitoring the fall in intraoperative PTH (IOPTH) following the removal of a parathyroid adenoma has proven to be useful for primary hyperparathyroidism in order to confirm completeness of surgery [88]. However, its role in 2HPT remains less well defined. Several studies have confirmed that a significant reduction in IOPTH levels compared to preoperative levels was highly predictive of postoperative success [89–97]. Furthermore, there is data supporting IOPTH as a valuable tool in intraoperative surgical decision-making by identifying patients with both supernumerary, ectopic, and fewer than four parathyroid glands [90, 93, 98]. Optimal timing of IOPTH measurement has ranged from 10 to 30 min after the removal of the hyperplastic parathyroid glands, and criteria for percentage reduction for determining success has ranged from 50 to 90% of preoperative levels [99, 100].

Because of the high success rate of surgery for refractory 2HPT without IOPTH monitoring, its value in guiding surgical approach and cost-effectiveness have been questioned [101–103]. Pitt concluded that in 33 consecutive patients with refractory 2HPT, IOPTH levels did predict outcome but did not alter surgical management in any patient [101]. Furthermore, IOPTH does have clear limitations. Roshon reported that IOPTH failed to predict persistent hypoparathyroidism [92]. Moor found that although IOPTH levels predicted early outcomes, they did not predict long-term outcomes and the likelihood of recurrence [104]. Several authors have noted that predicting failures were considerably more difficult than predicting successes based on IOPTH levels [90, 100]

IOPTH monitoring is a promising technique for patients with refractory 2HPT. It however, does not replace meticulous exploration of all potential sites of glandular hyperplasia and its true cost-effectiveness remains to be seen. In the case of recurrent or persistent disease, IOPTH may play a valuable role especially when used in conjunction with preoperative imaging modalities [69, 86, 105].

Recurrent and Persistent Secondary Hyperparathyroidism

A comprehensive understanding of normal surgical anatomy, parathyroid embryology, and pathology are the keys to initial success. Regardless of surgical approach, meticulous and deliberate exploration of all areas that may harbor parathyroid tissue is of paramount importance. It is not surprising that the identification of fewer than four parathyroid glands at the time of initial parathyroid exploration results in higher failure rates [28, 32, 106–109].

Revision surgery is the preferred method of managing recurrent or persistent refractory 2HPT. Although in experienced hands, reoperation of the neck can be safely performed, it is a difficult operation with potentially higher complications, such as recurrent laryngeal nerve injuries [23, 28]. Prior to reoperation, careful evaluation should attempt to locate the abnormal parathyroid gland. Multiple imaging techniques may be required and are often complementary [83–85]. Scintigraphy with or without CT co-apposition, ultrasound, CT scan with contrast, MRI, and highly selective venous sampling for parathyroid concentrations have all been employed. IOPTH is a valuable tool in confirming successful removal of recurrent disease and some surgeons have also incorporated intraoperative ultrasound and gamma cameras in selected patients [110].

There may be differing rates of recurrence depending upon the type of original operation, with higher likelihood in patients who underwent TPTX + AT [32, 33]. Several studies have also found that the likelihood of successful reoperation was higher when the original operation was SPTX [28, 46, 47]. When recurrence was due to hyperplastic parathyroid tissue at the autotransplanted site, eradication was difficult and occasionally required the destruction of forearm musculature.

For patients who have an identifiable lesion but where revision surgery is contraindicated, a variety of techniques have been described to obliterate the offending gland. These techniques include percutaneous ethanol injection, ultrasound guided laser ablation, and superselective embolization [111]. Most reports are small retrospective clinical studies and some have reported a high rate of significant complications. Percutaneous ethanol injection therapy is the technique most frequently reported [105]. The largest series was by Chen and colleagues who reported excellent results in 49 patients with recurrent or persistent HPTH, achieving success rate of greater than 90% [105]. The technique has promise but complications are of concern. In particular, the upper parathyroid glands are frequently situated immediately adjacent to the recurrent laryngeal nerves, which are at risk of injury with this procedure. A broader experience with long-term follow up is necessary before this can be recommended as the treatment of choice.

Calcimimetics and Refractory Hyperparathyroidism

The calcimimetic cinacalcet hydrochloride has been shown to be highly effective in lowering PTH levels in patients with 2HPT [112–119]. Unfortunately, for patients with refractory 2HPT, cinacalcet is required at least until renal transplantation. In the USA, most patients with ESRD are unlikely to receive a renal transplant and only about 50% of those on the waiting list will undergo transplantation within 3 years [117]. Thus, the need for cinacalcet in the absence of parathyroid surgery would be lifelong and expensive. An interesting cost analysis comparing parathyroidectomy and cinacalcet was conducted by Narayan and colleagues [117].

They projected that surgery would be more cost-effective if dialysis is required for greater than 7.25 months. These calculations used the US data and conclusions may differ in other countries.

In selected patients, medical therapy may be the only option. Tominaga et al. provided an excellent outline of indications for cinacalcet in the contemporary care of patients with refractory 2HPT [120]. These included patients at high surgical risk from anesthesia or revision surgery, inaccessible parathyroid glands, nonlocalizing parathyroid glands, or inability to remove all parathyroid tissue, such as parathyromatosis. Calcimimetics clearly show promise and are helpful in some patients but long-term clinical experience is limited.

Demographics of Refractory Hyperparathyroidism and Surgery

Considerable advances have been made over the past 20 years in the medical management of patients with refractory 2HPT and continue to play an essential role in conjunction with surgery in this patient population. However, it is unclear whether this has translated into a change in the surgical demographics [3, 7, 8]. Population studies have observed fluctuating rates of parathyroidectomy and differing rates throughout various countries [10]. Foley et al. looked at parathyroidectomy trends in hemodialysis patients from 1992 to 2002 in the USA and discovered a fall then rise in rates over that time [7]. The highest rates were seen in 1994 and 2002 while 1998 experienced the lowest rate. A follow-up study by the same investigators looking at trends to 2007 found gradually increasing rates of parathyroidectomy from 2005 to 2007 [8]. A study by Shen et al. analyzed 202 consecutive operations from 1988 to 2007 and compared differences between two decades. They observed that although medical management has improved, the surgical population remained unchanged with respect to biochemical and symptomatic indications for surgery [121].

Subtotal Parathyroidectomy and Relocation of Remnant: A Personal Approach to Refractory Secondary Hyperparathyroidism (J. Yoo)

Subtotal parathyroidectomy and relocation (SPARE) of the remnant is my personal surgical approach to address multiglandular disease, such as 2HPT. The operation begins with the standard exploration and identification of four or more hyperplastic parathyroid glands, with each being assessed for degree of hyperplasia based on size, nodularity, and firmness. Prior to the removal of any gland, I evaluate the vascular pedicle to each parathyroid gland. I then determine the anticipated length of the vascular pedicle and the viability of the parathyroid gland when it is isolated on its blood supply (Fig. 10.5). This is done with a view to relocate a remnant of one parathyroid gland (with its blood supply intact) to a new position superficial to the strap muscles. In the ideal situation, the most "normal" appearing gland can be

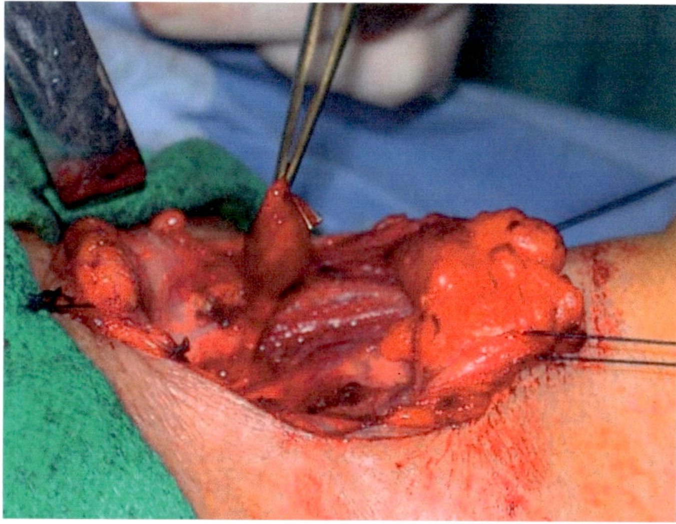

Fig. 10.5 Subtotal parathyroidectomy and relocation of the remnant: parathyroid isolated on vascular pedicle

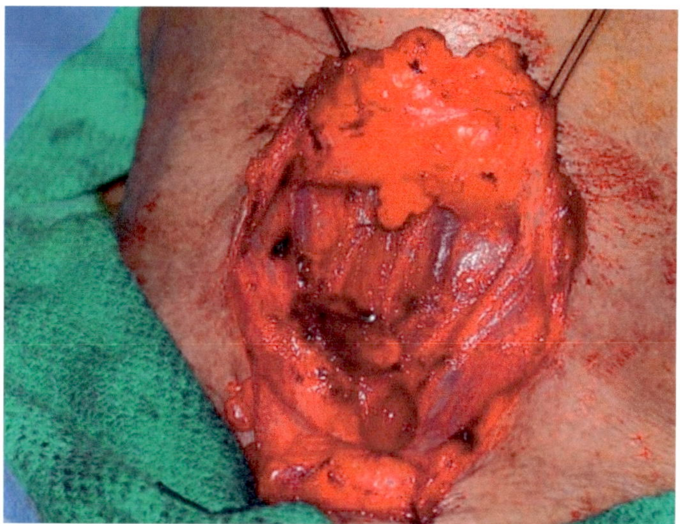

Fig. 10.6 Pedicled parathyroid remnant relocated between strap muscles and directly under the skin. Note the metal clip used to anchor and mark the remnant

carefully dissected keeping the attachments to its artery and vein. Once I am satisfied with the range of movement of one parathyroid gland on its vascular pedicle, the other three hyperplastic parathyroid glands are removed and confirmed by frozen section. The remaining parathyroid gland is then relocated to its new position superficial to the strap muscles (Fig. 10.6). The vascular pedicle length is usually long enough that the parathyroid gland can be brought directly between the divided strap muscle midline. On occasion a small opening can be created directly through the strap muscle so that the parathyroid gland can be brought through. As well, a portion of the thyroid gland may occasionally require removal in order to facilitate the repositioning of the remnant parathyroid gland. Once the parathyroid has been repositioned superficial to the strap muscles and immediately deep to the skin, a portion of this remaining parathyroid gland is removed and confirmed by frozen section. The viability of the parathyroid remnant is reassessed, and marked and anchored with large metal clips (usually two). The skin closure is carried out in the standard fashion and usually no drainage tube is inserted.

The SPARE operation was developed in order to incorporate many of the advantages of both traditional surgical techniques (SPTX and TPTX + AT) while eliminating most of the disadvantages of each. SPTX appears to have excellent initial success rates, lower recurrence rates, and the potential for earlier return of parathyroid homeostasis since the remnant parathyroid gland is kept viable on its blood supply. One important disadvantage of SPTX is the need to re-explore the thyroid compartment should the remnant become the source of recurrent hyperparathyroidism. The advantage of TPTX + AT is the elimination of neck re-exploration as compared to SPTX, since the forearm is the traditional site of implantation. However, unlike SPTX, transplanted parathyroid tissue requires additional time to recruit blood supply and regain function. The delay in parathyroid function is therefore expected to be longer than with SPTX. Furthermore, TPTX + AT may have higher rates of recurrence and parathyromatosis. Because of the high risk of severe hypoparathyroidism, we infrequently perform TPTX without AT.

The SPARE operation is therefore a modification of the traditional SPTX, where one hyperplastic parathyroid remnant is repositioned to a favorable location for easy retrieval or partial re-excision should the patient develop recurrent hyperparathyroidism. The remnant is situated directly under the skin flaps and remains viable throughout. In the event of a recurrence, the reoperation can be done under local anesthetic and does not require re-exploration of the thyroid compartment. The likelihood of recurrence or persistence due to ectopic or supernumerary glands should be similar for all surgical approaches, including the SPARE operation.

Tailored Parathyroidectomy for significant Renal 2HPT (J.E.M. Young)

For patients having a first operation for 2HPT, I do not do routine imaging prior to surgery. These patients require all four quadrant exploration with appropriate hemithymectomy, hemithyroidectomy, or both if necessary to remove both parathyroid glands on each side. These patients all have large glands measuring from 8 mm to 2–3 cm. These glands are usually easy to find and have characteristic appearances. I usually identify all four parathyroid glands before excising any, and if I plan on leaving a small fragment of one gland behind, it is usually the inferior gland.

I remove the major portion of the smallest inferior gland as the first part of the excision of abnormal tissue. I try and leave a well visualized 3 × 3 × 3 mm bit of parathyroid tissue marked with tiny metal clips. I then remove both upper parathyroid glands. It is important to note that leaving a portion of an upper parathyroid gland behind means a subsequent recurrence is much more difficult to treat surgically than a recurrence of a portion of an inferior gland (because of the upper gland's proximity to the recurrent laryngeal nerve). After removing both upper parathyroid glands and almost all of one of the inferior parathyroid glands, I now examine the remaining inferior parathyroid gland. If the remnant of the first surgically treated gland remains viable, I remove this entire contralateral inferior gland. If there is any question of viability of the small fragment I do a subtotal resection of the remaining inferior parathyroid gland and leave the most viable piece of either gland behind. In some circumstances I leave behind small pieces of both inferior parathyroid glands recognizing that either one may not survive. Each is marked with metal clips. In a situation where I am in doubt that I have preserved well–vascularized parathyroid remnants, I transplant a small portion of parathyroid tissue into the anterior, inner aspect of the left SCM muscle marking the tunnel with three metal clips and as well as cryopreserve a small portion of parathyroid gland. The parathyroid tissue is placed in 4 ½ cc of RPMI solution with ½ cc of DSMO, frozen with liquid nitrogen, and placed in deep freeze.

This operation of SPTX, as described above, is reserved for that group of renal patients with 2HPT in whom it is predicted that they will have a renal transplant, either cadaveric or live-related, in the near future.

For those patients with 2HPT with no planned renal transplant in the future, I do total parathyroidectomy of the detectable parathyroid tissue and do auto transplantation of a small bit of parathyroid tissue as noted above. Some parathyroid tissue is also cryopreserved.

SPTX as described can be done as an outpatient, whereas those patients treated with total parathyroidectomy will require admission to hospital and 3–10 days of high dose oral calcium, vitamin D, and intravenous calcium.

The success rate of this "tailored" approach, to patients depending on their likelihood of transplantation has been very high with only rare patients requiring reoperation 3–15 or more years later.

Conclusion

Parathyroidectomy remains the most reliable and effective means for managing refractory 2HPT. The operation can be performed safely and with high rates of success. However, in the minority of cases, the disorder remains problematic due to persistent or recurrent disease. New therapies like cinacalcet and other calcimimetics show promise for selected patients. Emerging technologies, such as IOPTH monitoring, better imaging modalities, and ablative procedures, may improve outcomes especially in patients with recurrent disease.

SPTX, TPTX+AT, and TPTX without AT are three surgical techniques for refractory 2HPT. Although controversy remains regarding the best approach, based on our overview of the literature and experience, our preference is to recommend subtotal parathyroidectomy in most cases. Only in rare instances where renal transplantation is not an option, would total parathyroidectomy without autotransplantation be considered. Regardless of the treatment approach adopted, a multidisciplinary approach that involves the surgeon, nephrologist, and endocrinologist will provide the optimal management of these complex patients.

References

1. Young EW, Albert JM, Satayathum S, et al. Predictors and consequences of altered mineral metabolism: the dialysis outcomes and practice patterns study. Kidney Int. 2005;67:1179–87.
2. Komaba H, Shiizaki K, Fukagawa M. Pharmacotherapy and interventional treatments for secondary hyperparathyroidism: current therapy and future challenges. Expert Opin Biol Ther. 2010;10(12):1729–42.
3. Jean G, Vanel T, Terrat JC, Chazot C. Prevention of secondary hyperparathyroidism in hemodialysis patients: the key role of native vitamin D supplementation. Hemodial Int. 2010;14(4): 486–91.
4. Yamada S, Taniguchi M, Tokumoto M, Tsuruya K, Hirakata H, Iida M. Early intervention with intravenous or pulse oral vitamin D therapy is more effective in the treatment of secondary hyperparathyroidism. Ther Apher Dial. 2010;14(4):424–31.
5. Joy MS, Karagiannis PC, Peyerl FW. Outcomes of secondary hyperparathyroidism in chronic kidney disease and the direct costs of treatment. J Manag Care Pharm. 2007;13(5):397–411.
6. Valderrabano F, Berthoux FC, Jones EH, Mehls O. Report on management of renal failure in Europe, XXV, 1994 end-stage renal disease and dialysis report. The EDTA-ERA Registry. European Dialysis and Transplant Association-European Renal Association. Nephrol Dial Transplant. 1996;11 suppl 1:2–21.
7. Foley RN, Li S, Liu J, Gilbertson DT, Chen SC, Collins AJ. The fall and rise of parathyroidectomy in U.S. hemodialysis patients, 1992 to 2002. J Am Soc Nephrol. 2005;16(1):210–8. Epub 2004 Nov 24.
8. Li S, Chen YW, Peng Y, Foley RN, St Peter WL. Trends in parathyroidectomy rates in US hemodialysis patients from 1992 to 2007. Am J Kidney Dis. 2011;57(4):602–11. Epub 2010 Dec 24.
9. Fraser WD. Hyperparathyroidism. Lancet. 2009;374(9684):145–58.
10. Tominaga Y, Matsuoka S, Uno N. Surgical and medical treatment of secondary hyperparathyroidism in patients on continuous dialysis. World J Surg. 2009;33:2335–42.
11. Block GA. Prevalence and clinical consequences of elevated Ca×P product in hemodialysis patients. Clin Nephrol. 2000;54:318–24.
12. National Kidney Foundation. K/DOQI clinical practice guidelines for bone metabolism and disease in chronic kidney disease. Am J Kidney Dis. 2003;42:S1–201.
13. Block GA, Klassen PS, Lazarus JM, et al. Mineral metabolism, mortality, and morbidity in the maintenance hemodialysis patients. J Am Soc Nephrol. 2004;15:2208–18.
14. Dussol B, Morand P, Martinat C, Lombard E, Portugal H, Brunet P, Berland Y. Influence of parathyroidectomy on mortality in hemodialysis patients: a prospective observational study. Ren Fail. 2007;29(5):579–86.
15. Trombetti A, Stoermann C, Robert JH, Herrmann FR, Pennisi P, Martin PY, Rizzoli R. Survival after parathyroidectomy in patients with end-stage renal disease and severe hyperparathyroidism. World J Surg. 2007;31(5):1014–21.

16. Packman KS, Demeure MJ. Indications for parathyroidectomy extent of treatment for patients with secondary hyperparathyroidism. Surg Clin North Am. 1995;75(3):465–82.
17. Jovanovic DB, Pejanovic S, Vukovic L, Djukanovic L, Jankovic R, Kalezic N, Paunovic I, Zivaljevic V. Ten years' experience in subtotal parathyroidectomy of hemodialysis patients. Ren Fail. 2005;27(1):19–24.
18. Tominaga Y, Matsuoka S, Uno N, et al. Removal of autografted parathyroid tissue from recurrent renal hyperparathyroidism in hemodialysis patients. World J Surg. 2010;34(6): 1312–7.
19. Tominaga Y, Kazuharu U, Haba T, et al. More than 1,000 cases of total parathyroidectomy with forearm autograft for renal hyperparathyroidism. Am J Kidney Dis. 2001;38(4):S168–71.
20. Rothmund M, Wagner PK, Schark C. Subtotal parathyroidectomy versus total parathyroidectomy and autotransplantation in secondary hyperparathyroidism: a randomized trial. World J Surg. 1991;15:745–50.
21. Hargrove GM, Pasieka JL, Hanley DA, et al. Short- and long-term outcome of total parathyroidectomy with immediate autografting versus subtotal parathyroidectomy in patients with end-stage renal disease. Am J Nephrol. 1999;19:559–64.
22. Stanbury SW, Lumb GA, Nicholson WF. Elective subtotal parathyroidectomy for renal hyperparathyroidism. Lancet. 1960;1:1793–8.
23. Seehofer D, Steinmüller T, Rayes N, Podrabsky P, Riethmüller J, Klupp J, Ulrich F, Schindler R, Frei U, Neuhaus P. Parathyroid hormone venous sampling before reoperative surgery in renal hyperparathyroidism: comparison with noninvasive localization procedures and review of the literature. Arch Surg. 2004;39(12):1331–8. Review.
24. Alveryd A. Parathyroid glands in thyroid surgery. Acta Chir Scand. 1968;389(Suppl):1–120.
25. Wells Jr SA, Gunnells JC, Shelburne JD, et al. Transplantation of the parathyroid glands in man: clinical indications and results. Surgery. 1975;78:34–44.
26. Tominaga Y. Surgical management of secondary hyperparathyroidism in uremia. Am J Med Sci. 1999;317(6):390–7.
27. Ogg CS. Total parathyroidectomy in the treatment of secondary (renal) hyperparathyroidism. Br Med J. 1967;4:331–4.
28. Stracke S, Keller F, Steinbach G, Henne-Bruns D, Wuerl P. Long-term outcome after total parathyroidectomy for the management of secondary hyperparathyroidism. Nephron Clin Pract. 2009;111(2):c102–9. Epub 2009 Jan 13.
29. Puccini M, Carpi A, Cupisti A, Caprioli R, Iacconi P, Barsotti M, Buccianti P, Mechanick J, Nicolini A, Miccoli P. Total parathyroidectomy without autotransplantation for the treatment of secondary hyperparathyroidism associated with chronic kidney disease: clinical and laboratory long-term follow-up. Biomed Pharmacother. 2010;64(5):359–62. Epub 2009 Oct 23.
30. Drakopoulos S, Koukoulaki M, Apostolou T, Pistolas D, Balaska K, Gavriil S, Hadjiconstantinou V. Total parathyroidectomy without autotransplantation in dialysis patients and renal transplant recipients, long-term follow-up evaluation. Am J Surg. 2009;198(2):178–83. Epub 2009 Feb 13.
31. Koonsman M, Hughes K, Dickerman R, et al. Parathyroidectomy in chronic renal failure. Am J Surg. 1994;168(6):631–4.
32. Richards ML, Wormuth J, Bingener J, et al. Parathyroidectomy in secondary hyperparathyroidism: is there an optimal operative management? Surgery. 2006;139:174–80.
33. Cattan P, Halimi B, Aidan K, et al. Reoperation for secondary uremic hyperparathyroidism: are technical difficulties influenced by initial surgical procedure? Surgery. 2000;127:562–5.
34. Schneider R, Waldmann J, Ramaswany A, et al. Frequency of ectopic and supranumerary intrathymic parathyroid glands in patients with renal hyperparathyroidism: analysis of 461 patients undergoing initial parathyroidectomy with bilateral cervical thymectomy. World J Surg. 2011;35:1260–5.
35. Uno N, Tominaga Y, Matsuoka S, et al. Incidence of parathyroid glands located in thymus in patients with renal hyperparathyroidism. World J Surg. 2008;32:2516–9.
36. Gomes EM, Nunes RC, Lacativa PG, et al. Ectopic and extranumerary parathyroid glands location in patients with hyperparathyroidism secondary to end stage renal disease. Acta Cir Bras. 2007;22(2):105–9.

37. Edis AJ, Levitt MD. Supernumerary parathyroid glands: implications for the surgical treatment of secondary hyperparathyroidism. World J Surg. 1987;11:398–401.
38. Marx SJ. Hyperparathyroid and hypoparathyroid disorders. N Engl J Med. 2000;343: 1863–75.
39. Torer N, Torun D, Torer H, et al. Predictors of early postoperative hypocalcemia in hemodialysis patients with secondary hyperparathyroidism. Transplant Proc. 2009;41(9):3642–6.
40. Coen G, Calabria S, Bellinghieri G, et al. Parathyroidectomy in chronic renal failure: short- and long-term results on parathyroid function, blood pressure and anemia. Nephron. 2001;88(2):149–55.
41. Nicholson ML, Veitch PS, Feehally J. Parathyroidectomy in chronic renal failure: comparison of three operative strategies. J R Coll Surg Edinb. 1996;41(6):382–7.
42. Wagner PK, Eckhardt J, Rothmund M. Subtotal parathyroidectomy versus total parathyroidectomy with autotransplantation in secondary hyperparathyroidism. A randomized study. Chirurg. 1991;62(3):189–94.
43. Alberston DA, Poole Jr GV, Myers RT. Subtotal parathyroidectomy versus total parathyroidectomy with autotransplantation for secondary hyperparathyroidism. Am Surg. 1985;51(1): 16–20.
44. Takagi H, Tominaga Y, Uchida K, Yamada N, Kawai M, Kano T, Morimoto T. Subtotal versus total parathyroidectomy with forearm autograft for secondary hyperparathyroidism in chronic. Ann Surg. 1984;200(1):18–23.
45. Gagne ER, Urena P, Leite-Silva S, et al. Short- and long-term efficacy of total parathyroidectomy with immediate autografting compared with subtotal parathyroidectomy in hemodialysis patients. J Am Soc Nephrol. 1992;3:1008–17.
46. Melck AL, Carty SE, Seethala RR, et al. Recurrent hyperparathyroidism and forearm parathyromatosis after total parathyroidectomy. Surgery. 2010;148(4):867–73.
47. Falvo L, Catania A, Sorrenti S, D'Andrea V, Santulli M, De Antoni E. Relapsing secondary hyperparathyroidism due to multiple nodular formations after total parathyroidectomy with autograft. Am Surg. 2003;69(11):998–1002.
48. Korzets Z, Magen H, Kraus L, et al. Total parathyroidectomy with autotransplantation in haemodialysed patients with secondary hyperparathyroidism: should it be abandoned ? Nephrol Dial Transplant. 1987;2:341–6.
49. Neyer U, Hoerandner H, Haid A, Zimmermann G, Niederle B. Total parathyroidectomy with autotransplantation in renal hyperparathyroidism: low recurrence after intra-operative tissue selection. Nephrol Dial Transplant. 2002;17(4):625–9.
50. Lando MJ, Hoover LA, Zuckerbraun L, Goodman D. Autotransplantation of parathyroid tissue into sternocleidomastoid muscle. Arch Otolaryngol Head Neck Surg. 1988;114(5):557–60.
51. Chou FF, Chi SY, Hsieh KC. Hypoparathyroidism after total parathyroidectomy plus subcutaneous autotransplantation for secondary hyperparathyroidism–any side effects? World J Surg. 2010;34(10):2350–4.
52. Yoon JH, Nam KH, Chang HS, Chung WY, Park CS. Total parathyroidectomy and autotransplantation by the subcutaneous injection technique in secondary hyperparathyroidism. Surg Today. 2006;36(4):304–7.
53. Echenique-Elizondo M, Díaz-Aguirregoitia FJ, Amondarain JA, Vidaur F. Parathyroid graft function after presternal subcutaneous autotransplantation for renal hyperparathyroidism. Arch Surg. 2006;141(1):33–8.
54. Kinnaert P, Salmon I, Decoster-Gervy C, Vienne A, De Pauw L, Hooghe L, Tielemans C. Long-term results of subcutaneous parathyroid grafts in uremic patients. Arch Surg. 2000;135(2):186–90.
55. Monchik JM, Bendinelli C, Passero Jr MA, Roggin KK. Subcutaneous forearm transplantation of autologous parathyroid tissue in patients with renal hyperparathyroidism. Surgery. 1999; 126(6):1152–8. discussion 1158–9.
56. Sun Y, Cai H, Bai J, Zhao H, Miao Y. Endoscopic total parathyroidectomy and partial parathyroid tissue autotransplantation for patients with secondary hyperparathyroidism: a new surgical approach. World J Surg. 2009;33(8):1674–9.

57. Barbaros U, Erbil Y, Yildirim A, Saricam G, Yazici H, Ozarmağan S. Minimally invasive video-assisted subtotal parathyroidectomy with thymectomy for secondary hyperparathyroidism. Langenbecks Arch Surg. 2009;394(3):451–5. Epub 2008 Aug 23.
58. Barczyński M, Cichoń S, Konturek A, Cichoń W. Minimally invasive video-assisted parathyroidectomy versus open minimally invasive parathyroidectomy for a solitary parathyroid adenoma: a prospective, randomized, blinded trial. World J Surg. 2006;30(5):721–31.
59. Mourad M, Ngongang C, Saab N, Coche E, Jamar F, Michel JM, Maiter D, Malaise J, Squifflet JP. Video-assisted neck exploration for primary and secondary hyperparathyroidism: initial experience. Surg Endosc. 2001;15(10):1112–5. Epub 2001 Jul 5.
60. Conzo G, Perna AF, Sinisi AA, Palazzo A, Stanzione F, Della Pietra C, Livrea A. Total parathyroidectomy without autotransplantation in the surgical treatment of secondary hyperparathyroidism of chronic kidney disease. J Endocrinol Invest. 2011. [Epub 2011 Mar 22].
61. Coulston JE, Egan R, Willis E, Morgan JD. Total parathyroidectomy without autotransplantation for renal hyperparathyroidism. Br J Surg. 2010;97(11):1674–9.
62. Chan HW, Chu KH, Fung SK, Tang HL, Lee W, Cheuk A, Yim KF, Tong MK, Lee KC. Prospective study on dialysis patients after total parathyroidectomy without autoimplant. Nephrology (Carlton). 2010;15(4):441–7.
63. Shih ML, Duh QY, Hsieh CB, Lin SH, Wu HS, Chu PL, Chen TY, Yu JC. Total parathyroidectomy without autotransplantation for secondary hyperparathyroidism. World J Surg. 2009;33(2):248–54.
64. Rayes N, Seehofer D, Schindler R, Reinke P, Kahl A, Ulrich F, Neuhaus P, Nüssler NC. Long-term results of subtotal vs total parathyroidectomy without autotransplantation in kidney transplant recipients. Arch Surg. 2008;143(8):756–61. discussion 761.
65. Lorenz K, Ukkat J, Sekulla C, Gimm O, Brauckhoff M, Dralle H. Total parathyroidectomy without autotransplantation for renal hyperparathyroidism: experience with a qPTH-controlled protocol. World J Surg. 2006;30(5):743–51.
66. Saunders RN, Karoo R, Metcalfe MS, Nicholson ML. Four gland parathyroidectomy without reimplantation in patients with chronic renal failure. Postgrad Med J. 2005;81(954):255–8.
67. Ockert S, Willeke F, Richter A, Jonescheit J, Schnuelle P, Van Der Woude F, Post S. Total parathyroidectomy without autotransplantation as a standard procedure in the treatment of secondary hyperparathyroidism. Langenbecks Arch Surg. 2002;387(5–6):204–9. Epub 2002 Aug 14.
68. Schlosser K, Veit JA, Witte S, Fernández ED, Victor N, Knaebel HP, Seiler CM, Rothmund M. Comparison of total parathyroidectomy without autotransplantation and without thymectomy versus total parathyroidectomy with autotransplantation and with thymectomy for secondary hyperparathyroidism: TOPAR PILOT-Trial. Trials. 2007;8:22.
69. Dotzenrath C, Cupisti K, Goretzki E, Mondry A, Vossough A, Grabensee B, Röher HD. Operative treatment of renal autonomous hyperparathyroidism: cause of persistent or recurrent disease in 304 patients. Langenbecks Arch Surg. 2003;387(9–10):348–54. Epub 2002 Dec 14.
70. Malmaeus J, Akerström G, Johansson H, Ljunghall S, Nilsson P, Selking O. Parathyroid surgery in chronic renal insufficiency. Subtotal parathyroidectomy versus total parathyroidectomy with autotransplantation to the forearm. Acta Chir Scand. 1982;148(3):229–38.
71. Wells Jr SA, Christiansen C. The transplanted parathyroid gland: evaluation of cryopreservation and other environmental factors which affect its function. Surgery. 1974;75(1):49–55.
72. Guerrero MA. Cryopreservation of parathyroid glands. Int J Endocrinol. 2010;2010:829540. Epub 2010 Dec 8.
73. Wagner PK, Seesko HG, Rothmund M. Replantation of cryopreserved human parathyroid tissue. World J Surg. 1991;15(6):751–5.
74. Borot S, Lapierre V, Carnaille B, Goudet P, Penfornis A. Results of cryopreserved parathyroid autografts: a retrospective multicenter study. Surgery. 2010;147(4):529–35. Epub 2010 Feb 12.
75. Guerrero MA, Evans DB, Lee JE, Bao R, Bereket A, Gantela S, Griffin GD, Perrier ND. Viability of cryopreserved parathyroid tissue: when is continued storage versus disposal indicated? World J Surg. 2008;32(5):836–9.

76. Cohen MS, Dilley WG, Wells Jr SA, Moley JF, Doherty GM, Sicard GA, Skinner MA, Norton JA, DeBenedetti MK, Lairmore TC. Long-term functionality of cryopreserved parathyroid autografts: a 13-year prospective analysis. Surgery. 2005;138(6):1033–40. discussion 1040–1.
77. Caccitolo JA, Farley DR, van Heerden JA, Grant CS, Thompson GB, Sterioff S. The current role of parathyroid cryopreservation and autotransplantation in parathyroid surgery: an institutional experience. Surgery. 1997;122(6):1062–7.
78. Lai EC, Ching AS, Leong HT. Secondary and tertiary hyperparathyroidism: role of preoperative localization. ANZ J Surg. 2007;77(10):880–2.
79. Vulpio C, Bossola M, De Gaetano A, Maresca G, Bruno I, Fadda G, Morassi F, Magalini SC, Giordano A, Castagneto M. Usefulness of the combination of ultrasonography and 99mTc-sestamibi scintigraphy in the preoperative evaluation of uremic secondary hyperparathyroidism. Head Neck. 2010;32(9):1226–35.
80. de la Rosa A, Jimeno J, Membrilla E, Sancho JJ, Pereira JA, Sitges-Serra A. Usefulness of preoperative Tc-mibi parathyroid scintigraphy in secondary hyperparathyroidism. Langenbecks Arch Surg. 2008;393(1):21–4. Epub 2007 Feb 9.
81. Papanikolaou V, Vrochides D, Imvrios G, Papagiannis A, Gakis D, Ouzounidis N, Giakoustidis D, Fouzas I, Antoniadis N, Ntinas A, Arsos G, Kardasis D, Takoudas D. Tc-99m sestamibi accuracy in detecting parathyroid tissue is increased when combined with preoperative laboratory values: a retrospective study in 453 Greek patients with chronic renal failure who underwent parathyroidectomy. Transplant Proc. 2008;40(9):3163–5.
82. Harris L, Yoo J, Driedger A, Fung K, Franklin J, Gray D, Holliday R. Accuracy of technetium-99m SPECT-CT hybrid images in predicting the precise intraoperative anatomical location of parathyroid adenomas. Head Neck. 2008;30(4):509–17.
83. Lomonte C, Buonvino N, Selvaggiolo M, Dassira M, Grasso G, Vernaglione L, Basile C. Sestamibi scintigraphy, topography, and histopathology of parathyroid glands in secondary hyperparathyroidism. Am J Kidney Dis. 2006;48(4):638–44.
84. Fuster D, Torregrosa JV, Setoain X, Domenech B, Campistol JM, Rubello D, Pons F. Localising imaging in secondary hyperparathyroidism. Minerva Endocrinol. 2008;33(3): 203–12.
85. Hindié E, Zanotti-Fregonara P, Just PA, Sarfati E, Mellière D, Toubert ME, Moretti JL, Jeanguillaume C, Keller I, Ureña-Torres P. Parathyroid scintigraphy findings in chronic kidney disease patients with recurrent hyperparathyroidism. Eur J Nucl Med Mol Imaging. 2010;37(3):623–34. Epub 2009 Nov 28.
86. Hessman O, Stålberg P, Sundin A, Garske U, Rudberg C, Eriksson LG, Hellman P, Akerström G. High success rate of parathyroid reoperation may be achieved with improved localization diagnosis. World J Surg. 2008;32(5):774–81. discussion 782–3.
87. Seehofer D, Rayes N, Klupp J, Nüssler NC, Ulrich F, Graef KJ, Schindler R, Steinmüller T, Frei U, Neuhaus P. Prevalence of thyroid nodules and carcinomas in patients operated on for renal hyperparathyroidism: experience with 339 consecutive patients and review of the literature. World J Surg. 2005;29(9):1180–4.
88. Carneiro-Pla D. Contemporary and practical uses of intraoperative parathyroid hormone monitoring. Endocr Pract. 2011;17 Suppl 1:44–53.
89. Hughes DT, Miller BS, Doherty GM, Gauger PG. Intraoperative parathyroid hormone monitoring in patients with recognized multiglandular primary hyperparathyroidism. World J Surg. 2011;35(2):336–41.
90. Freriks K, Hermus AR, de Sévaux RG, Bonenkamp HJ, Biert J, den Heijer M, Sweep FC, van Hamersvelt HW. Usefulness of intraoperative parathyroid hormone measurements in patients with renal hyperparathyroidism. Head Neck. 2010;32(10):1328–35.
91. Ikeda Y, Kurihara H, Morita N, Miyabe R, Takami H. The role of quick bio-intact PTH(1–84) assay during parathyroidectomy for secondary hyperparathyroidism. J Surg Res. 2007;141(2): 306–10. Epub 2007 Apr 6.
92. Roshan A, Kamath B, Roberts S, Atkin SL, England RJ. Intra-operative parathyroid hormone monitoring in secondary hyperparathyroidism: is it useful? Clin Otolaryngol. 2006;31(3): 198–203.

93. Barczy ski M, Cicho S, Konturek A, Cicho W. A randomised study on a new cost-effective algorithm of quick intraoperative intact parathyroid hormone assay in secondary hyperparathyroidism. Langenbecks Arch Surg. 2005;390(2):121–7. Epub 2005 Feb.
94. Seehofer D, Rayes N, Klupp J, Steinmüller T, Ulrich F, Müller C, Schindler R, Frei U, Neuhaus P. Predictive value of intact parathyroid hormone measurement during surgery for renal hyperparathyroidism. Langenbecks Arch Surg. 2005;390(3):222–9. Epub 2005 Feb 22.
95. Weber T, Zeier M, Hinz U, Schilling T, Büchler MW. Impact of intraoperative parathyroid hormone levels on surgical results in patients with renal hyperparathyroidism. World J Surg. 2005;29(9):1176–9.
96. Lokey J, Pattou F, Mondragon-Sanchez A, Minuto M, Mullineris B, Wambergue F, Foissac-Geroux P, Noel C, de Sagazan HL, VanHille P, Proye CA. Intraoperative decay profile of intact (1–84) parathyroid hormone in surgery for renal hyperparathyroidism–a consecutive series of 80 patients. Surgery. 2000;128(6):1029–34.
97. Chou FF, Lee CH, Chen JB, Hsu KT, Sheen-Chen SM. Intraoperative parathyroid hormone measurement in patients with secondary hyperparathyroidism. Arch Surg. 2002;137(3): 341–4.
98. Irvin III GL, Molinari AS, Figueroa C, Carneiro DM. Improved success rate in reoperative parathyroidectomy with intraoperative PTH assay. Ann Surg. 1999;229(6):874–8. discussion 878–9.
99. Riss P, Kaczirek K, Heinz G, Bieglmayer C, Niederle B. A "defined baseline" in PTH monitoring increases surgical success in patients with multiple gland disease. Surgery. 2007;142(3):398–404.
100. Kaczirek K, Riss P, Wunderer G, Prager G, Asari R, Scheuba C, Bieglmayer C, Niederle B. Quick PTH assay cannot predict incomplete parathyroidectomy in patients with renal hyperparathyroidism. Surgery. 2005;137(4):431–5.
101. Pitt SC, Panneerselvan R, Chen H, Sippel RS. Secondary and tertiary hyperparathyroidism: the utility of ioPTH monitoring. World J Surg. 2010;34(6):1343–9.
102. Gasparri G, Camandona M, Bertoldo U, Sargiotto A, Papotti M, Raggio E, Nati L, Martino P, Felletti G, Mengozzi G. The usefulness of preoperative dual-phase 99mTc MIBI-scintigraphy and IO-PTH assay in the treatment of secondary and tertiary hyperparathyroidism. Ann Surg. 2009;250(6):868–71.
103. Müller-Stich BP, Brändle M, Binet I, Warschkow R, Lange J, Clerici T. To autotransplant simultaneously or not—can intraoperative parathyroid hormone monitoring reliably predict early postoperative parathyroid hormone levels after total parathyroidectomy for hyperplasia? Surgery. 2007;142(1):47–56.
104. Moor JW, Roberts S, Atkin SL, England RJ. Intraoperative parathyroid hormone monitoring to determine long-term success of total parathyroidectomy for secondary hyperparathyroidism. Head Neck. 2011;33(3):293–6.
105. Chen HH, Lin CJ, Wu CJ, Lai CT, Lin J, Cheng SP, Yang TL. Chemical ablation of recurrent and persistent secondary hyperparathyroidism after subtotal parathyroidectomy. Ann Surg. 2011;253(4):786–90.
106. Verdonck J, Geuens G, Delaere P, Vander Poorten V, Evenepoel P, Debruyne E. Surgical findings and post-operative parathormone levels in patients with secondary hyperparathyroidism. B-ENT. 2009;5(3):143–8.
107. Gasparri G, Camandona M, Abbona GC, Papotti M, Jeantet A, Radice E, Mullineris B, Dei Poli M. Secondary and tertiary hyperparathyroidism: causes of recurrent disease after 446 parathyroidectomies. Ann Surg. 2001;233(1):65–9.
108. Kinnaert P, Nagy N, Decoster-Gervy C, De Pauw L, Salmon I, Vereerstraeten P. Persistent hyperparathyroidism requiring surgical treatment after kidney transplantation. World J Surg. 2000;24(11):1391–5.
109. Donckier V, Decoster-Gervy C, Kinnaert P. Long-term results after surgical treatment of renal hyperparathyroidism when fewer than four glands are identified at operation. J Am Coll Surg. 1997;184(1):70–4.

110. Casella C, di Fabio F, Pata G, Salerni B. Methods of intraoperative localization in the surgery treatment of persistent and recurrent secondary hyperparathyroidism. Ann Ital Chir. 2006;77(6):473–7. discussion 478–9.
111. Carrafiello G, Lagana D, Mangini M, Dionigi G, Rovera F, Carcano G, Cuffari S, Fugazzola C. Treatment of secondary hyperparathyroidism with ultrasonographically guided percutaneous radiofrequency thermoablation. Surg Laparosc Endosc Percutan Tech. 2006;16(2): 112–6.
112. Al-Hilali N, Hussain N, Kawy YA, Al-Azmi M. A novel dose regimen of cinacalcet in the treatment of severe hyperparathyroidism in hemodialysis patients. Saudi J Kidney Dis Transpl. 2011;22(3):448–55.
113. Guerra R, Auyanet I, Fernández EJ, Pérez MÁ, Bosch E, Ramírez A, Suria S, Checa MD. Hypercalcemia secondary to persistent hyperparathyroidism in kidney transplant patients: analysis after a year with cinacalcet. J Nephrol. 2011;24(1):78–82.
114. Mittman N, Desiraju B, Meyer KB, Chattopadhyay J, Avram MM. Treatment of secondary hyperparathyroidism in ESRD: a 2-year, single-center crossover study. Kidney Int Suppl. 2010;117:S33–6.
115. Ichii M, Ishimura E, Okuno S, Chou H, Kato Y, Tsuboniwa N, Nagasue K, Maekawa K, Yamakawa T, Inaba M, Nishizawa Y. Decreases in parathyroid gland volume after cinacalcet treatment in hemodialysis patients with secondary hyperparathyroidism. Nephron Clin Pract. 2010;115(3):c195–202. Epub 2010 Apr 23.
116. Yokoyama K. Clinical issues regarding cinacalcet hydrochloride in Japan. Ther Apher Dial. 2009;13 Suppl 1:S12–4.
117. Narayan R, Perkins RM, Berbano EP, Yuan CM, Neff RT, Sawyers ES, Yeo FE, Vidal-Trecan GM, Abbott KC. Parathyroidectomy versus cinacalcet hydrochloride-based medical therapy in the management of hyperparathyroidism in ESRD: a cost utility analysis. Am J Kidney Dis. 2007;49(6):801–13.
118. Torres PU. Cinacalcet HCl: a novel treatment for secondary hyperparathyroidism caused by chronic kidney disease. J Ren Nutr. 2006;16(3):253–8.
119. Cunningham J, Danese M, Olson K, Klassen P, Chertow GM. Effects of the calcimimetic cinacalcet HCl on cardiovascular disease, fracture, and health-related quality of life in secondary hyperparathyroidism. Kidney Int. 2005;68(4):1793–800.
120. Tominaga Y, Matsuoka S, Uno N, Sato T. Parathyroidectomy for secondary hyperparathyroidism in the era of calcimimetics. Ther Apher Dial. 2008;12 Suppl 1:S21–6.
121. Shen WT, Kebebew E, Suh I, Duh QY, Clark OH. Two hundred and two consecutive operations for secondary hyperparathyroidism: has medical management changed the profiles of patients requiring parathyroidectomy? Surgery. 2009;146(2):296–9. Epub 2009 Jun 26.

Chapter 11
Tertiary Hyperparathyroidism Pathogenesis, Clinical Features, and Medical Management

D. Sudhaker Rao and Dolores Shoback

Keywords Tertiary hyperparathyroidism • Refractory hyperparathyroidism • Parathyroidectomy • Vitamin D • Calcitriol • Cinacalcet • Phosphate binders • Brown tumors • Marrow fibrosis

Introduction

Hypersecretion of parathyroid hormone (PTH) occurs in three distinct forms. Sporadic primary hyperparathyroidism is the most common (see Chaps. 5 and 6). Tertiary hyperparathyroidism [1–3], the subject of this chapter, is the least common (Table 11.1). Secondary hyperparathyroidism caused by a pathologic process outside the parathyroid glands (e.g., kidney failure, phosphate wasting, and so forth) is discussed fully in Chap. 7 and is referred to in the current chapter in the context of "refractory" secondary hyperparathyroidism. Secondary hyperparathyroidism shares many pathogenic, clinical, biochemical, radiological, and bone histological features of tertiary hyperparathyroidism, except that with the development of hypercalcemia the classification changes from secondary to tertiary hyperparathyroidism [4].

The term tertiary hyperparathyroidism should be reserved for the rare occurrence of truly autonomous PTH secretion associated with hypercalcemia—the result of the development of adenomatous changes and nodules against the background of chronic

D.S. Rao, MBBS, FACP, FACE (✉)
Bone & Mineral Metabolism, Bone & Mineral Research Laboratory,
Henry Ford Medical Center, New Center One, Henry Ford Hospital,
Suite# 800, 3031 W. Grand Blvd, Detroit, MI 48202, USA
e-mail: srao1@hfhs.org

D. Shoback, MD
Endocrine Research Unit, San Francisco Department of Veterans Affairs Medical Center,
University of California, San Francisco, CA, USA
e-mail: dolores.shoback@ucsf.edu

A.A. Khan and O.H. Clark (eds.), *Handbook of Parathyroid Diseases:
A Case-Based Practical Guide*, DOI 10.1007/978-1-4614-2164-1_11,
© Springer Science+Business Media, LLC 2012

Table 11.1

Classification of hyperparathyroidism
Primary hyperparathyroidism
Sporadic
Familial syndromes
Isolated familial
Hyperparathyroidism-jaw tumor syndrome
MEN I and II syndromes
Secondary hyperparathyroidism (nonrenal)
Vitamin D deficiency/insufficiency
Calcium malabsorption
Hypophosphatemic disorders
Secondary hyperparathyroidism (renal)
Early secondary hyperparathyroidism (most common ~75%)
Refractory secondary hyperparathyroidism (second most common <20%)
Tertiary hyperparathyroidism (least common <5%)

and prolonged secondary hyperparathyroidism often of several years' duration [3, 4]. Historically, this descriptive term is attributed to the late Dr. Walter St. Goar, in the context of discussing a patient in the Case Records of the Massachusetts General Hospital. Regrettably, the term is often misused to refer to secondary hyperparathyroidism, in the context of chronic kidney disease (CKD), when serum PTH levels are moderately high. Tertiary hyperparathyroidism should be restricted to those patients in whom *hypercalcemia* has developed as a consequence of parathyroid gland autonomy. Some experts recommend abandoning the term "tertiary" altogether and using the descriptor "hypercalcemic secondary hyperparathyroidism." The authors prefer the term tertiary hyperparathyroidism to distinguish the clinical entity because it requires specific, often urgent management decisions.

Earlier in the transformation of secondary to tertiary hyperparathyroidism is what has been termed "refractory secondary hyperparathyroidism" characterized by marked elevations in serum PTH levels (intact PTH >1,000 pg/ml or >106 pmol/L) [4]. In this chapter, we discuss both the rare tertiary hyperparathyroidism, as defined above, and the more common refractory secondary hyperparathyroidism as part of a continuum of the same pathogenic mechanisms, differing only in the degree of PTH hypersecretion and the presence or absence of hypercalcemia [5].

Etiology and Pathogenesis

Tertiary hyperparathyroidism always results from the chronic relentless stimulus to PTH secretion, and it occurs almost exclusively in patients with CKD on maintenance dialysis and, less frequently, after renal transplantation [3, 4]. By definition, therefore, tertiary hyperparathyroidism is almost always preceded by a prolonged period of secondary hyperparathyroidism. In its classic form, PTH secretion has reached "a point of no return" and, thus, is no longer under the usual constraints of suppression by high serum calcium (Ca) levels [5]. In addition, associated vitamin D and or calcitriol deficiencies, hyperphosphatemia (an inevitable consequence of renal failure), and the loss of the normal proliferative control mechanisms in parathyroid cells contribute to the evolution of tertiary hyperparathyroidism [1–4]. Consequently, the parathyroid cell mass is greatly increased with characteristic monoclonal nodular areas in the background of diffuse hyperplasia [2–4]. Hypercalcemia, a direct consequence of unrestrained hypersecretion of PTH, is a cardinal feature of tertiary hyperparathyroidism. It is important and necessary to distinguish hypercalcemia due to tertiary hyperparathyroidism from postrenal transplant hypercalcemia, which occurs in almost all transplant recipients. Tertiary hyperparathyroidism also occurs occasionally in two other situations: in patients with prolonged vitamin D deficiency due to unrecognized malabsorption [6] and in patients on long-term oral phosphate (P) therapy for hypophosphatemic disorders [7, 8].

Autonomous secondary hyperparathyroidism, which encompasses both refractory secondary and tertiary hyperparathyroidism [5], occurs because of disturbed feedback relationships (see Chapter 1 on PTH Secretion and Synthesis) leading to excess PTH secretion and parathyroid cell proliferation [1, 9]. These unique pathogenic features help to distinguish tertiary from both the primary and the "usual" earlier secondary hyperparathyroid states (see Chaps. 5–7). The changes in the parathyroid glands at the cellular and molecular levels sustain the greatly increased rate of PTH secretion. The two most common causes for PTH hypersecretion in CKD are hyperphosphatemia and calcitriol deficiency. However, for reasons that are not entirely clear, some patients go on to develop autonomous parathyroid hyperplasia with nodular or adenomatous transformation [2–4], a state from which the parathyroid gland is unable to recover.

Teleologically, one would expect involution of the enlarged parathyroid glands with optimal control of serum P levels and the use of calcitriol or its analogues, but this is rarely achieved in clinical practice. Reduced expression of the calcium-sensing (CaSR) and the vitamin D receptors (VDRs) has been demonstrated in these enlarged parathyroid glands both in experimental animal and human studies [10]. Other molecular abnormalities include overexpression of cell-cycle proteins, oncogenes involved in the multiple endocrine neoplasia type 1, and mutations in tumor-suppressor genes involved in tumorigenesis of sporadic primary parathyroid adenomas [2]. As a result of these molecular defects and because of continued stimulus from hyperphosphatemia, the size(s) of the parathyroid gland(s) is enormously increased—often several-fold and up to 25-fold over normal in some series. Reductions in VDR and CaSR expression, which appear to be necessary and sufficient for shifting the Ca–PTH set-point relationship, are more pronounced in the nodular compared to the internodular areas of these enlarged parathyroid glands [3, 4, 10]. This mechanism has been proposed to explain the lack of predictable responses to medical therapy with calcitriol and its analogues or with cinacalcet (see below).

Hyperphosphatemia leads to parathyroid cell proliferation and reduced expression of CaSR and VDR [1, 9–11]. In addition, hyperphosphatemia independently lowers the serum Ca, further exacerbating PTH hypersecretion [3, 4]. Even in patients with severe hypophosphatemia, due to either genetic disorders or tumor-induced osteomalacia, long-term oral phosphate therapy leads to hyperparathyroidism and can produce hypercalcemic secondary hyperparathyroidism, a scenario mimicking tertiary hyperparathyroidism [7, 8]. Finally, prolonged and severe vitamin D deficiency can evolve from an initial state of hypocalcemic secondary hyperparathyroidism, associated with osteomalacia, to hypercalcemic secondary hyperparathyroidism or even tertiary hyperparathyroidism in exceedingly rare cases, often restricted to case reports [6].

Clinical Presentation

The clinical features of tertiary hyperparathyroidism include bone pain, fractures, pruritis, muscle weakness, as well as symptoms of hypercalcemia. A typical patient has been on maintenance dialysis for at least 5 years and has variable symptoms related to hypercalcemia. However, it is often difficult to separate symptoms of hypercalcemia from those related to the underlying CKD. Bone pain and tenderness (either localized or diffuse) are characteristic and almost always associated with proximal or generalized muscle weakness. In those with poorly controlled serum P, intense pruritus is common. Corneal calcification, often referred to as band keratopathy, is characteristically seen in patients with chronically elevated serum Ca×P products. Pathologic fractures, in contrast to fragility fractures, are seen at the sites of brown tumors in more severe cases. Cortical thinning in the shafts of the long bones, a unique feature of PTH-mediated bone loss, is the rule, rather than an exception. Subcutaneous calcification, a consequence of poorly controlled serum P levels with resulting elevations in the Ca-P product, can be palpable in some patients (Figs. 11.1 and 11.2). In others, the uncommon complication of calciphylaxis may develop with deposition of Ca-P crystals in blood vessels and subsequent inflammation and small

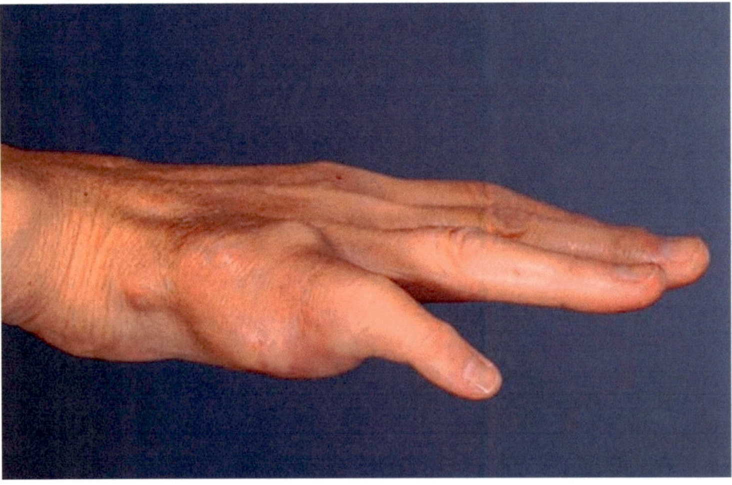

Fig. 11.1 Visible and palpable soft tissue calcifications (see an X-ray of hands in Fig. 11.2)

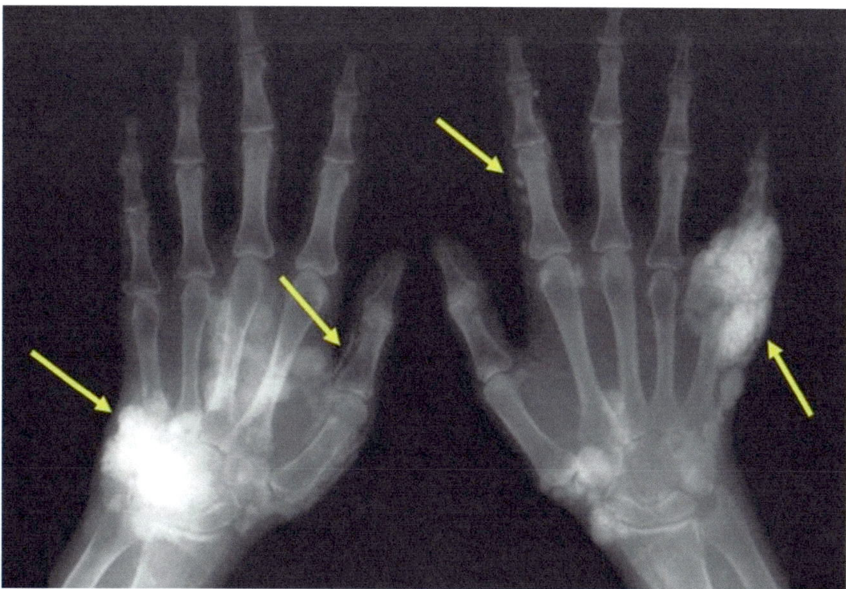

Fig. 11.2 Extensive soft tissue and vascular calcifications from the same patient as in Fig. 11.1

Table 11.2

Laboratory features of renal secondary and tertiary hyperparathyroid states

Variable	Early	Refractory	Tertiary
Serum calcium	Low/normal	Normal	High
Serum phosphate	High	High	High
Total alkaline phosphatase	Normal/high	High	High
Bone-specific alkaline phosphatase	Normal/high	High	High
Intact PTH (pg/ml)	<500	≥1,000	≥1,000
Bone biopsy	Variable	High turnover	High turnover
Marrow fibrosis	Variable	Mild to moderate	Moderate to extensive

vessel occlusion. Necrosis, gangrene, and secondary infection can develop as well as myopathy and rhabdomyolysis. Other risk factors to the development of calciphylaxis include diabetes, obesity, protein C and protein S deficiencies, as well as drugs, such as glucocorticoids. Calciphylaxis can be fatal, and therefore, close monitoring of serum Ca and P in patients with tertiary hyperparathyroidism is necessary.

Biochemical findings of tertiary hyperparathyroidism are noted in Table 11.2. Besides hypercalcemia, a necessary condition for the diagnosis of tertiary hyperparathyroidism, hyperphosphatemia of varying degrees is present, except in those rare patients with hypophosphatemic disorders or vitamin D deficiency. Serum PTH levels are very high, often >1,000 pg/ml (>106 pmol/L), with elevations in serum total and bone-specific alkaline phosphatase levels. The magnitude of elevations in serum PTH levels is always much greater in patients on dialysis, although one of the authors (DSR) has seen a few patients with tertiary hyperparathyroidism due to chronic vitamin D depletion with serum PTH levels >1,000 pg/ml (>106 pmol/L). In contrast, serum PTH levels in tertiary hyperparathyroidism due to oral P therapy rarely exceed 500 pg/ml (>53 pmol/L) [7, 8].

Evaluation of a Patient with Tertiary Hyperparathyroidism

The evaluation begins with a careful history and physical examination, and a review of the dialysis or transplant program records, which is crucial in planning investigative and therapeutic strategies. Obtaining information on the type of renal disease (glomerular versus tubulo-interstitial), duration (both pre- and on dialysis), and previous parathyroid surgeries is critical. A complete review of the medications may uncover drugs which can also elevate serum Ca & PTH, such as hydrochlorothiazide or lithium. Although the diagnostic approach to tertiary hyperparathyroidism was relatively straightforward prior to the 1970s, it is often challenging in current practice. Patients are treated with a variety of vitamin D metabolites, and phosphate binders are often interrupted because of elevations in serum levels of Ca, P, and Ca×P product. Consequently, it is often difficult to rely on the current serum PTH or alkaline phosphatase (total or bone specific) levels, which may be affected by these therapeutic maneuvers. Accurate records of the types, doses, and duration of recent therapies should be obtained. Physical examination should include assessment of bone pain and tenderness, and skeletal and soft tissue abnormalities (Figs. 11.1 and 11.2). Pseudoclubbing of the digits due to resorption of the terminal phalanges (Figs. 11.3 and 11.4), palpable soft tissue swelling due to calcium deposits (Figs. 11.1 and 11.2), and palpable bone deformities due to brown tumors, when present, are pathognomonic and indicative of more severe forms of secondary hyperparathyroidism—tertiary or refractory secondary hyperparathyroidism [5]. Corneal calcifications are best assessed by an experienced clinician or referred to an ophthalmologist for a slit lamp examination. When present, it is almost always an indication for surgery. Careful assessment of proximal lower extremity muscle strength is recommended and can easily be evaluated by observing the ability of a patient to rise from a sitting position with hands folded across the chest. Proximal myopathy is a feature of more severe hyperparathyroidism. Occasionally, patients are referred for evaluation because of ulcerating nonhealing skin lesions due to calciphylaxis, a serious life-threatening condition that often requires immediate parathyroidectomy.

Appropriate imaging studies to ascertain the effects of chronic excess PTH secretion include anteroposterior X-ray views of both hands and the pelvis, where the early signs of hyperparathyroidism are easily discernable (Figs. 11.4–11.9). Since the earliest radiological signs of excess PTH are first seen in phalanges of hands and symphysis pubis, other X-rays may not be necessary in the initial evaluation of the patient. In selected cases, site-specific X-rays may be helpful to exclude brown tumors, which are usually seen in patients with evidence of significant subperiosteal bone resorption on X-rays. Serum total and bone-specific alkaline phosphatase levels are almost always elevated in patients with tertiary and refractory secondary hyperparathyroidism and serve as useful biochemical clues for selecting patients for further imaging.

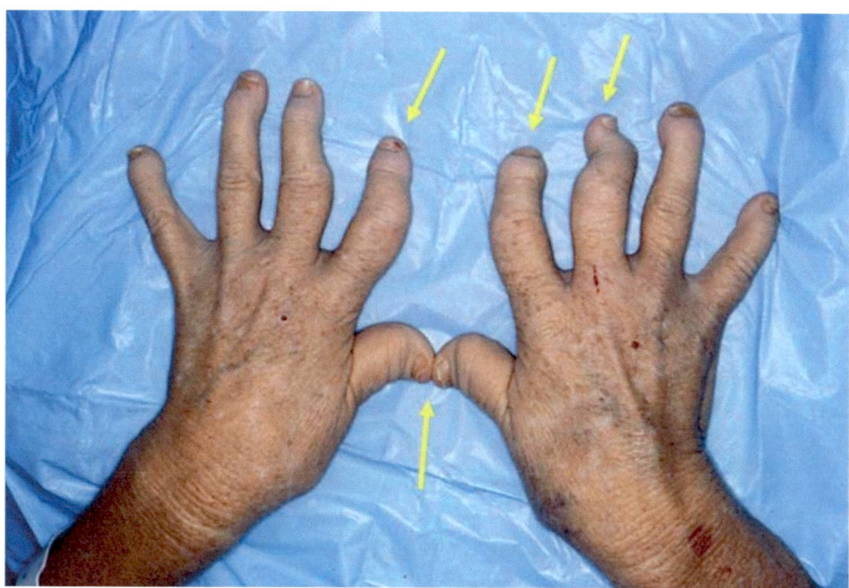

Fig. 11.3 Pseudoclubbing due to resorption of terminal digital bones due to severe refractory hyperparathyroidism

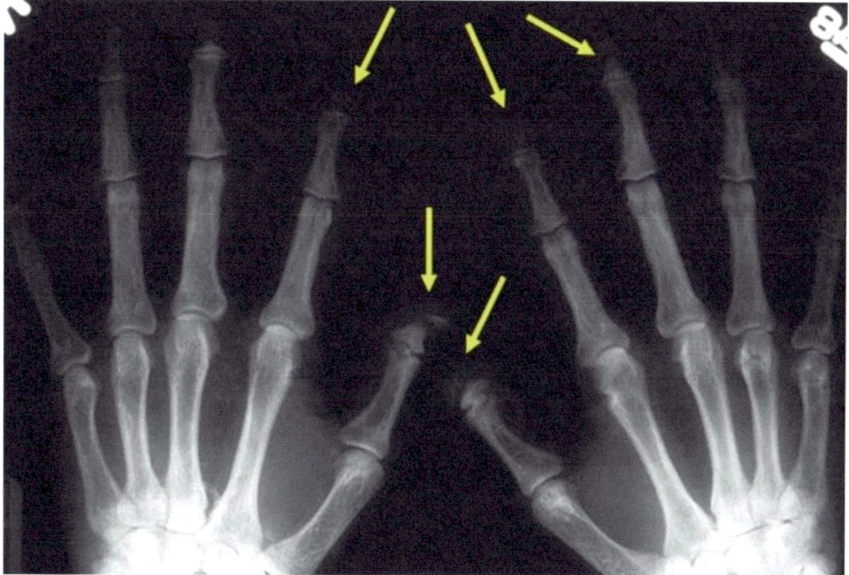

Fig. 11.4 X-ray of hands from the patient in Fig. 11.3. Not the loss of terminal digital bones resulting in "pseudoclubbing"

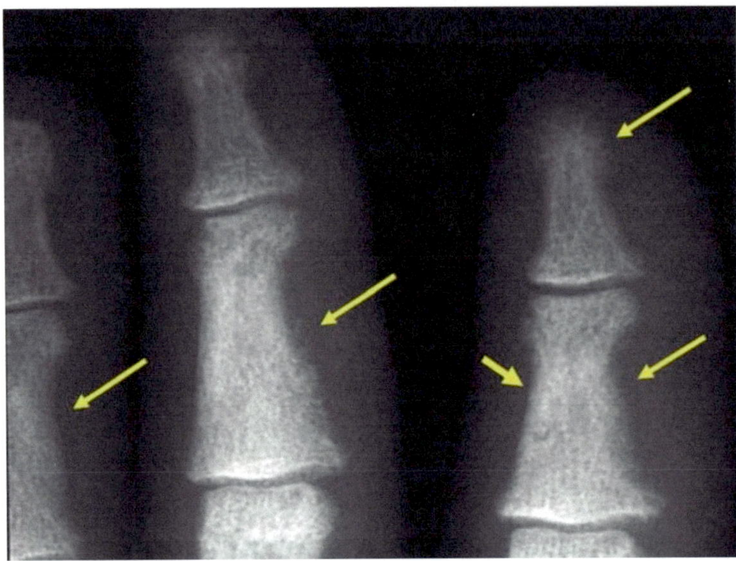

Fig. 11.5 Scalloping subperiosteal bone resorption in the middle phalanges (*thin long arrows*). Note the loss of cortical details (*short thick arrow*) and "penciling" of the terminal phalanges (*thin long arrow*) due to severe refractory hyperparathyroidism

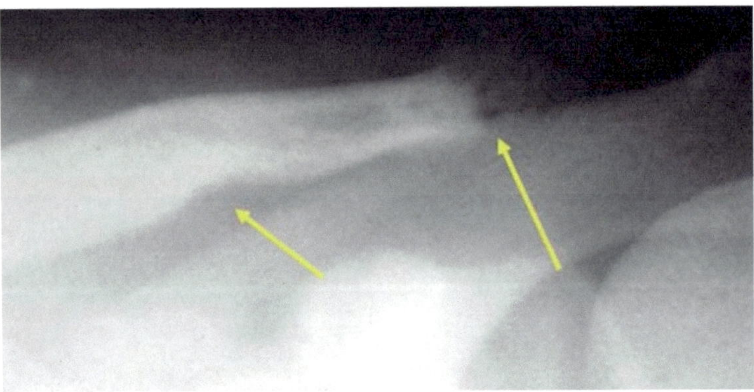

Fig. 11.6 Scalloping bone resorption in the clavicle. Note the resorption of the lateral end and the "thumb print impression"-type resorption of the inferior aspect of the clavicle (*arrows*) due to severe refractory hyperparathyroidism

Since bone mineral density is inevitably reduced in patients with tertiary hyperparathyroidism, we do not recommend its routine measurement. However, a bone biopsy, following in vivo double-tetracycline labeling, is very useful in characterizing the exact bone histology, assessing the severity of PTH's effects on bone histology and marrow fibrosis (Figs. 11.10–11.12), and predicting response to parathyroidectomy [12]. Regrettably, very few clinicians take advantage of this simple diagnostic

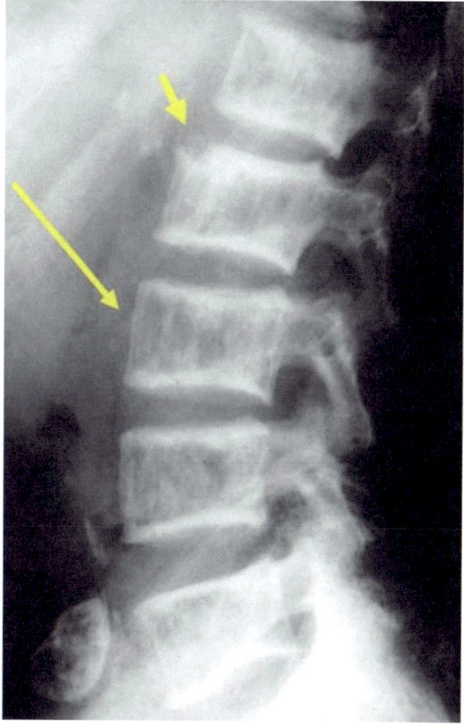

Fig. 11.7 Sclerotic vertebrae ("Rugger Jersey" Spine) with erosions (*short arrow*), and cystic changes within the vertebrae (*long arrow*) due to severe tertiary hyperparathyroidism

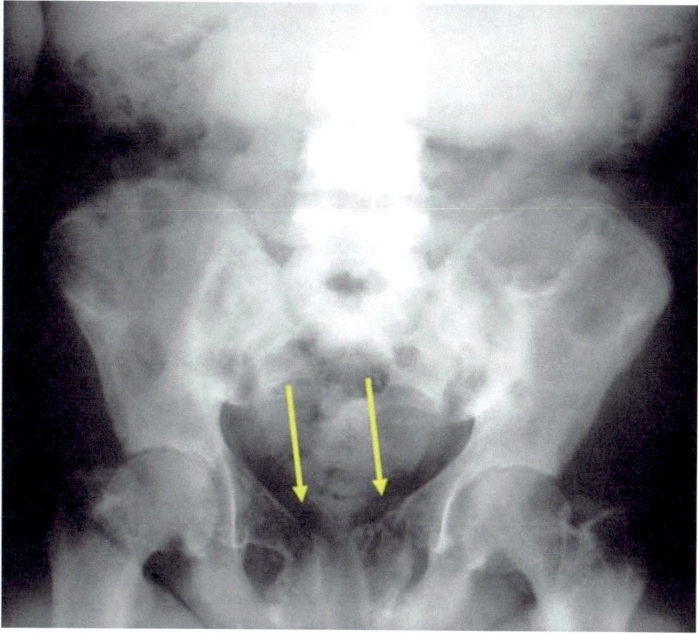

Fig. 11.8 Cystic expansile lesions in both superior pubic rami with widened symphysis pubis due to severe tertiary hyperparathyroidism (*arrows*)

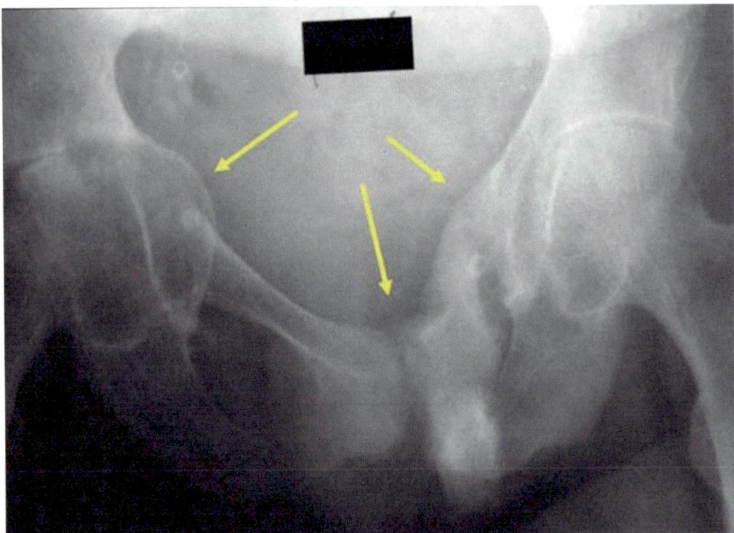

Fig. 11.9 Deformed pelvis resulting from distorted symphysis pubis and protrusio acetabuli due to severe tertiary hyperparathyroidism (*arrows*)

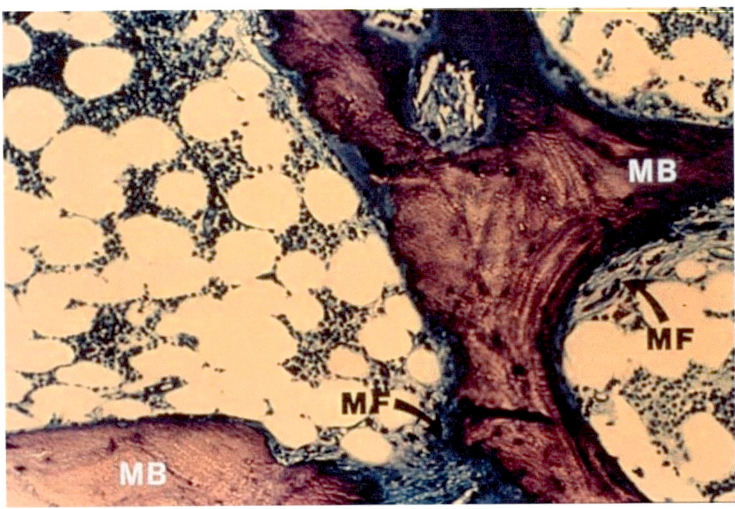

Fig. 11.10 Renal osteodystrophy (ROD) showing peritrabecular fibrosis (MF) along with normal mineralized bone (MB). An area of intratrabecular resorption is seen at the top (Rao, DS et al. N Engl J Med. Reprinted with permission. Copyright © 1993 Massachusetts Medical Society. All rights reserved)

procedure, and instead rely heavily on biochemical measurements, which are at best difficult to interpret and at worst misleading. A properly in vivo tetracycline-labeled and analyzed bone biopsy can provide the necessary information essential in the management of the patient with renal osteodystrophy.

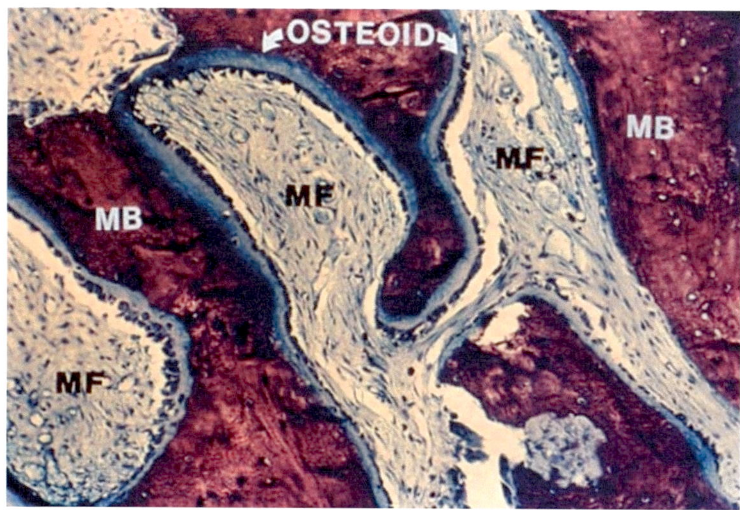

Fig. 11.11 Renal osteodystrophy (ROD) showing severe bone marrow fibrosis occupying the entire marrow space, a process that leads to erythropoietin resistance. Note the increased osteoid surface and thickness, often misinterpreted as "high turnover osteomalacia" or "hyperosteiodosis." However, tetracycline double labeling was present in >70% of the surfaces, and bone formation was increased, thus excluding osteomalacia in this patient (Rao, DS et al. N Engl J Med. Reprinted with permission. Copyright © 1993 Massachusetts Medical Society. All rights reserved)

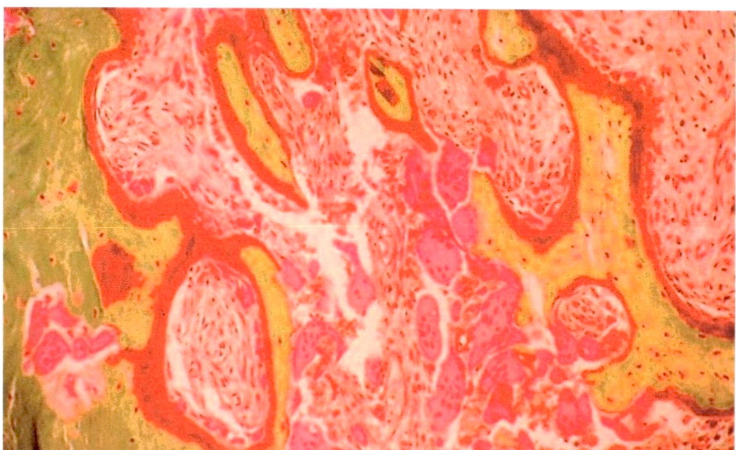

Fig. 11.12 Renal osteodystrophy (ROD) with streaming osteoclasts and marrow fibrosis occupying almost the entire marrow space. No discernable hematopoietic cells are seen. Note the increased osteoid surface and thickness (*red*), but osteomalacia is excluded by the presence of double-tetracycline labeling and increased bone formation rate. The green areas represent mineralized bone. Also, note the increased number of osteocytes (*red dots* within the green areas) indicative of a high turnover state that facilitates the recruitment of osteoblasts, which ultimately become osteocytes in the mineralized bone

Medical Management

As CKD progresses, abnormalities in phosphate handling, calcitriol synthesis, and the control of secretion and proliferation of parathyroid cells fuel the transition of secondary hyperparathyroidism to refractory secondary and eventually to tertiary hyperparathyroidism in a subset of patients on dialysis. This transition is often accompanied by a distinct parathyroid pathology—that of nodular hyperplasia on the background of diffuse hyperplasia [4, 13, 14]. At this stage, effective medical management and dietary strategies are challenging to implement and have limited success in terms of outcomes.

Physicians treating patients with CKD at different stages, both pre- and postdialysis, use the following approaches in an attempt to alter the abnormal pathophysiology described above and improve clinical outcomes. These include dietary phosphate restriction, phosphate binders, vitamin D sterols, and the calcimimetic, cinacalcet [15]. Each approach addresses one or more of the mineral and hormonal abnormalities in patients with CKD. The National Kidney Foundation (NKF) has developed the Kidney Disease Outcomes Quality Initiative (K-DOQI) guidelines for practitioners to direct their management of the mineral and hormonal alterations in patients with CKD [16]. These include the following specific targets for these parameters: (1) intact PTH, 150–300 pg/ml (15.9–31.8 pmol/L); (2) serum Ca, 8.4–9.5 mg/dl (2.10–2.37 mmol/L); (3) serum P, 3.5–5.5 mg/dl (1.13–1.78 mmol/L); and (4) $Ca \times P$ product, <55 mg^2/dl^2 (<4.44 $mmol^2/L^2$). Needless to say, it is challenging to reach and then maintain these biochemical targets in patients with secondary hyperparathyroidism on dialysis, despite the variety and potency of available therapies. Currently, it is estimated that <10% of patients on dialysis meet all four of these target end points [16].

Phosphate Binders

Once refractory secondary hyperparathyroidism develops, patients usually have either failed or failed to comply with recommended strategies to control serum P levels. Nevertheless, all the management approaches should be carefully reconsidered and attempted, as appropriate in a given patient, before referring for parathyroidectomy. As noted above, management begins with a careful review of the timing and dosing of prior therapeutic interventions to which the patient has been exposed.

Abnormalities in renal P clearance and hyperphosphatemia are addressed by prescribing a phosphate-restricted diet and phosphate binders. Avoiding calcium-containing phosphate binders (calcium acetate or carbonate) is advised in order to prevent further rises in serum Ca and the risk of vascular, valvular, and soft tissue calcifications in patients with tertiary hyperparathyroidism. Ectopic calcification may increase the risk of vascular complications in these high-risk patients. Preferred phosphate binders are the non-Ca-containing options which include sevelamer hydrochloride (800–1,600 mg three times daily with meals, depending on the serum P level) [17] and lanthanum carbonate (1,500–3,000 mg divided into doses with meals) [18]. These options are recommended and are titrated in order to achieve the target serum P concentration as advised by the NKF-K/DOQI guidelines [15]. Unfortunately, poor dietary compliance is often the cause of poorly controlled serum P levels and hyperphosphatemia. In such patients, it is essential to aggressively pursue phosphate lowering strategies in order to reduce the serum $Ca \times P$ product and avoid parathyroidectomy. Usually, such patients have been on dialysis for 10–20 or more years and have significant comorbidity, such as cardiovascular disease, nutritional compromise, fractures, bone pain, and myopathy. This places these individuals with tertiary hyperparathyroidism at high risk for parathyroidectomy.

Vitamin D and Its Analogues

The mainstay of medical therapy for secondary hyperparathyroidism is calcitriol or an activated vitamin D analogue [19–21]. The patient presenting with tertiary hyperparathyroidism, however, usually has been receiving daily oral calcitriol or intravenous calcitriol or paricalcitol with dialysis, often for many years, and has become progressively resistant to those therapies. Once persistent hypercalcemia develops, calcitriol or vitamin D analogue therapy is generally held. Rechallenging of the patient with tertiary hyperparathyroidism with an activated form of vitamin D (calcitriol or another compound in Table 11.3)—even in low doses—must be performed with caution and with close monitoring of serum Ca and P. Calcitriol therapy often further increases serum Ca and P levels, and usually has to be stopped. Rarely can the titration regimens, detailed in Table 11.3, be employed in patients with refractory secondary or tertiary hyperparathyroidism. Thus, calcitriol and vitamin D analogues, which are invaluable therapeutic strategies to suppress PTH secretion in patients with CKD, are challenging to administer in those with tertiary hyperparathyroidism. The complications of hypercalcemia and hyperphosphatemia result from increased intestinal absorption of calcium and phosphate.

Considerable research has been directed toward identifying noncalcemic analogues of calcitriol to control secondary hyperparathyroidism without further increasing hypercalcemia, hyperphosphatemia, and raising the $Ca \times P$ product further [19–21]. Unfortunately, none of the analogues currently available in the USA (paricalcitol and doxercalciferol) are ideal and able to meet the treatment goals completely. This is especially true if upward dose titrations are needed to lower intact PTH levels to achieve the NKF-K/DOQI target (see Table 11.3). Paricalcitol is less hypercalcemic both in animal models and in human studies compared to calcitriol [19–21]; however, with dose escalation, the same concerns of hypercalcemia become apparent. Although doxercalciferol requires hepatic 25-hydroxylation to become 1,25-dihydroxyvitamin D2 and achieve its inhibitory effect on PTH secretion, this agent too has the same narrow therapeutic window as calcitriol in patients with refractory secondary or tertiary hyperparathyroidism. Other vitamin D analogues, available outside the USA, may be better able to accomplish PTH suppression without raising serum Ca and P levels in tertiary hyperparathyroidism, and more data are needed in this group of patients.

Table 11.3 Vitamin D and its analogues used in the treatment of mineral abnormalities and secondary hyperparathyroidism in patients with CKD

Analogue	Compound	Dosing
Calcitriol[a]	1 alpha, 25 dihydroxyvitamin D3	Oral: 0.25–1.0 mcg/day or every other day or three times/week; supplied as 0.25 or 0.5 mcg capsules and oral solution (1 mcg/ml); increase dose by 0.25 mcg/day every 4–8 weeks; usual doses: 0.5–1.0 mcg/day
		Intravenous: 1.0 (0.02 mcg/kg) to 2.0 mcg by injection given with dialysis three times weekly; dose increases of 0.5–1.0 mcg recommended at 2–4-week intervals; dose range: 0.5–4 mcg
Doxercalciferol[b]	1 alpha hydroxyvitamin D2	Oral: 10 mcg/three times weekly at dialysis; can be titrated by 2.5 mcg at 8-week intervals if PTH >300 pg/ml; maximum dose: 20 mcg/three times weekly
		Intravenous: 4 mcg given three times weekly at the end of dialysis; increase based on PTH >300 pg/ml and other parameters by 1 to 2 mcg/dose at 8-week intervals
Paricalcitol[c]	19-nor-1 alpha, 25 dihydroxy vitamin D2	Oral: 1 to 2 mcg/day or 2–4 mcg three times weekly (depending on the initial PTH value—either below or above 500 pg/ml and the serum Ca and P concentrations)
		Intravenous: 0.04 mcg/kg to 0.1 mcg/kg (2.8–7 mcg) as bolus every other day with dialysis; may be increased by 2–4 mcg at 2–4 week intervals[d]
Alfacalcidiol[e–g]	1 alpha hydroxyvitamin D3	Oral: 1.0 mcg/day is usual initial dose with increases of 0.5 mcg/day every 2–4 weeks; usual dose: 1 to 2 mcg/day
		Intravenous: 1 mcg per dialysis (two or three times weekly); dosage increases of 1 mcg every week as necessary; maintenance dose: 6 mcg/week
Maxacalcitol[e]	22-oxa-1 alpha, 25-dihydroxyvitamin D3 or 22 oxa-calcitriol[g]	Consult prescribing information
Falecalcitriol[e]	1 alpha, 25 dihydroxy-26,27-F6 Vitamin D3[g]	Consult prescribing information

[a]Dosing adapted from Rocaltrol Prescribing Information at http://www.rocheusa.com for oral formulations and from Calcijex Prescribing Information at http://www.rxabbott.com for the intravenous formulation

[b]Dosing adapted from Hectoral Prescribing Information for oral and intravenous formulations at http://www.hectorol.com/healthcare

[c]Dosing adapted from Zemplar Prescribing Information at http://www.rxabbott.com

[d]An alternative intravenous dosing regimen (three times weekly) is recommended as follows: 2.5–5 mcg for PTH levels of 300–600 pg/ml; 6–10 mcg for PTH levels of 600–1,000 pg/ml; and 10–15 mcg for PTH levels >1,000 pg/ml (g)

[e]Not approved for use in the USA

[f]Dosing information adapted from http://www.drugs.com/mmx/one-alpha.html

[g]For dosing information, consult recommendations and regulatory information available in country where prescribed

Although therapy with vitamin D analogues is challenging in patients with refractory secondary or tertiary hyperparathyroidism, activated forms of vitamin D can be combined, often quite advantageously, with the calcimimetic agent cinacalcet (described below) in order to lower the serum Ca and PTH levels and the $Ca \times P$ product in patients with tertiary hyperparathyroidism. The calcemic effects of calcitriol or its analogues are counteracted by the serum Ca-lowering actions of cinacalcet. In this manner, substantial PTH lowering can be achieved without raising serum Ca levels.

Cinacalcet

Identification of the CaSR as a critical molecule in the control of PTH secretion and parathyroid cell proliferation opened up opportunities for developing compounds capable of interacting with this receptor to control parathyroid function [20, 22, 23]. Cinacalcet, one such agent, is an allosteric modulator of the CaSR that interacts with the receptor to enhance its sensitivity to ambient serum Ca. This facilitates inhibition of PTH secretion and cell growth through the CaSR—two critical cellular functions that are overactive in advanced CKD. Although CaSR expression appears to be downregulated in the parathyroid glands removed at surgery from patients with advanced CKD (i.e., patients with refractory secondary and tertiary hyperparathyroidism), calcimimetic therapy can still suppress PTH secretion [4, 13, 15, 22, 23]. As noted above, cinacalcet can be combined with vitamin D analogues in patients with severe and autonomous forms of hyperparathyroidism in an effort to forestall surgery and improve clinical status.

Several placebo-controlled trials have established the safety and efficacy of cinacalcet in patients with uremic secondary hyperparathyroidism [24–26]. Most patients in these trials, however, did not have tertiary hyperparathyroidism but were enrolled because of *uncontrolled* secondary hyperparathyroidism. The majority were taking phosphate binders (93%) and activated vitamin D or its analogues (66%) prior to enrollment into and during the study [24]. Therefore, to some extent, their hyperparathyroidism had resisted standard medical management to achieve NKF-K/DOQI goals.

In reporting combined data from two of these pivotal trials, Block et al. [24] noted that 43% of patients ($N=371$) treated with once-daily doses of cinacalcet (30–180 mg) for 26 weeks achieved a reduction in PTH levels from an average baseline of 642 ± 18 pg/ml to ≤ 250 pg/ml (≤ 26.5 pmol/L) (the primary endpoint of the study)—compared to only 5% of placebo-treated patients ($N=370$). In a subgroup analysis of patients with severe secondary hyperparathyroidism and baseline PTH levels > 800 pg/ml (> 84.8 pmol/L), 63% of those treated with cinacalcet experienced a 30% or greater decrement in PTH vs. only 7% of placebo-treated patients. Further analysis showed that the likelihood of achieving serum PTH levels of 250 pg/ml (26.5 pmol/L) or lower, if the initial serum Ca levels were > 10.2 mg/dl, was 9.4-fold greater (CI: 3.5–25.5) if patients were given cinacalcet vs. placebo.

Longer duration of dialysis (>5 years) or higher baseline serum P levels (>6.0 mg/dl) or Ca×P products (>60 mg^2/dl^2) did not block responsiveness to cinacalcet. In the entire group of patients, average serum Ca and P levels fell by 6.8 and 8.4%, respectively, with a fall in the Ca×P product of 14.6%—changes all representing significant improvements vs. treatment with placebo [24]. The safety profile of this agent was acceptable overall with nausea and vomiting occurring in ~30% of cinacalcet-treated patients, compared to 16–19% for these side effects in placebo-treated patients [24]. Hypocalcemia (defined as serum Ca<7.5 mg/dl) was observed in ~5% of cinacalcet-treated vs. 1% in placebo-treated patients [24] but would be unlikely in a patient with tertiary hyperparathyroidism. Thus, the observed biochemical and hormonal changes due to cinacalcet, if large enough and sustainable in patients with tertiary hyperparathyroidism, would be expected to produce improved clinical outcomes, but this has not been demonstrated in prospective studies.

Data on the long-term biochemical control of secondary hyperparathyroidism as well as any improvements in quality of life, skeletal and cardiovascular complications, and mortality due to therapy with cinacalcet are extremely limited. In studies of 6 months' duration, 46–65% of patients receiving cinacalcet achieved NKF-K/DOQI targets for serum Ca, P, and PTH and Ca×P product—significantly better than the percentages of placebo-treated patients at these targets (10–30%) [25]. Open-label extensions of the initial clinical trials showed that >50% of patients maintained serum PTH levels in the NKF-K/DOQI target range at 52 and 100 weeks of therapy with cinacalcet [26]. Thus, while placebo-controlled trial data on the chronic administration of cinacalcet to patients with tertiary hyperparathyroidism are unavailable, this agent still remains the most plausible, mechanistically sound way to attempt to control the biochemical and hormonal derangements in these patients without surgery.

Cinacalcet has been tested in several small studies of patients with persistent hypercalcemic hyperparathyroidism after renal transplantation [27–31]. In that population, persisting hyperparathyroidism and hypercalcemia have been implicated in declining graft function, progressive bone demineralization, and ectopic calcifications. Cinacalcet therapy is effective at significantly lowering serum PTH and Ca levels in these patients, although it is not FDA approved for this indication. Cinacalcet has also been used to lower serum PTH and Ca levels in patients with CKD who have refractory hyperparathyroidism—after parathyroidectomy—due to either graft hyperfunction or the presence of ectopic or supernumerary parathyroid tissue [32, 33]. Limited experience has been reported on the use of cinacalcet in patients with two of the most dreaded complications of hyperparathyroidism: calciphylaxis [34, 35] and parathyromatosis [36, 37]. Fortunately, both are rare conditions with the latter occurring as a complication of prior surgery during which spillage of parathyroid tissue occurred. No doubt, larger published experience will emerge regarding management of these patient populations over time. At present, it is clear that targeting the CaSR remains a critical component of the medical armamentarium to control overactive parathyroid tissue in patients with CKD.

Summary

In conclusion, tertiary hyperparathyroidism is an end result of chronic excessive demands on the parathyroid glands to secrete hormone and to grow, imposed by an altered homeostatic system. These demands can be met initially by increased secretion by each cell, but cannot be sustained indefinitely, without proliferation and expansion of cell mass, eventually leading to gland enlargement and autonomy. In some ways, tertiary hyperparathyroidism is analogous to endemic goiter due to prolonged and severe iodine deficiency. The goiter rarely involutes with iodine replacement. In fact, many patients develop hyperthyroidism with iodine supplementation due to underlying autonomous function!

Most patients have characteristic clinical, biochemical, radiological, and bone histological features. Most do not respond adequately to medical therapy, but it is well-worth a trial with calcitriol or its analogues and cinacalcet. Post parathyroidectomy, these patients often experience "bone hunger," which may be prolonged. An experienced team approach is essential to avoid peri- and postoperative problems.

References

1. Parfitt AM. Parathyroid growth: normal and abnormal. In: Bilezikian JP, Levine MA, Marcus R, editors. The parathyroids: basic and clinical concepts. New York: Academic; 2001. p. 293–330.
2. Arnold A, Brown MF, Urena P, Gaz RD, Sarfati E, Drueke T. Monoclonality of parathyroid tumors in chronic renal failure and in primary hyperparathyroid hyperplasia. J Clin Invest. 1995;95:2047–53.
3. Drueke TB. The pathogenesis of parathyroid gland hyperplasia in chronic renal failure. Kidney Int. 1995;48:259–72.
4. Goodman WG, Quarles LD. Development and progression of secondary hyperparathyroidism in chronic kidney disease: lessons from molecular genetics. Kidney Int. 2008;74:276–88.
5. Indridason OS, Quarles DL. Tertiary hyperparathyroidism and refractory secondary hyperparathyroidism. In: Favus MJ, editor. Primer on the metabolic bone diseases and disorders of mineral metabolism. Chicago: Lippincott Williams & Wilkins; 1999. p. 198–202.
6. Bolla G, Disdler P, Harle JR, et al. Hyperparathyroidie tertiaire revelatrice d'une maladie coeliaque de l'adulte. Presse Med. 1994;23:346–8.
7. Savio RM, Gosnell JE, Posen S, Reeve TS, Delbridge LW. Parathyroidectomy for tertiary hyperparathyroidism associated with X-linked dominant hypophosphatemic rickets. Arch Surg. 2004;139:218–22.
8. Mchenry CR, Mostafavi K, Murphy TA. Tertiary hyperparathyroidism attributable to long-term oral phosphate therapy. Endocr Pract. 2006;12:294–8.
9. Parfitt AM, Wang Q, Palnitkar S. Rates of cell proliferation in adenomatous, suppressed, and normal parathyroid tissue: implications for pathogenesis. J Clin Endocrinol Metab. 1998;83:863–9.
10. Grzela T, Chudzinski W, Lasiecka Z, et al. The calcium-sensing receptor and vitamin D receptor expression in tertiary hyperparathyroidism. Int J Mol Med. 2006;17:779–83.
11. Wang Q, Palnitkar S, Parfitt AM. Parathyroid cell proliferation in the rat: effect of age and of phosphate administration and recovery. Endocrinology. 1996;137:4558–62.
12. Al BW, Martin KJ. Role of bone biopsy in renal osteodystrophy. Saudi J Kidney Dis Transpl. 2009;20:12–9.

13. Drueke T, Martin D, Rodriguez M. Can calcimimetics inhibit parathyroid hyperplasia? Evidence from preclinical studies. Nephrol Dial Transplant. 2007;22:1828–39.
14. Martin KJ, Gonzalez EA. Metabolic bone disease in chronic kidney disease. J Am Soc Nephrol. 2007;18:875–85.
15. Cozzolino M, Galassi A, Pasho S, Fallabrino G, Gallieni M, Brancaccio D. Preventive measures and new pharmacological approaches of calcium and phosphate disorders. Contrib Nephrol. 2008;161:234–9.
16. Eknoyan G, Levin A, Levin NW, National Kidney Foundation. K/DOQI clinical practice guidelines for bone metabolism and disease in chronic kidney disease. Kidney disease outcomes quality initiative. Am J Kidney Dis. 2003;42 Suppl 3:S-1–201.
17. Prescribing information for renagel, http://www.renagel.com. Accessed 3 Aug 2009.
18. Prescribing information for fosrenol, http://www.fosrenol.com .Accessed 3 Aug 2009.
19. Andress DL, Vitamin D. Treatment in chronic kidney disease. Semin Dial. 2005;18:315–21.
20. Hudson JQ. Secondary hyperparathyroidism in chronic kidney disease: focus on clinical consequences and vitamin D therapies. Ann Pharmacother. 2006;40:1584–93.
21. Brown AJ, Slatopolsky E. Drug insight: vitamin D analogs in the treatment of secondary hyperparathyroidism in patients with chronic kidney disease. Nat Clin Pract Endocrinol Metab. 2007;3:134–44.
22. Brown EM. Clinical lessons from the calcium-sensing receptor. Nat Clin Pract Endocrinol Metab. 2007;3:122–33.
23. Shahapuni I, Monge M, Oprisiu R, et al. Drug Insight: renal indications of calcimimetics. Nat Clin Pract Nephrol. 2006;2:316–25.
24. Block GA, Martin KJ, de Francisco AL, et al. Cinacalcet for secondary hyperparathyroidism in patients receiving hemodialysis. N Engl J Med. 2004;350:1516–25.
25. Moe SM, Chertow GM, Coburn JW, et al. Achieving NKF-K/DOQI bone metabolism and disease treatment goals with cinacalcet HCl. Kidney Int. 2005;67:760–71.
26. Moe SM, Cunningham J, Bommer J, et al. Long-term treatment of secondary hyperparathyroidism with the calcimimetic cinacalcet HCl. Nephrol Dial Transplant. 2005;20:2186–93.
27. Kruse AE, Eisenberger U, Frey FJ, Mohaupt MG. The calcimimetic cinacalcet normalizes serum calcium in renal transplant patients with persistent hyperparathyroidism. Nephrol Dial Transplant. 2005;20:1311–4.
28. Apostolou T, Kollia K, Damianou L, et al. Hypercalcemia due to resistant hyperparathyroidism in renal transplant patients treated with the calcimimetic agent cinacalcet. Transplant Proc. 2006;38:3514–6.
29. Szwarc I, Argiles A, Garrigue V, et al. Cinacalcet chloride is efficient and safe in renal transplant recipients with posttransplant hyperparathyroidism. Transplantation. 2006;82:675–80.
30. El-Amm JM, Doshi MD, Singh A, et al. Preliminary experience with cinacalcet use in persistent secondary hyperparathyroidism after kidney transplantation. Transplantation. 2007;83:546–9.
31. Serra AL, Braun SC, Starke A, et al. Pharmacokinetics and pharmacodynamics of cinacalcet in patients with hyperparathyroidism after renal transplantation. Am J Transplant. 2008;8:803–10.
32. Dorsch O. Use of cinacalcet in a patient on long-term dialysis with end-stage renal failure and refractory secondary hyperparathyroidism. Nephrol Dial Transplant. 2007;22:637–40.
33. Lomonte C, Antonelli M, Losurdo N, Marchio G, Giammaria B, Basile C. Cinacalcet is effective in relapses of secondary hyperparathyroidism after parathyroidectomy. Nephrol Dial Transplant. 2007;22:2056–62.
34. Robinson MR, Augustine JJ, Korman NJ. Cinacalcet for the treatment of calciphylaxis. Arch Dermatol. 2007;143:152–4.
35. Mohammed IA, Sekar V, Bubtana AJ, Mitra S, Hutchison AJ. Proximal calciphylaxis treated with calcimimetic "Cinacalcet". Nephrol Dial Transplant. 2008;23:387–9.
36. Daphnis E, Stylianou K, Katsipi I, et al. Parathyromatosis and the challenge of treatment. Am J Kidney Dis. 2006;48:502–5.
37. Unbehaun R, Lauerwald W. Successful use of cinacalcet HCl in a patient with end-stage renal failure and refractory secondary hyperparathyroidism due to parathyromatosis. Clin Nephrol. 2007;67:188–92.

Chapter 12
Surgical Treatment of Persistent Hyperparathyroidism After Renal Transplantation

Frederic Triponez and Pieter Evenepoel

Keywords Indications and timing for parathyroidectomy in tertiary hyperparathyroidism • Renal transplantation • Tertiary HPT pathophysiology • Clinical features and medical management • Thymectomy • Parathyroid graft function and survival • Cryopreservation • Intraoperative PTH monitoring in tertiary hyperparathyroidism.

Patient

The patient is a 35-year-old man with polycystic kidney disease. He has been on dialysis for 5 years and received a kidney graft 3 months ago. During the course of dialysis, he presented severe secondary hyperparathyroidism (HPT) (parathyroid hormone [PTH]) up to 100 times the upper limit of normal without hypercalcemia and with two parathyroid glands measuring more than 1 cm at ultrasound examination. He did not undergo parathyroidectomy (PTX) because the secondary HPT could be controlled with vitamin D analogues and calcimimetics. Three months after kidney transplantation, he presents with tertiary HPT with hypercalcemia, 10.4 mg/dl (2.6 mmol/l), and high levels of PTH (30 times the upper limit of normal). His bone density scan shows osteopenia.

F. Triponez, MD (✉)
Thoracic and endocrine surgery, University Hospital of Geneva, 1211 Geneva, Switzerland
e-mail: frederic.triponez@hcuge.ch

P. Evenepoel
Department of Medicine, Division of Nephrology,
University of Leuven, Leuven, Belgium
e-mail: pieter.evenepoel@uz.kuleuven.ac.be

A.A. Khan and O.H. Clark (eds.), *Handbook of Parathyroid Diseases:*
A Case-Based Practical Guide, DOI 10.1007/978-1-4614-2164-1_12,
© Springer Science+Business Media, LLC 2012

Questions
1. What are the indications for PTX in patients after kidney transplantation?
2. Are there other therapeutic options?
3. When is the ideal time for a PTX completed after a kidney transplantation?
4. Which investigations are recommended preoperatively?
5. Which operation should be performed?
6. What are the expected symptomatic and metabolic benefits of PTX?
7. What are the risks of PTX?

Pathophysiology of Tertiary HPT After Renal Transplantation

Secondary HPT is a common sequela of chronic renal failure. The pathogenesis is complex but involves hypocalcemia, hyperphosphatemia, and low 1,25 vitamin D (calcitriol) [1–3] (see Chap. 9 of this book).

Successful kidney transplantation corrects the physiologic and metabolic abnormalities responsible for secondary HPT [4, 5]. PTH levels show a biphasic decline after successful renal transplantation: a rapid drop (by approximately 50%) during the first 3–6 months, attributed to a reduction of the parathyroid functional mass [5], followed by a more gradual decline [6]. The long life span of parathyroid cells (approximately 20 years) [7] contributes to the very slow involution of the hyperplastic parathyroid glands after renal transplantation. As a result, elevated intact PTH levels persist in more than 25% of patients 1 year after transplantation, despite the presence of normal renal function [6, 8]. This condition is often referred to as tertiary or autonomous HPT [9]. The term autonomous HPT refers to a specific functional state of the parathyroid glands: being relatively nonresponsive to negative feedback mechanisms.

Prolonged renal failure before and during dialysis, as well as high serum PTH, calcium, phosphorus, and/or alkaline phosphatase levels at the time of kidney transplantation, is associated with tertiary HPT [1, 6]. These findings, and the observation of large parathyroid glands by ultrasonography [10], predict the severity of posttransplant HPT. Renal graft function is also an important determinant of posttransplant PTH serum levels [6]. Immunosuppressive drugs, including steroids, also contribute to tertiary HPT [11, 12]. Finally, low 25(OH)VitD3 [8] and calcitriol levels [12, 13] and diminished expression of vitamin D and calcium-sensing receptor [14] are involved in the pathogenesis of tertiary HPT after renal transplantation.

Clinical Implications of Tertiary HPT

Tertiary HPT is present after transplantation in patients with hypercalcemia and hypophosphatemia and can adversely affect bone density. High PTH concentrations stimulate the renal production of calcitriol which in turn increases intestinal calcium absorption and improves the skeletal mobilization of calcium. Correction of uremia and normalization of serum phosphorus levels are additional factors contributing to the resolution of the skeletal resistance to PTH, thus facilitating the release of calcium due to osteoclastic bone resorption [15]. Finally, resorption of soft tissue calcifications can also contribute to posttransplantation hypercalcemia [15]. Hypercalcemia and high levels of PTH can lead to muscle weakness, fatigue, constipation, depression, and other symptoms. Moreover, adverse cardiovascular events are more likely in patients on dialysis [16].

Hypophosphatemia occurs in up to 90% of renal-transplant recipients and is linked to dysregulation of renal tubular phosphate reabsorption. Tertiary HPT, immunosuppressive drugs, and diuretics are all involved in the pathogenesis of urinary phosphorus wasting and posttransplant hypophosphatemia or "tertiary hyperphosphatoninism" [17]. A major consequence of persistent renal phosphorus wasting after renal transplantation is a progressive decrease in bone mineral density (BMD) which contributes to the increased fracture risk in these patients.

Prospective studies have shown a rapid rate of bone loss during the first 6 months after renal transplantation (about 1.5% per month at the lumbar spine) [15]. Limited data is available regarding posttransplant bone morphology. Most studies reflect a decrease in bone formation in the face of persistently elevated bone resorption. This imbalance, together with a prolonged mineralization lag time, contributes to the progressive loss of bone mass. Thus, renal-transplant recipients are at increased risk of fractures because of immunosuppressive drugs (particularly corticosteroids), renal phosphorus wasting, hypophosphatemia, and a relative deficiency of calcitriol [6, 11, 18, 19]. Elevated blood PTH levels also independently adversely influence bone density [15, 20–22].

Medical Management of Persistent Hyperparathyroidism After Renal Transplantation

Because patients with tertiary HPT following renal transplantation have hypercalcemia and hypophosphatemia, "conventional" strategies (phosphate binders, calcium supplements, and vitamin D) are not indicated in most patients. Treatment of hypophosphatemia by oral phosphate administration accentuates hyperphosphaturia and may support the development of nephrocalcinosis. Renal-transplant candidates with severe secondary HPT, therefore, benefit from PTX before transplantation [6].

Cinacalcet, a calcimimetic agent, is now available for treating patients with secondary HPT. Calcimimetics allosterically modulate the Ca-sensing receptor (CaSR), increasing its sensitivity to extracellular Ca and thereby lowering PTH secretion from the parathyroid gland [23]. Cinacalcet is expensive (the additional cost per month per patient is estimated to vary from about $300 [30 mg] to $1,800 [180 mg]) [24, 25] and has not been approved for the treatment of tertiary HPT in most countries, leaving PTX as the only therapeutically effective option for these patients [16].

Indication and Timing of Posttransplant PTX

The selection of patients with tertiary HPT for PTX should be based on clinical and metabolic criteria, including persistent hypercalcemia, persistent hypercalciuria, renal phosphorus wasting, high bone turnover, and pruritus. However, no evidence-based guidelines have been published. For most clinicians, tertiary HPT with hypercalcemia is the main indication, although the absolute calcium level varies in different medical centers. Parathyroid gland volume is an additional indication. In one study, 90% of parathyroid glands weighing more than 500 mg contained hyperplastic nodules [26]. Apoptosis is unlikely to occur in nodular hyperplasia because of low vitamin D receptor expression [27]. Thus, after renal transplantation, patients with tertiary HPT and one or more parathyroid glands that weigh an estimated 500 mg or more have little chance of tertiary HPT regression.

In most medical centers, a delay of 1 year is recommended after kidney transplantation in order for the hyperplastic parathyroid glands to regress. In some centers, however, PTX is recommended at 3 months because most patients should have recovered normal parathyroid function by this time [4, 6]. Earlier PTX may lessen the detrimental metabolic effects of tertiary HPT [28].

Preoperative Imaging

Few studies have focused on the specificity and sensitivity of preoperative imaging studies in patients with tertiary HPT after renal transplantation. In one study, preoperative sestamibi scans failed to localize all the abnormal parathyroid glands in all 41 patients with secondary HPT and tertiary HPT, and only localized mediastinal parathyroid tumors in 3 of 8 patients [29]. Combining sestamibi, ultrasound, and magnetic resonance imaging (MRI) made it possible to localize the parathyroid glands in 63.2% of patients, according to Kebebew et al. [30], who concluded that these imaging techniques are not very useful in patients having an initial parathyroid operation. Other surgeons, conversely, and particularly those adhering to a focused surgical approach are rather enthusiastic about the added value of these techniques [31–33].

Ectopic parathyroid glands are found in about 30% of patients with renal HPT [34, 35]. Unfortunately, most ectopic glands are small intrathymic nests of parathyroid cells and are not likely to be identified by any imaging technique. Sestamibi and ultrasound tend to identify the largest parathyroid glands [36–39].

Preoperative imaging techniques provide some useful information about both the parathyroid and the thyroid glands, but cannot be recommended routinely based on scientific evidence and should be used selectively. The two most useful imaging techniques are neck ultrasound and sestamibi scintigraphy which can be used as an indication of the location and size of the biggest parathyroid glands. However, these imaging techniques only very rarely identify all parathyroid glands and, in our opinion, should not be used to direct the extent of PTX in tertiary HPT. In reoperative

PTX for tertiary HPT, we suggest to begin with neck ultrasound and sestamibi scintigraphy and, if these two studies are negative, to pursue with MRI, fine needle aspiration of a suspicious nodule with PTH measurement in the aspirated fluid. We reserve highly selective venous sampling for patients with persistent or recurrent secondary HPT or tertiary HPT and with negative noninvasive localization studies [30, 34, 39–42].

Surgical Treatment of Persistent Hyperparathyroidism After Renal Transplantation

Extent of Surgery

McPhaul first reported in 1964 that tertiary HPT could be successfully managed with subtotal PTX [43]. Because kidney-transplant recipients often have or may develop reduced kidney function, the recommended surgical approach is bilateral neck exploration and subtotal PTX or total PTX with autotransplantation [30, 35, 44–46]. This is the same treatment that is recommended by most parathyroid experts for patients with refractory secondary HPT [47–49].

No studies have directly compared the efficacy of subtotal PTX with total PTX+ autotransplantation for tertiary HPT. Retrospective studies suggest that the results between these two approaches are similar in tertiary HPT [35, 45, 46, 50, 51]. Both approaches aim at removing most of the parathyroid gland tissue (the "subtotal" approach). We prefer a subtotal PTX rather than total PTX with autotransplantation because of concern about hypoparathyroidism if parathyroid autograft does not function. During the operation, the most normal parathyroid gland should be biopsied first and marked with a clip and, if viable, the other parathyroid glands should be removed.

A more selective approach ("focused") is recommended by some experts on the basis of preoperative criteria (the results of localizing techniques) or intraoperative criteria (findings from macroscopic evaluation during bilateral neck exploration and intraoperative PTH (IOPTH) monitoring) [31–33, 52, 53]. The reason for this is that up to one-third of such patients with tertiary HPT are described as having a single- or double-parathyroid adenoma. Although this observation conflicts with the general belief that all four parathyroid glands are hyperplastic in tertiary HPT [54], these investigators report a success rate of greater than 90% when judged by postoperative symptom relief and normal calcium levels. They, therefore, suggest that when used selectively, up to one-third of patients with tertiary HPT could undergo less than subtotal PTX and have a success rate similar to that of patients who had a subtotal approach. However, the follow-up times were less than 6 months in three of these studies [31–33]. More importantly, postoperative PTH levels and renal function at follow-up were not reported, yet both are important in order to conclude that PTX is successful.

There are no prospective studies to our knowledge comparing both approaches ("focused" vs. "subtotal") in patients with tertiary HPT. However, there is good evidence that in patients with refractory secondary HPT a less-than-subtotal PTX increases the risk of failure and persistent or recurrent HPT [46, 55]. A retrospective analysis of 83 parathyroidectomies performed in 74 patients in Lille and San Francisco showed that a less-than-subtotal PTX was associated with 5.2 times (95% CI 1.4–20) increased risk of failure or recurrent HPT compared with subtotal PTX in patients with tertiary HPT [56]. We, therefore, recommend a subtotal approach as the standard surgical operation for patients with tertiary HPT.

Cryopreservation

Cryopreservation of hyperplastic parathyroid tissue resected during PTX for possible subsequent autotransplantation has been used to correct postoperative hypoparathyroidism. Although the rationale of this practice is sound, its implementation in daily practice may be hampered by logistic problems related to the freezing and storage of the tissue, as well as licensing requirements. Skepticism also remains about the functional capacity of the cryopreserved parathyroid glands [57]. A recent study reported that 46% of grafts functioned appropriately and 23% functioned partially after reimplantation [58]. These results by experts in the field are probably better than what occurs at other medical centers. As hypoparathyroidism can be observed after PTX and is increasingly acknowledged to confer health risks, more efforts are warranted to optimize the practice of cryopreservation.

Role of Simultaneous Thymectomy

In autopsy series, about 13% of individuals have more than four parathyroid glands [59], whereas in surgical series of parathyroidectomies for renal HPT or for familial HPT up to 30% of individuals have more than four parathyroid glands [34, 35, 60]. Most of the ectopic or supernumerary glands are found within the thymus. These ectopic parathyroid glands are usually responsible for recurrent HPT in patients with continuous stimuli to the parathyroid cells due to either renal insufficiency or genetic mutation. Some surgeons routinely perform an upper bilateral thymectomy in order to decrease the rate of recurrent or persistent HPT if renal function declines. The associated thymectomy slightly increases the risk of hypoparathyroidism and possibly the risk of injury to the recurrent laryngeal nerve, although the latter has never been demonstrated in this setting. In surgery for thyroid cancer, the association of thymectomy to the central neck dissection has been demonstrated to significantly increase the risk of hypoparathyroidism [61]. Other surgeons do not routinely remove the upper thymus in patients with tertiary HPT and good renal function.

In general, we recommend a thymectomy when an inferior gland is not found in its orthotopic location, when an intrathymic gland has been suggested by preoperative localizing techniques, and in most other patients with a higher risk of recurrent HPT (in patients with decreased renal function and in young patients with a long life expectancy).

Utility of Intraoperative PTH Monitoring

IOPTH monitoring has been reported to have an accuracy rate of >95% in patients with primary HPT [62–64]. However, it is not as accurate in patients with multiple abnormal parathyroid glands [65]. The accuracy of IOPTH in patients with renal HPT varies considerably [31, 50, 66–72]. IOPTH has often been reported independently of renal function (in patients on dialysis and in patients after kidney transplantation), and few articles have focused on patients with tertiary HPT. Only two studies, to our knowledge, have considered renal function when analyzing the accuracy of IOPTH monitoring; both showed a high positive predictive value (predicting cure when the patient is cured), but a poor negative predictive value (predicting insufficient resection in the patient with persistent HPT) [69, 72].

Three recent studies, two from the same group using the same patient population, showed that accuracy of IOPTH monitoring increased when the newest whole-PTH assay was used [50, 73, 74].

Given the low rate of treatment failure when a bilateral neck exploration is routinely performed, the overall clinical value of IOPTH monitoring remains controversial.

Surgical Complications

Sixteen of the forty-one studies on tertiary HPT reported the complication rate after surgery [3]. Transient hypocalcemia, the most common complication, ranged in frequency from less than 10% in studies using subtotal PTX to 100% of cases of total PTX plus autotransplantation. In patients after total PTX+ autotransplantation, the autotransplanted parathyroid tissue usually recovers its function a few months after PTX. Definitive hypoparathyroidism was reported in 0–10% of patients and appears more frequent after total PTX+ autotransplantation than after subtotal PTX.

Paralysis of the recurrent laryngeal nerve is another serious complication of PTX, but is usually transient. The rate of persistent recurrent laryngeal nerve palsy during an initial parathyroid exploration is estimated to be around 1% in experienced hands [75]. Other rarer complications can occur that are either directly related to the surgery, like wound infection, bleeding, or wound dehiscence, or potentially related to the hypoparathyroidism or hypocalcemia, like cardiac arrhythmia and cardiac failure, gout or pseudogout, pancreatitis, and renal failure.

Overall, PTX is a safe operation with an overall low complication rate; however, many patients who require PTX for tertiary HPT have numerous comorbidities.

Outcome

Calcium and Bone Metabolism

Most studies use biochemical criteria, such as the normalization of the serum calcium level and/or a decline of the PTH level, to define whether PTX has been successful. On the basis of these measures, most series report success rates between 70 and 100%.

Calcium levels decrease to below target levels after PTX in many patients. This is usually due, at least in the short term, to an increased shift of calcium from the circulation to the bone tissues (referred to as the "hungry bone" syndrome) [76]. In order to maintain the calcium levels within the normal range, many patients need intravenous calcium substitution soon after PTX. Oral calcium supplements are started as soon as the patient is able to swallow and the dose is progressively increased as necessary. Patients are advised to take the oral calcium salts separate from meals to enhance bioavailability. In most patients, active vitamin D supplements are started in the perioperative period in order to increase the absorption of calcium [77, 78]. Serum-ionized calcium and/or total calcium have to be monitored regularly, e.g., every 6–12 h for the first day or until the patient's calcium level is stable. After discharge, follow-up visits are mandatory because vitamin D and oral calcium supplements may need frequent adjustments to maintain the serum calcium level within the normal range.

There is little information related to the ideal range of PTH after kidney transplantation; however, PTH levels >200 pg/ml (21.5 pmol/l) correlated with low bone density in one study and with high turnover bone disease in another study. Clinicians should strive to maintain serum levels of calcium, phosphorus, and PTH within the targets put forward by the National Kidney Foundation for the different stages of chronic kidney disease [1]. The persisting stimulus created by ongoing uremia in patients with suboptimal renal function is likely to result in hypertrophy and hyperplasia of the remaining parathyroid tissue. Consequently, HPT may eventually be hypothesized to recur in the long term and the recurrence rate may be higher in patients with diminished renal function [56].

The 5-year survival rate for first cadaver kidney grafts is 67.1%, and only 79.8% of patients have a functioning kidney graft at 5 years. At 10 years, these rates decrease to 36.7 and 57.5%, respectively [79]. Thus, 20.2% of kidney-transplant recipients resume dialysis at 5 years and 42.5% at 10 years. Overall, about one-third of patients who receive a kidney transplant are at risk of redeveloping renal failure within 5 years after receiving the transplant, along with a return of the detrimental metabolic factors causing secondary HPT.

Serum phosphorus levels significantly increase after surgery, most probably as a result of decreased renal phosphorus wasting. This increase occurs despite increased bone deposition underlining the magnitude of renal phosphorus wasting in patients with tertiary HPT.

Serum alkaline phosphatase levels temporarily increase after PTX in patients with tertiary HPT [80–83]. Increased bone formation after PTX has been documented by bone histomorphometric studies showing an increase of the osteoblast surface after PTX. This increase reached a maximum at week 1 in cancellous bone and at week 4 in cortical bone [84]. Thereafter, a progressive decline toward normal levels was observed [51, 52, 68, 83].

Only three studies on PTX for tertiary HPT have reported the long-term effects on BMD [29, 85, 86]. The two most recent ones reported a mean increase of 7.1% of BMD 23 months after PTX [85] and 9.5% of BMD 37 months after PTX [86], respectively, when PTX was associated with optimal medical management (bone sparing immunosuppression, calcium and vitamin D supplementation).

Graft Function/Graft Survival

In contrast to older studies [87, 88], recent investigations generally show an increase in blood creatinine levels after PTX [83, 89–92]. The reason for the discrepancy might be that in the older studies only patients with severe hypercalcemia were referred for PTX. Because severe hypercalcemia impairs the GFR as a result of inducing renal vasoconstriction and nephrocalcinosis, when hypercalcemia in these patients is corrected, graft function may improve. The renal function deterioration in the early postoperative period may be related to the hemodynamic effects of PTH. Indeed, PTH has vasodilatory effects on preglomerular vessels at the same time as efferent arterioles are constricted, presumably secondary to renin release [93]. When these effects are reversed, renal function may deteriorate acutely. In the long term, however, these hemodynamic changes may help attenuate the progression of renal failure, as has been shown in an animal model [94]. To our knowledge, only one study reported a decreased graft survival after PTX, and since only a 10% graft survival was reported at 6 years [90], it is hard to believe that these poor results can be explained by PTX alone. Overall, there appears to be no difference in the overall graft survival between patients who underwent PTX between 1966 and 1997 [44] and those who did so after 1998 [83, 92].

Blood Pressure and Serum Lipids

Although still a controversial issue, most studies have reported a decrease in blood pressure [89, 91, 95, 96] and in serum lipid profiles after PTX, some of them involving renal-transplant recipients [91, 94, 97].

The blood pressure lowering effect of PTX is most probably related to the normalization of the serum calcium and/or PTH levels. Hypercalcemia may induce hypertension through an increase in cardiac output or peripheral vascular resistance, or both, or through an increased release or action, or both, of pressor substances such as catecholamines and renin.

Decreased activity of the lipoprotein lipase [98] and hepatic lipase [99] has been implicated in the pathogenesis of dyslipidemia related to HPT. These changes in lipase metabolism were corrected by PTX and calcium-channel blockade. Finally, insulin has been shown to correct the disturbed metabolism of triglyceride-rich particles, thereby indicating that the effect of PTH at least partially involves inhibition of insulin secretion or interference with its peripheral action [100].

Conclusion

PTX provides metabolic benefits in patients with tertiary HPT after renal transplantation. In general, the goals of PTX are to prevent or reverse the negative consequences of tertiary HPT, especially on bone density and the cardiovascular system. Because renal function unfortunately often deteriorates after renal transplantation (overall median graft survival is approximately 15 years), a subtotal PTX or total PTX with autotransplantation is currently believed to be the best surgical approach.

PTX is safe and the results are excellent when the operation is performed by an experienced surgeon. Frequent monitoring of the serum calcium level with appropriate administration of calcium and vitamin D is required in the early post-PTX period to avoid severe hypocalcemia. Although renal function deteriorates immediately after PTX, overall graft survival is similar to that of controls.

References

1. National Kidney Foundation. K/DOQI clinical practice guidelines for bone metabolism and disease in chronic kidney disease. Am J Kidney Dis. 2003;42(4 Suppl 3):S1–201.
2. Slatopolsky E. The role of calcium, phosphorus and vitamin D metabolism in the development of secondary hyperparathyroidism. Nephrol Dial Transplant. 1998;13 Suppl 3:3–8.
3. Triponez F, Clark OH, Vanrenthergem Y, Evenepoel P. Surgical treatment of persistent hyperparathyroidism after renal transplantation. Ann Surg. 2008;248(1):18–30.
4. Messa P, Sindici C, Cannella G, et al. Persistent secondary hyperparathyroidism after renal transplantation. Kidney Int. 1998;54(5):1704–13.
5. Bonarek H, Merville P, Bonarek M, et al. Reduced parathyroid functional mass after successful kidney transplantation. Kidney Int. 1999;56(2):642–9.
6. Evenepoel P, Claes K, Kuypers D, et al. Natural history of parathyroid function and calcium metabolism after kidney transplantation: a single-centre study. Nephrol Dial Transplant. 2004;19(5):1281–7.
7. Parfitt AM. Hypercalcemic hyperparathyroidism following renal transplantation: differential diagnosis, management, and implications for cell population control in the parathyroid gland. Miner Electrolyte Metab. 1982;8(2):92–112.
8. Reinhardt W, Bartelworth H, Jockenhovel F, et al. Sequential changes of biochemical bone parameters after kidney transplantation. Nephrol Dial Transplant. 1998;13(2):436–42.

9. Castleman B, Kibbee BU. Case records of the Massachusetts General Hospital: case 46–1963. N Engl J Med. 1963;269:97–101.
10. Clark OH, Stark DA, Duh QY, et al. Value of high resolution real-time ultrasonography in secondary hyperparathyroidism. Am J Surg. 1985;150(1):9–17.
11. Dumoulin G, Hory B, Nguyen NU, et al. No trend toward a spontaneous improvement of hyperparathyroidism and high bone turnover in normocalcemic long-term renal transplant recipients. Am J Kidney Dis. 1997;29(5):746–53.
12. Torres A, Rodriguez AP, Concepcion MT, et al. Parathyroid function in long-term renal transplant patients: importance of pre-transplant PTH concentrations. Nephrol Dial Transplant. 1998;13 Suppl 3:94–7.
13. Caravaca F, Fernandez MA, Cubero J, et al. Are plasma 1,25-dihydroxyvitamin D3 concentrations appropriate after successful kidney transplantation? Nephrol Dial Transplant. 1998;13 Suppl 3:91–3.
14. Drueke TB. Primary and secondary uraemic hyperparathyroidism: from initial clinical observations to recent findings. Nephrol Dial Transplant. 1998;13(6):1384–7.
15. Torres A, Lorenzo V, Salido E. Calcium metabolism and skeletal problems after transplantation. J Am Soc Nephrol. 2002;13(2):551–8.
16. Evenepoel P. Calcimimetics in chronic kidney disease: evidence, opportunities and challenges. Kidney Int. 2008;74(3):265–75.
17. Evenepoel P, Naesens M, Claes K, et al. Tertiary 'hyperphosphatoninism' accentuates hypophosphatemia and suppresses calcitriol levels in renal transplant recipients. Am J Transplant. 2007;7(5):1193–200.
18. Setterberg L, Sandberg J, Elinder CG, Nordenstrom J. Bone demineralization after renal transplantation: contribution of secondary hyperparathyroidism manifested by hypercalcaemia. Nephrol Dial Transplant. 1996;11(9):1825–8.
19. Cunningham J. Pathogenesis and prevention of bone loss in patients who have kidney disease and receive long-term immunosuppression. J Am Soc Nephrol. 2007;18(1):223–34.
20. Rojas E, Carlini RG, Clesca P, et al. The pathogenesis of osteodystrophy after renal transplantation as detected by early alterations in bone remodeling. Kidney Int. 2003;63(5):1915–23.
21. Carlini RG, Rojas E, Weisinger JR, et al. Bone disease in patients with long-term renal transplantation and normal renal function. Am J Kidney Dis. 2000;36(1):160–6.
22. Dissanayake IR, Epstein S. The fate of bone after renal transplantation. Curr Opin Nephrol Hypertens. 1998;7(4):389–95.
23. Nagano N. Pharmacological and clinical properties of calcimimetics: calcium receptor activators that afford an innovative approach to controlling hyperparathyroidism. Pharmacol Ther. 2006;109(3):339–65.
24. Moe SM, Cunningham J, Bommer J, et al. Long-term treatment of secondary hyperparathyroidism with the calcimimetic cinacalcet HCl. Nephrol Dial Transplant. 2005;20(10):2186–93.
25. Shahapuni I, Monge M, Oprisiu R, et al. Drug Insight: renal indications of calcimimetics. Nat Clin Pract Nephrol. 2006;2(6):316–25.
26. Tominaga Y, Numano M, Tanaka Y, et al. Surgical treatment of renal hyperparathyroidism. Semin Surg Oncol. 1997;13(2):87–96.
27. Taniguchi M, Tokumoto M, Matsuo D, et al. Persistent hyperparathyroidism in renal allograft recipients: vitamin D receptor, calcium-sensing receptor, and apoptosis. Kidney Int. 2006;70(2):363–70.
28. Gwinner W, Suppa S, Mengel M, et al. Early calcification of renal allografts detected by protocol biopsies: causes and clinical implications. Am J Transplant. 2005;5(8):1934–41.
29. Milas M, Weber CJ. Near-total parathyroidectomy is beneficial for patients with secondary and tertiary hyperparathyroidism. Surgery. 2004;136(6):1252–60.
30. Kebebew E, Duh QY, Clark OH. Tertiary hyperparathyroidism: histologic patterns of disease and results of parathyroidectomy. Arch Surg. 2004;139(9):974–7.
31. Thanasoulis L, Bingener J, Sirinek K, Richards M. A successful application of the intraoperative parathyroid hormone assay in tertiary hyperparathyroidism. Am Surg. 2007;73(3):281–3.

32. Nichol PF, Mack E, Bianco J, et al. Radioguided parathyroidectomy in patients with secondary and tertiary hyperparathyroidism. Surgery. 2003;134(4):713–7.

33. Pellitteri PK. Directed parathyroid exploration: evolution and evaluation of this approach in a single-institution review of 346 patients. Laryngoscope. 2003;113(11):1857–69.

34. Pattou FN, Pellissier LC, Noel C, et al. Supernumerary parathyroid glands: frequency and surgical significance in treatment of renal hyperparathyroidism. World J Surg. 2000;24(11): 1330–4.

35. Triponez F, Dosseh D, Hazzan M, et al. Subtotal parathyroidectomy with thymectomy for autonomous hyperparathyroidism after renal transplantation. Br J Surg. 2005;92(10):1282–7.

36. Lo CY, Lang BH, Chan WF, et al. A prospective evaluation of preoperative localization by technetium-99 m sestamibi scintigraphy and ultrasonography in primary hyperparathyroidism. Am J Surg. 2007;193(2):155–9.

37. Muros MA, Bravo Soto J, Lopez Ruiz JM, et al. Two-phase scintigraphy with technetium 99m-sestamibi in patients with hyperparathyroidism due to chronic renal failure. Am J Surg. 2007;193(4):438–42.

38. Perie S, Fessi H, Tassart M, et al. Usefulness of combination of high-resolution ultrasonography and dual-phase dual-isotope iodine 123/technetium Tc 99 m sestamibi scintigraphy for the preoperative localization of hyperplastic parathyroid glands in renal hyperparathyroidism. Am J Kidney Dis. 2005;45(2):344–52.

39. Guillem P, Vlaeminck-Guillem V, Dracon M, et al. L'imagerie preoperatoire des hyperparathyroidies des insuffisants renaux a-t-elle un interet en pratique clinique? Ann Chir. 2006;131(1):27–33.

40. Seehofer D, Steinmuller T, Rayes N, et al. Parathyroid hormone venous sampling before reoperative surgery in renal hyperparathyroidism: comparison with noninvasive localization procedures and review of the literature. Arch Surg. 2004;139(12):1331–8.

41. Wells Jr SA, Debenedetti MK, Doherty GM. Recurrent or persistent hyperparathyroidism. J Bone Miner Res. 2002;17 Suppl 2:N158–62.

42. Caron NR, Sturgeon C, Clark OH. Persistent and recurrent hyperparathyroidism. Curr Treat Options Oncol. 2004;5(4):335–45.

43. McPhaul JJ, McIntosh D, Hammond W, Park O. Autonomous secondary (renal) parathyroid hyperplasia. N Engl J Med. 1964;271:1342.

44. Kerby JD, Rue LW, Blair H, et al. Operative treatment of tertiary hyperparathyroidism: a single-center experience. Ann Surg. 1998;227(6):878–86.

45. Tominaga Y, Uchida K, Haba T, et al. More than 1,000 cases of total parathyroidectomy with forearm autograft for renal hyperparathyroidism. Am J Kidney Dis. 2001;38(4 Suppl 1): S168–71.

46. Gasparri G, Camandona M, Abbona GC, et al. Secondary and tertiary hyperparathyroidism: causes of recurrent disease after 446 parathyroidectomies. Ann Surg. 2001;233(1):65–9.

47. Sancho JJ, Sitges-Serra A. Surgical Approach to Secondary Hyperparathyroidism. In: Clark OH, Duh QY, editors. Textbook of endocrine surgery, vol. 50. San Francisco: W. B. Saunders; 1997. p. 403–9.

48. Rothmund M, Wagner PK, Schark C. Subtotal parathyroidectomy versus total parathyroidectomy and autotransplantation in secondary hyperparathyroidism: a randomized trial. World J Surg. 1991;15(6):745–50.

49. Tominaga Y, Johansson H, Takagi H. Secondary hyperparathyroidism: pathophysiology, histopathology, and medical and surgical management. Surg Today. 1997;27(9):787–92.

50. Kaczirek K, Prager G, Riss P, et al. Novel parathyroid hormone (1–84) assay as basis for parathyroid hormone monitoring in renal hyperparathyroidism. Arch Surg. 2006;141(2): 129–34.

51. Sitges-Serra A, Caralps-Riera A. Hyperparathyroidism associated with renal disease. Pathogenesis, natural history, and surgical treatment. Surg Clin North Am. 1987;67(2):359–77.

52. Nichol PF, Starling JR, Mack E, et al. Long-term follow-up of patients with tertiary hyperparathyroidism treated by resection of a single or double adenoma. Ann Surg. 2002;235(5): 673–8.

53. Kilgo MS, Pirsch JD, Warner TF, Starling JR. Tertiary hyperparathyroidism after renal transplantation: surgical strategy. Surgery. 1998;124(4):677–83.
54. Krause MW, Hedinger CE. Pathologic study of parathyroid glands in tertiary hyperparathyroidism. Hum Pathol. 1985;16(8):772–84.
55. Tominaga Y, Katayama A, Sato T, et al. Re-operation is frequently required when parathyroid glands remain after initial parathyroidectomy for advanced secondary hyperparathyroidism in uraemic patients. Nephrol Dial Transplant. 2003;18 Suppl 3:iii65–70.
56. Triponez F, Kebebew E, Dosseh D, et al. Less-than-subtotal parathyroidectomy increases the risk of persistent/recurrent hyperparathyroidism after parathyroidectomy in tertiary hyperparathyroidism after renal transplantation. Surgery. 2006;140(6):990–7.
57. Saxe AW, Gibson GW, Kay S. Characterization of a simplified method of cryopreserving human parathyroid tissue. Surgery. 1990;108(6):1033–8. discussion 1038–9.
58. Cohen MS, Dilley WG, Wells Jr SA, et al. Long-term functionality of cryopreserved parathyroid autografts: a 13-year prospective analysis. Surgery. 2005;138(6):1033–40.
59. Akerstrom G, Malmaeus J, Bergstrom R. Surgical anatomy of human parathyroid glands. Surgery. 1984;95(1):14–21.
60. Punch JD, Thompson NW, Merion RM. Subtotal parathyroidectomy in dialysis-dependent and post-renal transplant patients. A 25-year single-center experience. Arch Surg. 1995;130(5):538–42.
61. Pereira JA, Jimeno J, Miquel J, et al. Nodal yield, morbidity, and recurrence after central neck dissection for papillary thyroid carcinoma. Surgery. 2005;138(6):1095–100. discussion 1100–1.
62. Irvin 3rd GL, Prudhomme DL, Deriso GT, et al. A new approach to parathyroidectomy. Ann Surg. 1994;219(5):574–9.
63. Johnson LR, Doherty G, Lairmore T, et al. Evaluation of the performance and clinical impact of a rapid intraoperative parathyroid hormone assay in conjunction with preoperative imaging and concise parathyroidectomy. Clin Chem. 2001;47(5):919–25.
64. Westerdahl J, Bergenfelz A. Sestamibi scan-directed parathyroid surgery: potentially high failure rate without measurement of intraoperative parathyroid hormone. World J Surg. 2004;28(11):1132–8.
65. Haciyanli M, Lal G, Morita E, et al. Accuracy of preoperative localization studies and intraoperative parathyroid hormone assay in patients with primary hyperparathyroidism and double adenoma. J Am Coll Surg. 2003;197(5):739–46.
66. Lokey J, Pattou F, Mondragon-Sanchez A, et al. Intraoperative decay profile of intact (1–84) parathyroid hormone in surgery for renal hyperparathyroidism—a consecutive series of 80 patients. Surgery. 2000;128(6):1029–34.
67. Chou FF, Lee CH, Chen JB, et al. Intraoperative parathyroid hormone measurement in patients with secondary hyperparathyroidism. Arch Surg. 2002;137(3):341–4.
68. Seehofer D, Rayes N, Klupp J, et al. Predictive value of intact parathyroid hormone measurement during surgery for renal hyperparathyroidism. Langenbecks Arch Surg. 2005;390(3): 222–9.
69. Kaczirek K, Riss P, Wunderer G, et al. Quick PTH assay cannot predict incomplete parathyroidectomy in patients with renal hyperparathyroidism. Surgery. 2005;137(4):431–5.
70. Haustein SV, Mack E, Starling JR, Chen H. The role of intraoperative parathyroid hormone testing in patients with tertiary hyperparathyroidism after renal transplantation. Surgery. 2005;138(6):1066–71.
71. Lorenz K, Dralle H. Will intra-operative measurement of parathyroid hormone alter the surgical concept of renal hyperparathyroidism? Langenbecks Arch Surg. 2005;390(4):277–9.
72. Triponez F, Dosseh D, Hazzan M, et al. Accuracy of intra-operative PTH measurement during subtotal parathyroidectomy for tertiary hyperparathyroidism after renal transplantation. Langenbecks Arch Surg. 2006;391(6):561–5.
73. Bieglmayer C, Kaczirek K, Prager G, Niederle B. Parathyroid hormone monitoring during total parathyroidectomy for renal hyperparathyroidism: pilot study of the impact of renal function and assay specificity. Clin Chem. 2006;52(6):1112–9.

74. Yamashita H, Gao P, Cantor T, et al. Comparison of parathyroid hormone levels from the intact and whole parathyroid hormone assays after parathyroidectomy for primary and secondary hyperparathyroidism. Surgery. 2004;135(2):149–56.

75. Dralle H, Sekulla C, Haerting J, et al. Risk factors of paralysis and functional outcome after recurrent laryngeal nerve monitoring in thyroid surgery. Surgery. 2004;136(6):1310–22.

76. Moore C, Lampe H, Agrawal S. Predictability of hypocalcemia using early postoperative serum calcium levels. J Otolaryngol. 2001;30(5):266–70.

77. Cozzolino M, Gallieni M, Corsi C, et al. Management of calcium refilling post-parathyroidectomy in end-stage renal disease. J Nephrol. 2004;17(1):3–8.

78. Sheikh MS, Ramirez A, Emmett M, et al. Role of vitamin D-dependent and vitamin D-independent mechanisms in absorption of food calcium. J Clin Invest. 1988;81(1):126–32.

79. U.S. Renal Data System, USRDS 2004 Annual Data Report: Atlas of End-Stage Renal Disease in the United States, National Institutes of Health, National Institute of Diabetes and Digestive and Kidney Diseases, Bethesda, MD. Available at http://www.usrds.org/atlas.htm. 2004, June 15, 2005.

80. Mazzaferro S, Chicca S, Pasquali M, et al. Changes in bone turnover after parathyroidectomy in dialysis patients: role of calcitriol administration. Nephrol Dial Transplant. 2000;15(6):877–82.

81. Coen G, Mazzaferro S, De Antoni E, et al. Procollagen type 1 C-terminal extension peptide serum levels following parathyroidectomy in hyperparathyroid patients. Am J Nephrol. 1994;14(2):106–12.

82. Urena P, Prieur P, Petrover M. [Alkaline phosphatase of bone origin in hemodialyzed patients. 110 assays]. Presse Med. 1996;25(29):1320–5.

83. Evenepoel P, Claes K, Kuypers DR, et al. Parathyroidectomy after successful kidney transplantation: a single centre study. Nephrol Dial Transplant. 2007;22(6):1730–7.

84. Yajima A, Inaba M, Ogawa Y, et al. Significance of time-course changes of serum bone markers after parathyroidectomy in patients with uraemic hyperparathyroidism. Nephrol Dial Transplant. 2007;22(6):1645–57.

85. Abdelhadi M, Nordenstrom J. Bone mineral recovery after parathyroidectomy in patients with primary and renal hyperparathyroidism. J Clin Endocrinol Metab. 1998;83(11):3845–51.

86. Collaud S, Staub-Zahner T, Trombetti A, et al. Increase in bone mineral density after successful parathyroidectomy for tertiary hyperparathyroidism after renal transplantation. World J Surg. 2008;32(8):1795–801.

87. David DS, Sakai S, Brennan BL, et al. Hypercalcemia after renal transplantation. Long-term follow-up data. N Engl J Med. 1973;289(8):398–401.

88. Geis WP, Popovtzer MM, Corman JL, et al. The diagnosis and treatment of hyperparathyroidism after renal homotransplantation. Surg Gynecol Obstet. 1973;137(6):997–1010.

89. Rostaing L, Moreau-Gaudry X, Baron E, et al. Changes in blood pressure and renal function following subtotal parathyroidectomy in renal transplant patients presenting with persistent hypercalcemic hyperparathyroidism. Clin Nephrol. 1997;47(4):248–55.

90. Lee PP, Schiffmann L, Offermann G, Beige J. Effects of parathyroidectomy on renal allograft survival. Kidney Blood Press Res. 2004;27(3):191–6.

91. Evenepoel P, Claes K, Kuypers D, et al. Impact of parathyroidectomy on renal graft function, blood pressure and serum lipids in kidney transplant recipients: a single centre study. Nephrol Dial Transplant. 2005;20(8):1714–20.

92. Schwarz A, Rustien G, Merkel S, et al. Decreased renal transplant function after parathyroidectomy. Nephrol Dial Transplant. 2007;22(2):584–91.

93. Massfelder T, Parekh N, Endlich K, et al. Effect of intrarenally infused parathyroid hormone-related protein on renal blood flow and glomerular filtration rate in the anaesthetized rat. Br J Pharmacol. 1996;118(8):1995–2000.

94. Ogata H, Ritz E, Odoni G, et al. Beneficial effects of calcimimetics on progression of renal failure and cardiovascular risk factors. J Am Soc Nephrol. 2003;14(4):959–67.

 95. Odenwald T, Nakagawa K, Hadtstein C, et al. Acute blood pressure effects and chronic hypotensive action of calcimimetics in uremic rats. J Am Soc Nephrol. 2006;17(3):655–62.
 96. Almirall J, Lopez T, Comerma I, et al. Effect of parathyroidectomy on blood pressure in dialysis patients. Nephron. 2002;92(2):495–6.
 97. Shigematsu T, Caverzasio J, Bonjour JP. Parathyroid removal prevents the progression of chronic renal failure induced by high protein diet. Kidney Int. 1993;44(1):173–81.
 98. Akmal M, Kasim SE, Soliman AR, Massry SG. Excess parathyroid hormone adversely affects lipid metabolism in chronic renal failure. Kidney Int. 1990;37(3):854–8.
 99. Klin M, Smogorzewski M, Ni Z, et al. Abnormalities in hepatic lipase in chronic renal failure: role of excess parathyroid hormone. J Clin Invest. 1996;97(10):2167–73.
100. Roullet JB, Lacour B, Yvert JP, Drueke T. Correction by insulin of disturbed TG-rich LP metabolism in rats with chronic renal failure. Am J Physiol. 1986;250(4 Pt 1):E373–6.

Chapter 13
Bone Density and Fracture Risk in Primary Hyperparathyroidism

E. Michael Lewiecki and Paul D. Miller

Keywords Bone turnover • Bone density • Assessment of skeletal strength • Areal and volumetric BMD • Histomorphometry • Bone geometry • Fracture risk and management • Normocalcemic hyperparathyroidism • PTHrP • QCT • Fracture risk

A healthy and active 58 year-old estrogen deficient postmenopausal woman tripped on a garden hose, fracturing her right wrist after landing on her outstretched arm. She was treated in the local hospital emergency department with a cast, followed up in the office by her family physician, and had an uneventful recovery. Three months later, laboratory studies done after a routine medical examination showed an elevated serum calcium of 11.2 mg/dL (reference range 8.4–10.4) [2.8 mmol/L, reference range 2.1–2.6]. Further evaluation of hypercalcemia showed a high serum parathyroid hormone (PTH) of 78 pg/mL (reference range 10–65) [8.2 pmol/L, reference range 1.1–6.8], a serum phosphate level at the low end of the normal range, and serum 25-hydroxyvitamin D level of 22 ng/mL [55 nmol/L]. Bone mineral density (BMD) testing by dual-energy X-ray absorptiometry (DXA) revealed a T-score of −1.8 at L1 to L4, −1.2 at the left femoral neck, and −2.6 at the left distal one-third radius. There was no history of kidney stones. The 24-h urinary calcium excretion was 235 mg (normal less than 250 mg). What is the cause of skeletal disease in this patient, what are its consequences, and how should she be managed?

E.M. Lewiecki, MD, FACP, FACE (✉)
New Mexico Clinical Research & Osteoporosis Center,
300 Oak Street NE, Albuquerque, NM 87106, USA
e-mail: lewiecki@aol.com

P.D. Miller, MD
Colorado Center for Bone Research, Lakewood, CO, USA

A.A. Khan and O.H. Clark (eds.), *Handbook of Parathyroid Diseases:
A Case-Based Practical Guide*, DOI 10.1007/978-1-4614-2164-1_13,
© Springer Science+Business Media, LLC 2012

Introduction

Since the advent of autoanalyzers for biochemical screening in the 1970s, osteitis fibrosa cystica has become a rare finding, with about 80% of PHPT in Western countries now being identified through routine laboratory testing in patients without well-defined skeletal symptoms [1]. These patients most often have mild or sometimes intermittent hypercalcemia. It is important to distinguish between PHPT and familial hypocalciuric hypercalcemia (FHH). Patients with FHH typically have inappropriately normal PTH levels, although 10–20% have been reported to have absolute elevation of serum PTH [2]. FHH is associated with normal parathyroid glands, and does not require surgery or medical treatment. It is differentiated from PHPT by performing a 24-h measurement of urine calcium and creatinine and determining the ratio of the clearance of calcium to the clearance of creatinine. Data compiled from five studies showed that a ratio of less than 0.01 had a sensitivity of 85%, a specificity of 88%, and a positive predictive value of 85% to detect FHH; a ratio of greater than 0.02 essentially ruled out the possibility of FHH [3]. In the same review, about 12% of patients with PHPT had a ratio below 0.01 and 49% had a ratio above 0.02, with the remainder between the two values. The clinical utility of urinary calcium/creatinine clearance ratios is described in more detail in the chapter on diagnosis. This is an important differential diagnosis in order to avoid an unnecessary neck exploration. Some patients with normal serum calcium and inappropriately high PTH levels are being detected in the evaluation for factors contributing to osteoporosis. These patients have been classified as having "normocalcemic primary hyperparathyroidism," a disorder associated with substantial skeletal involvement that may represent the earliest form of primary hyperthyroidism. In a longitudinal cohort study of 37 such patients (age 32–78, median 58 years; 95% female) followed for 1–8 years (median 3 years), 7 (19%) became hypercalcemic, all within the first 3 years of observation [4]. Three of the hypercalcemic patients had parathyroid surgery, with excision of a single parathyroid adenoma in two and excision of two hyperplastic glands in the third. Four normocalcemic patients also had surgery, with a single adenoma excised in one patient, a single hyperplastic gland excised in two others, and two hyperplastic glands removed from the fourth.

Patients with PHPT and skeletal disease usually come to clinical attention in one of the following three ways—(1) when a bone density test is done or a fracture occurs in a patient with known PHPT; (2) hypercalcemia and/or elevated PTH is found in the course of evaluating a patient with known skeletal disease; or (3) hypercalcemia is discovered in the evaluation of a patient with renal stone disease. This chapter explores the pathophysiology of skeletal disease in PHPT, its effect on bone mineral density (BMD) and fracture risk, and implications for clinical management.

Pathophysiology

Bone remodeling (turnover) is a physiological process that occurs on the surface of trabecular bone as discrete bone resorption pits (Howship lacunae) and in cortical bone as cylindrical tunnels (Haversian systems). In postmenopausal women, there is an elevated rate of bone remodeling, with bone resorption exceeding bone formation, as assessed by bone turnover markers [5] and transiliac double-tetracycline-labeled bone biopsy [6]. This is associated with bone loss [7], reduced BMD, skeletal fragility, and increased risk of fracture [8]. High remodeling rates weaken bone due to the local effect of greater number and size of Howship lucanae and Haversion systems acting as "stress risers" (focal areas of weakness that may be sites of microfracture initiation), and the systemic skeletal effect of reduced mineralization of bone matrix [9]. In PHPT, there is an increase in bone turnover, with elevated biochemical markers of bone resorption and formation compared to controls [10–12]. Coupling between bone resorption and formation remains in balance with PHPT, in contrast to the excess of resorption over formation that occurs with PMO. At the cellular level, the increase in bone resorption is seen as an increased number of osteoclasts and extension of resorption surfaces while the increase in bone formation is associated with an increase in the number of osteoblasts, increased osteoid surfaces, and increased mineral apposition rate. Two-dimensional (2-D) histomorphometric analyses of transiliac bone biopsy specimens in patients with PHPT have consistently shown reduction in cortical width and an increase in cortical porosity with preservation or enhancement of trabecular bone structure (e.g., trabecular volume, width, separation, and number) [13–23]. This is remarkably different than the findings in women with PMO, who typically have deficits in both bone compartments, with a reduction in trabecular volume as well as a decrease in cortical thickness [24]. Histomorphometric studies in postmenopausal women with mild PHPT suggest that the salutary effect of PTH on trabecular bone structure may be at least in part due to prolongation of the duration of the active bone formation phase in individual remodeling units [14]. There are limitations, however, in the assessment of skeletal structure with two-dimensional histomorphometry due to the small sample size analyzed in comparison to the total bone biopsy volume [25]. Three-dimensional histomorphometry with microcomputed tomography overcomes this limitation by allowing analysis of the entire biopsy specimen. This has confirmed preservation of trabecular bone microarchitecture in women and men with PHPT [26]. The material properties of bone have been evaluated by quantitative backscattered electron imaging. Using this technique with iliac crest bone biopsy specimens in patients with PHPT, reduced mineralization density has been observed [27]. This finding is consistent with the high bone turnover state of hyperparathyroidism, which results in "younger" bone with less time to become fully mineralized.

At the molecular level, PTH and its evolutionary cousin, PTH-related peptide (PTHrP), exert their skeletal effects through the PTH-1 receptor (also known as the PTH-PTHrP receptor), a G protein-coupled protein on the cell surface of osteoblasts and osteoblast precursors. Binding to the receptor by peptide sequences at the N-terminal of these hormones triggers a cascade of intracellular signaling that includes activation of cyclic AMP-dependent protein kinase A, calcium-dependent protein kinase C signaling pathways, MAP kinase and phosholipase A and D pathways, and stimulation of intracellular synthesis of insulin-like growth factor I (IGF-I) [28]. PTH also downregulates sclerostin, an inhibitor of Wnt (the mammalian homologue of wingless in Drosophila) signaling, an important pathway for bone formation [29].

The result is stimulation of osteoblast differentiation, activity, and life span resulting in an increase in bone formation. A secondary consequence of these events is increased osteoblastic expression of receptor activator of nuclear factor kappa B ligand (RANKL), which binds to its receptor (RANK) on the surface of osteoclasts and osteoclast precursors [30]. RANKL increases bone resorption by increasing the differentiation, activity, and life span of osteoclasts. PTH also decreases extracellular excretion of osteoprotegerin (OPG), a soluble cytokine that binds to RANKL, preventing its binding to RANK and counterbalancing the bone resorbing effect of RANKL. The net skeletal effect of PTH elevation is the result of the complex interaction of direct and indirect effects mediated through multiple signaling pathways, such as the Wnt-β-catenin pathway, with intermediate molecules that include bone morphogenetic proteins and IGF-I. The consequent regulation of bone formation and resorption varies according to factors that include bone type (trabecular vs. cortical) and the pattern of PTH elevation (continuous vs. intermittent) [31].

Assessment of Skeletal Strength

Areal BMD. Skeletal health in PHPT is most often measured with DXA, a technology that measures areal BMD (i.e., bone density in a two-dimensional projection of bone, expressed as g/cm^2) at the lumbar spine, hip, and forearm. The pattern of bone density in PHPT is strikingly different than postmenopausal osteoporosis (PMO). The typical, but certainly not invariable, finding in PMO is bone loss that predominates at skeletal sites that are rich in trabecular bone, with BMD lowest in the lumbar spine, relatively well-preserved in the distal one-third radius, and intermediate at the hip. The reverse pattern is often seen with PHPT, with BMD lowest at the distal one-thrid radius, preservation of BMD at the lumbar spine, and intermediate at the hip (Fig. 13.1) [16, 19], consistent with a catabolic effect of PTH on cortical bone and an anabolic effect on trabecular bone. The observed reduction in DXA-measured BMD at cortical skeletal sites (e.g., distal one-third radius) in PHPT may in part be an "artifact" of the increase in bone diameter, which could lead to decrease in areal BMD (bone mineral content [BMC]/bone area [cm^2]), even if the BMC remained the same [32]. In a report of 10 years' follow-up of a prospective observational study in 121 patients (30 men and 91 women) with PHPT that included a cohort of 52 who were asymptomatic and elected not to have parathyroid surgery, most were found to have stable BMD at the lumbar spine, hip, and radius [33]. However, 11 of the 52 (21%) had a BMD decrease of more than 10% recorded at one or more of these skeletal sites, with 10 of the 11 being women and 5 becoming postmenopausal during the study. The onset of menopause was the only factor, other than baseline serum calcium, that was associated with bone loss ($P=0.006$). A subsequent report described an additional 5 years of observation in 116 of the original group of patients having at least 1 follow-up BMD measurement [34]. In patients not having surgery, lumbar spine BMD remained stable while BMD at cortical skeletal sites decreased significantly (mean decrease of 10% at the femoral neck and mean decrease of 35% at the distal one-third radius) in patients observed for

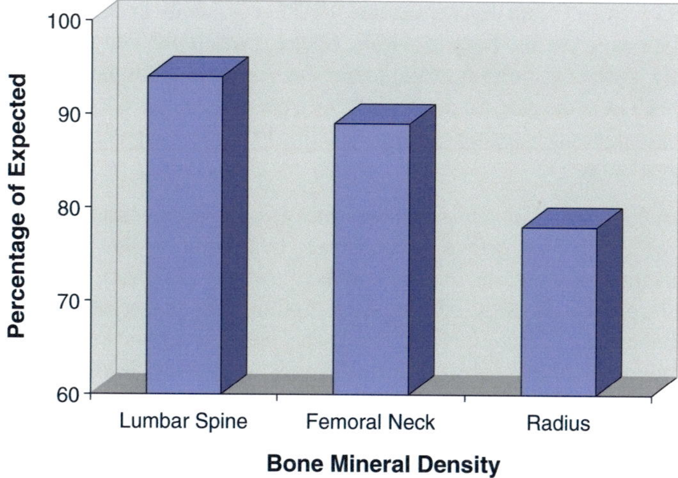

Fig. 13.1 Pattern of bone mineral density at three skeletal sites in patients with primary hyperparathyroidism. Bone density testing shows a divergence from expected values at each skeletal site (p = 0.0001) compared to a reference population matched for age, sex, and ethnicity. [Adapted from ref 19, Silverberg SJ et al.]

15 years. Over the entire follow-up period, 37% of patients not having parathyroidectomy showed evidence of disease progression (defined as one or more new criteria for surgery [35]), representing a substantial increase over the 25% rate of progression reported during the first 10 years [33].

Since most patients with PHPT are postmenopausal women [36–38], bone loss may occur due to excess PTH and/or estrogen deficiency. In clinical practice, it is advisable to measure BMD at three skeletal sites (lumbar spine, hip, distal one-third radius) in patients with PHPT in order to capture the full range of possible bone loss and to measure BMD regularly in those who choose not to have surgery, particularly postmenopausal women [32].

Volumetric BMD. Peripheral quantitative computed tomography (pQCT) has been used to measure volumetric BMD (vBMD) in patients with PHPT. This has shown a somewhat different pattern of bone density than seen with areal BMD by DXA. In a study of 36 women (mean age 60.50±10.80 years) with PHPT compared to 100 normal controls matched for age, sex, and body size, vBMD at the radius was measured by pQCT [39]. It was found that there was a significant vBMD reduction at a predominately trabecular region of the radius (4% proximal from the ulnar styloid) as well as at a cortical portion of radius (20% proximal from the ulnar styloid). This suggests that PHPT may have a catabolic effect on trabecular as well as cortical bone, and is consistent with the finding that patients with PHPT appear to have increased risk of fracture at trabecular as well as cortical skeletal sites. Areal BMD by DXA in the same patients showed a decrease in BMD at the one-third radius but no significant difference in BMD at the lumbar spine. Another study examined vBMD at a weight-bearing bone, the tibia, in 28 postmenopausal women (mean age

58.85±8.71 years) with hypercalcemic PHPT compared to 56 healthy controls matched for age, sex, and body size [40]. Again, it was found that vBMD was low in the mostly trabecular portion of the bone (4% proximal from the distal end of the tibia) as well as at the cortical portion (20% proximal from the distal end of the tibia) compared to controls, supporting the notion that PHPT is catabolic to both trabecular and cortical bone.

Histomorphometry. Conventional two-dimensional bone histomorphometry in patients with PHPT has shown an increase in bone turnover that is consistent with the observation of increases in bone turnover markers [11], with cortical thinning, increased cortical porosity, endosteal resorption, and preservation of trabecular bone volume and connectivity [41]. A 3-D analysis of transiliac bone biopsies using microcomputed tomography (micro CT) technology in 29 women with PHPT (7 premenopausal, 22 postmenopausal) compared to 20 controls (15 premenopausal, 5 postmenopausal) and in 15 men with PHPT showed a high correlation with conventional histomorphometry [26]. It was concluded that trabecular bone microarchitecture is preserved in patients with mild PHPT. Quantitative backscattered electron imaging (qBEI) was used to evaluate trabecular BMD distribution (BMDD) in iliac crest bone biopsies in 51 patients (16 men, 35 women) with mild PHPT [27]. The observed reduction in average mineralization density and increase in the heterogeneity of the degree of mineralization were consistent with reduced mean age of bone tissue and previous observations of high bone turnover in patients with PHPT.

Bone geometry. QCT has been utilized to assess geometric properties of bone in patients with PHPT. A cross-sectional study compared 36 women with PHPT to 100 healthy controls; pQCT of the radius showed a statistically significant 20% reduction in vBMD ($P<0.01$) at a predominantly trabecular region of interest (ROI) and a statistically significant 5% reduction at a predominantly cortical ROI ($P<0.01$) [39]. In these same patients, areal BMD measured by DXA in the women with PHPT was similar at the lumbar spine but decreased at the distal one-third radius compared to controls. The findings of this study suggest that PHPT may have a catabolic effect on both trabecular and cortical bone, although the effect on trabecular bone may not be detected with measurement of areal BMD by DXA. In comparison to controls, the patients with PHPT had a greater radius endosteal circumference (+11%, $P<0.01$) and periosteal circumference (+4%, $P<0.01$). In another study, 52 women with normocalcemic or hypercalcemic PHPT were compared to 56 matched controls; pQCT of the tibia showed differences in trabecular and cortical volumetric BMD consistent with a catabolic effect on both types of bone in patients with either type of PHPT [40]. Endosteal circumference of the tibia was greater with PHPT, but there was no difference in periosteal circumference compared to controls.

Post-parathyroidectomy: Surgical treatment of PHPT is associated with an increase in BMD at the lumbar spine [42, 43], hip [42, 43], and forearm [42–44]. BMD increases are greatest and most rapid at the lumbar spine and hip, and least and slowest at the radius. In a study of 34 patients with PHPT treated with parathyroidectomy and followed for 4 years after surgery, the lumbar spine mean BMD increase was 8.2% at 1 year ($P<0.005$) and 12.8% at 4 years ($P<0.001$), with similar increases at the femoral neck, while there was a more modest BMD increase at the radius that did not reach statistical significance until 3 years after surgery (4.0%, $P < 0.05$) [42]. In a randomized controlled clinical trial of parathyroidectomy ($n = 25$) versus non-surgical medical follow-up ($n = 28$) in patients with mild PHPT, parathyroidectomy was associated with a significant BMD increase at the femoral neck (group difference of 0.8% per year, $P = 0.01$) and total hip (group difference of 1.0% per year, $P = 0.001$), but not the lumbar spine (group difference of 0.6% per year) or forearm (group difference of 0.2% per year), compared to no surgery, after at least 24 months of follow-up [45]. In the longest (up to 15 years of follow-up) published prospective observational study of patients with and without parathyroidectomy for mild PHPT, there was a sustained increase in BMD at the lumbar spine, femoral neck, and one-third distal radius in those having surgery, as compared to stability (lumbar spine) or loss (femoral neck, distal one-third radius) of BMD in patients not having surgery [34].

Fracture Risk

While the relationship between BMD and fracture risk is well-established in "healthy" postmenopausal women [46], it is not clear whether that same relationship is present in premenopausal women or men with PHPT [47]. The reduction in bone strength that might be expected with cortical thinning and increased cortical porosity in PHPT may be at least partially attenuated by an increase in bone diameter associated with endosteal resorption and periosteal apposition observed in longitudinal studies of patients with untreated PHPT [48, 49], since small increases in bone size result in large increases in bone strength [50]. At skeletal sites constituted by a mix of trabecular and cortical bone (e.g., spine, hip), the contribution to bone strength imparted by preservation or enhancement of trabecular structure, combined with cortical thinning and expansion of cortical diameter to bone strength, is complex.

There is evidence that PHPT is associated with an overall increase in fracture risk, with a generally consistent pattern of increased risk of forearm fractures, most but not all studies showing an increased risk of vertebral fractures, and only marginal evidence for effects on hip fracture risk [51]. In a population-based study of 407 patients (314 women, 93 men, mean age at diagnosis 57.8 years) in Rochester, Minnesota, with PHPT diagnosed between 1965 and 1992, 471 fractures occurred during 5,766 person-years of follow-up [52]. Fracture rates were significantly higher at multiple skeletal sites in those with PHPT compared to the expected risk from gender- and age-specific incidence rates for the general population using standardized incidence ratios (SIRs) (Table 13.1). Fracture risk was increased at the spine (SIR 3.2, 95% confidence interval [CI] 2.5–4.0), distal forearm (SIR 2.2, 95% CI 1.6–2.9), ribs (SIR 2.7, 95% CI 2.1–3.5), pelvis (SIR 2.1, 95% CI 1/1–3.5), and all fractures (SIR 1.3, 95% CI 1.1–1.5). There was a marginal increase in hip fracture risk (SIR 1.4, 95% CI 1.0–2.0). A multivariate analysis for predictors of vertebral, distal forearm, or proximal femur fractures due to mild/moderate trauma in these

Table 13.1 Predictors of risk for vertebral, distal forearm, and proximal femur fractures in patients ($N=407$) with primary hyperparathyroidism [Adapted from Ref [52], Khosla et al. J Bone Miner Res. 1999]

Variable	Relative hazard	95% confidence interval
Univariate model		
Age (per decade increase)	1.7	1.2 to 1.9
Female	2.9	1.6 to 5.3
Highest serum calcium (per mg/dL increase)	1.2	0.9 to 1.6
Multivariate model		
Age (per decade increase)	1.6	1.4 to 1.9
Female	2.3	1.2 to 4.1

patients showed that increased age (relative hazard [RH] 1.6; 95% CI 1.4–1.9) and female gender (RH 2.3, 95% CI 1.2–4.1) were independent predictors of elevated fracture risk. Parathyroid surgery appeared to be protective for fractures, although the number of patients having surgery was small (23%). In contrast, an earlier study in the USA reported no increase in vertebral fracture risk with PHPT [53]. In a Danish study of 674 patients (501 women, 173 men, median age 61 years) with PHPT, all of whom eventually had parathyroid surgery, preoperative fracture risk was elevated at the spine (relative risk [RR] 3.5, 95% CI 1.3–9.7), lower leg and ankles (RR 2.3, 95% CI 1.2–4.3), nondistal forearm (RR 4.0, 95% CI 1.5–10.6), and for all fractures (RR 1.8, 95% CI 1.3–2.3) compared to matched controls from the national patient register [54]. There was no difference in femoral neck fractures (RR 1.4, 0.8–2.7). After parathyroid surgery, fracture risk was no different than controls (RR 1.0, 95% CI 0.8–1.3). Another Danish controlled-cohort study in 3,213 patients with PHPT (60% having parathyroid surgery and 40% not) followed for a median time of 6.1 years after diagnosis showed that parathyroid surgery reduced the risk of hip and upper arm fractures by about 50% [55]. In a population-based prospective study of 1,373 Swedish women hospitalized with a diagnosis of PHPT followed for a mean of 17 years with 23,341 person-years of observation, there was no increase in hip fracture risk compared to the background population [56]. Parathyroid surgery had no influence on hip fracture risk. The same study also evaluated 551 men with PHPT followed for a mean of 16.5 years with 9,091 person-years of observation. In this cohort, there was an increased risk of femoral neck fractures (RR 2.73, 95% CI 1.18–5.39), although the significance of this finding is uncertain due to the small number of fractures [8]. In an Italian study of 98 post-menopausal women with PHPT who were divided into "mild" and "nonmild" cohorts according to published guidelines [57], it was found that vertebral fracture risk was increased in those with mild PHPT, even when lumbar spine BMD was well-preserved [58]. The repeated and unexpected finding that vertebral fracture risk is elevated in PHPT suggests that factors other than BMD may be important determinants of bone strength in these patients.

Given the complexity of skeletal effects of chronic exposure to elevated PTH levels, uncertain relationship between BMD and fracture risk with PHPT, discordant findings on fracture risk at different skeletal sites before and after surgery, and limitations of study design, severity of disease, and patient selection in many reports, further study is indicated. Well-designed prospective clinical trials with skeletal end points provide a better understanding of the natural history of PHPT and the effect of parathyroid surgery on skeletal health. The preponderance of evidence to date suggests that PHPT is associated with increased fracture risk at both trabecular and cortical skeletal sites, despite the frequent observation that the catabolic effects of prolonged PTH elevation are seen in cortical but not trabecular bone, and that parathyroid surgery reduces fracture risk, at least at some skeletal sites. It has been hypothesized that the finding of increased risk of vertebral fractures with PHPT may be due to surveillance bias (i.e., patients with PHPT being more likely than the general population to have spine X-rays in the evaluation of back pain), thinning of the cortical envelope of vertebral bodies, or high bone turnover [47].

Treatment

Prior to the widespread use of multichannel biochemical screening that included measurement of serum calcium, the management of PHPT was straightforward, since virtually all patients were symptomatic with kidney stones, bone disease, or manifestations of severe hypercalcemia that required parathyroid surgery. Surgery is associated with improvement in BMD and reduction in fracture risk. Since most patients diagnosed with PHPT are asymptomatic [59] and new options for nonsurgical management are becoming available, evaluation and treatment require more careful consideration. Although the definitive treatment of PHPT remains parathyroid surgery and current guidelines include a recommendation for surgery when the T-score is −2.5 or less, some patients with PHPT do not meet the criteria for parathyroidectomy [60] or choose not to have surgery that is offered. Once the diagnosis of PHPT is made, evaluation should include a search for other factors that may contribute to poor skeletal health, much the same as with the evaluation of osteoporosis [61–66]. Treatment should then be directed to maintaining a healthy lifestyle (e.g., regular physical activity, good nutrition, avoidance of cigarette smoking, moderation of alcohol intake, and minimizing exposure to drugs known to have adverse skeletal effects), avoiding drugs known to cause hypercalcemia (e.g., thiazide diuretics, lithium), correcting all modifiable risk factors for bone loss and fracture, and using pharmacological agents when appropriate. Since most patients with PHPT are postmenopausal women, many of the studies of medical treatment of PHPT have focused on this population.

The case presented at the beginning of this chapter is a postmenopausal woman with a fragility fracture of the forearm who was found to have PHPT. The DXA study showed a T-score value that was consistent with a diagnosis of osteoporosis in a pattern of skeletal distribution typical of PHPT (lower BMD at the 33% radius than the lumbar spine and hip). It is likely that she has osteoporosis secondary to PHPT, with postmenopausal estrogen deficiency probably being a contributing factor. Parathyroid surgery is indicated once other etiologies of hypercalcemia, including FHH, are excluded.

Summary

PHPT is associated with elevated bone turnover, modest reduction in BMD, and increased fracture risk. Areal BMD measured by DXA shows a pattern of bone loss that predominately affects cortical skeletal sites while vBMD measured by pQCT shows loss of trabecular and cortical bone mass, suggesting a catabolic action with both types of bone. PHPT is associated with cortical thinning due to endosteal resorption with an increase in endosteal circumference. At some skeletal sites, there is a compensatory periosteal expansion that may attenuate the loss of bone strength caused by the cortical thinning. Conventional histomorphometry and three-dimensional micro CT show preservation of trabecular microarchitecture. Increased fracture rates with PHPT have been observed at trabecular skeletal sites, such as the spine, as well as cortical sites, such as the forearm. In studies of patients with PHPT who do not have surgery, BMD has decreased or remained stable. It is plausible that the skeletal effects of PHPT may be influenced by factors that include the duration of disease, magnitude of hypercalcemia and/or PTH elevation, age, sex, and hormonal status. Further study is needed to better define these relationships. Parathyroidectomy, the definitive treatment for PHPT in patients who meet guidelines for surgery [60], results in lower bone turnover, increased BMD (more at trabecular than cortical skeletal sites), and reduction of fracture risk. Some pharmacological agents, especially bisphosphonates and calcimimetics, have a potential role in the management of patients with PHPT who are not candidates for surgery.

References

1. Silverberg SJ, Bilezikian JP. Evaluation and management of primary hyperparathyroidism. J Clin Endocrinol Metab. 1996;81(6):2036–40.
2. Marx SJ. Familial hypocalciuric hypercalcemia. N Engl J Med. 1980;303:810–1.
3. Fuleihan GE. Familial benign hypocalciuric hypercalcemia. J Bone Miner Res. 2002; 17:N51–6.
4. Lowe H, McMahon DJ, Rubin MR, Bilezikian JP, Silverberg SJ. Normocalcemic primary hyperparathyroidism: further characterization of a new clinical phenotype. J Clin Endocrinol Metab. 2007;92(8):3001–5.
5. Garnero P, Hausherr E, Chapuy M-C, et al. Markers of bone resorption predict hip fracture in elderly women: the EPIDOS prospective study. J Bone Miner Res. 1996;11:1531–8.
6. Parfitt AM, Villanueva AR, Foldes J, Rao DS. Relations between histologic indices of bone formation: implications for the pathogenesis of spinal osteoporosis. J Bone Miner Res. 1995; 10(3):466–73.
7. Bauer DC, Sklarin PM, Stone KL, et al. Biochemical markers of bone turnover and prediction of hip bone loss in older women: the study of osteoporotic fractures. J Bone Miner Res. 1999; 14(8):1404–10.
8. Garnero P. Markers of bone turnover for the prediction of fracture risk. Osteoporos Int. 2000;11 Suppl 6:S55–65.
9. Raisz LG. Pathogenesis of osteoporosis: concepts, conflicts, and prospects. J Clin Invest. 2005; 115(12):3318–25.

10. Christiansen P, Steiniche T, Brixen K, et al. Primary hyperparathyroidism: biochemical markers and bone mineral density at multiple skeletal sites in Danish patients. Bone. 1997;21(1):93–9.

11. Valdemarsson S, Lindergard B, Tibblin S, Bergenfelz A. Increased biochemical markers of bone formation and resorption in primary hyperparathyroidism with special reference to patients with mild disease. J Intern Med. 1998;243(2):115–22.

12. Katagiri M, Ohtawa T, Fukunaga M, Harada T. Evaluation of bone loss and the serum markers of bone metabolism in patients with hyperparathyroidism. Surg Today. 1995;25(7):598–604.

13. Parisien M, Silverberg SJ, Shane E, et al. The histomorphometry of bone in primary hyperparathyroidism: preservation of cancellous bone structure. J Clin Endocrinol Metab. 1990; 70(4):930–8.

14. Dempster DW, Parisien M, Silverberg SJ, et al. On the mechanism of cancellous bone preservation in postmenopausal women with mild primary hyperparathyroidism. J Clin Endocrinol Metab. 1999;84(5):1562–6.

15. Steiniche T, Christiansen P, Vesterby A, et al. Primary hyperparathyroidism: bone structure, balance, and remodeling before and 3 years after surgical treatment. Bone. 2000;26(5):535–43.

16. Parisien M, Cosman F, Mellish RW, et al. Bone structure in postmenopausal hyperparathyroid, osteoporotic, and normal women. J Bone Miner Res. 1995;10(9):1393–9.

17. Parisien M, Mellish RW, Silverberg SJ, et al. Maintenance of cancellous bone connectivity in primary hyperparathyroidism: trabecular strut analysis. J Bone Miner Res. 1992;7(8):913–9.

18. Eriksen EF, Mosekilde L, Melsen F. Trabecular bone remodeling and balance in primary hyperparathyroidism. Bone. 1986;7(3):213–21.

19. Silverberg SJ, Shane E, de la Cruz L, et al. Skeletal disease in primary hyperparathyroidism. J Bone Miner Res. 1989;4(3):283–91.

20. Christiansen P, Steiniche T, Vesterby A, Mosekilde L, Hessov I, Melsen F. Primary hyperparathyroidism: iliac crest trabecular bone volume, structure, remodeling, and balance evaluated by histomorphometric methods. Bone. 1992;13(1):41–9.

21. van Doorn L, Lips P, Netelenbos JC, Hackeng WH. Bone histomorphometry and serum concentrations of intact parathyroid hormone (PTH(1–84)) in patients with primary hyperparathyroidism. Bone Miner. 1993;23(3):233–42.

22. Vogel M, Hahn M, Delling G. Trabecular bone structure in patients with primary hyperparathyroidism. Virchows Arch. 1995;426(2):127–34.

23. Uchiyama T, Tanizawa T, Ito A, Endo N, Takahashi HE. Microstructure of the trabecula and cortex of iliac bone in primary hyperparathyroidism patients determined using histomorphometry and node-strut analysis. J Bone Miner Metab. 1999;17(4):283–8.

24. Barger-Lux MJ, Recker RR. Bone microstructure in osteoporosis: transilial biopsy and histomorphometry. Top Magn Reson Imaging. 2002;13(5):297–305.

25. Muller R, Van CH, Van DB, et al. Morphometric analysis of human bone biopsies: a quantitative structural comparison of histological sections and micro-computed tomography. Bone. 1998;23(1):59–66.

26. Dempster DW, Muller R, Zhou H, et al. Preserved three-dimensional cancellous bone structure in mild primary hyperparathyroidism. Bone. 2007;41(1):19–24.

27. Roschger P, Dempster DW, Zhou H, et al. New observations on bone quality in mild primary hyperparathyroidism as determined by quantitative backscattered electron imaging. J Bone Miner Res. 2007;22(5):717–23.

28. Dempster DW, Cosman F, Parisien M, Shen V, Lindsay R. Anabolic actions of parathyroid hormone on bone. Endocr Rev. 1993;14:690–709.

29. Bellido T, Ali AA, Gubrij I, et al. Chronic elevation of parathyroid hormone in mice reduces expression of sclerostin by osteocytes: a novel mechanism for hormonal control of osteoblastogenesis. Endocrinology. 2005;146(11):4577–83.

30. Fu Q, Jilka RL, Manolagas SC, O'Brien CA. Parathyroid hormone stimulates receptor activator of NFkappaB ligand and inhibits osteoprotegerin expression via protein kinase A activation of cAMP-response element-binding protein. J Biol Chem. 2002;277(50):48868–75.

31. Canalis E, Giustina A, Bilezikian JP. Mechanisms of anabolic therapies for osteoporosis. N Engl J Med. 2007;357(9):905–16.

32. Miller PD, Bilezikian JP. Bone densitometry in asymptomatic primary hyperparathyroidism. J Bone Miner Res. 2002;17:N98–102.
33. Silverberg SJ, Shane E, Jacobs TP, Siris E, Bilezikian JP. A 10-year prospective study of primary hyperparathyroidism with or without parathyroid surgery. N Engl J Med. 1999;341:1249–55.
34. Rubin MR, Bilezikian JP, McMahon DJ, et al. The natural history of primary hyperparathyroidism with or without parathyroid surgery after 15-years. J Clin Endocrinol Metab. 2008;93(9):3462–70.
35. Consensus Development Conference Panel. Diagnosis and management of asymptomatic primary hyperparathyroidism: consensus development conference statement. Ann Intern Med. 1991;114:593–7.
36. Wermers RA, Khosla S, Atkinson EJ, et al. Incidence of primary hyperparathyroidism in Rochester, Minnesota, 1993–2001: an update on the changing epidemiology of the disease. J Bone Miner Res. 2006;21(1):171–7.
37. Silverberg SJ. Natural history of primary hyperparathyroidism. Endocrinol Metabol Clin North Am. 2000;29(3):451–64.
38. Palmer M, Jakobsson S, Akerstrom G, Ljunghall S. Prevalence of hypercalcaemia in a health survey: a 14-year follow-up study of serum calcium values. Eur J Clin Invest. 1988;18(1):39–46.
39. Chen Q, Kaji H, Iu MF, et al. Effects of an excess and a deficiency of endogenous parathyroid hormone on volumetric bone mineral density and bone geometry determined by peripheral quantitative computed tomography in female subjects. J Clin Endocrinol Metab. 2003;88(10):4655–8.
40. Charopoulos I, Tournis S, Trovas G, et al. Effect of primary hyperparathyroidism on volumetric bone mineral density and bone geometry assessed by peripheral quantitative computed tomography in postmenopausal women. J Clin Endocrinol Metab. 2006;91(5):1748–53.
41. Eriksen EF. Primary hyperparathyroidism: lessons from bone histomorphometry. J Bone Miner Res. 2002;17:N95–7.
42. Silverberg SJ, Gartenberg F, Jacobs TP, et al. Increased bone mineral density after parathyroidectomy in primary hyperparathyroidism. J Clin Endocrinol Metab. 1995;80:729–34.
43. Christiansen P, Steiniche T, Brixen K, et al. Primary hyperparathyroidism: effect of parathyroidectomy on regional bone mineral density in Danish patients: a three-year follow-up study. Bone. 1999;25(5):589–95.
44. Leppla DC, Snyder W, Pak CY. Sequential changes in bone density before and after parathyroidectomy in primary hyperparathyroidism. Invest Radiol. 1982;17(6):604–6.
45. Rao DS, Phillips ER, Divine GW, Talpos GB. Randomized controlled clinical trial of surgery versus no surgery in patients with mild asymptomatic primary hyperparathyroidism. J Clin Endocrinol Metab. 2004;89(11):5415–22.
46. Marshall D, Johnell O, Wedel H. Meta-analysis of how well measures of bone mineral density predict occurrence of osteoporotic fractures. BMJ. 1996;312(7041):1254–9.
47. Bilezikian JP. Bone strength in primary hyperparathyroidism. Osteoporos Int. 2003;14 Suppl 5:113–7.
48. Parfitt AM. Parathyroid hormone and periosteal bone expansion. J Bone Miner Res. 2002;17(10):1741–3.
49. Adami S, Braga V, Squaranti R, Rossini M, Gatti D, Zamberlan N. Bone measurements in asymptomatic primary hyperparathyroidism. Bone. 1998;22(5):565–70.
50. Seeman E, Duan Y, Fong C, Edmonds J. Fracture site-specific deficits in bone size and volumetric density in men with spine or hip fractures. J Bone Miner Res. 2001;16(1):120–7.
51. Khosla S, Melton III LJ. Fracture risk in primary hyperparathyroidism. J Bone Miner Res. 2002;17:N103–7.
52. Khosla S, Melton III LJ, Wermers RA, Crowson CS, O'Fallon WM, Riggs BL. Primary hyperparathyroidism and the risk of fracture: a population-based study. J Bone Miner Res. 1999;14(10):1700–7.
53. Wilson RJ, Rao S, Ellis B, Kleerekoper M, Parfitt AM. Mild asymptomatic primary hyperparathyroidism is not a risk factor for vertebral fractures. Ann Intern Med. 1988;109:959–62.

54. Vestergaard P, Mollerup CL, Frokjaer VG, Christiansen P, Blichert-Toft M, Mosekilde L. Cohort study of risk of fracture before and after surgery for primary hyperparathyroidism. BMJ. 2000;321(7261):598–602.

55. Vestergaard P, Mosekilde L. Parathyroid surgery is associated with a decreased risk of hip and upper arm fractures in primary hyperparathyroidism: a controlled cohort study. J Intern Med. 2004;255(1):108–14.

56. Larsson K, Ljunghall S, Krusemo UB, Naessen T, Lindh E, Persson I. The risk of hip fractures in patients with primary hyperparathyroidism: a population-based cohort study with a follow-up of 19 years. J Intern Med. 1993;234(6):585–93.

57. Bilezikian JP, Potts Jr JT. Asymptomatic primary hyperparathyroidism: new issues and new questions – bridging the past with the future. J Bone Miner Res. 2002;17:N57–67.

58. De GS, Romagnoli E, Diacinti D, D'Erasmo E, Minisola S. The risk of fractures in postmeno-pausal women with primary hyperparathyroidism. Eur J Endocrinol. 2006;155(3):415–20.

59. Bilezikian JP, Silverberg SJ. Clinical practice. Asymptomatic primary hyperparathyroidism. N Engl J Med. 2004;350(17):1746–51.

60. Bilezikian JP, Khan AA, Potts Jr JT. Guidelines for the management of asymptomatic primary hyperparathyroidism: summary statement from the third international workshop. J Clin Endocrinol Metab. 2009;94(2):335–9.

61. Favus MJ. Postmenopausal osteoporosis and the detection of so-called secondary causes of low bone density. J Clin Endocrinol Metab. 2005;90(6):3800–1.

62. Tannenbaum C, Clark J, Schwartzman K, et al. Yield of laboratory testing to identify secondary contributors to osteoporosis in otherwise healthy women. J Clin Endocrinol Metab. 2003;87:4431–7.

63. Fitzpatrick LA. Secondary causes of osteoporosis. Mayo Clin Proc. 2002;77(5):453–68.

64. Compston J. Secondary causes of osteoporosis in men. Calcif Tissue Int. 2001;69(4):193–5.

65. Orlic ZC, Raisz LG. Causes of secondary osteoporosis. J Clin Densitom. 1999;2(1):79–92.

66. Harper KD, Weber TJ. Secondary osteoporosis – diagnostic considerations. Endocrinol Metabol Clin North Am. 1998;27(2):325–48.

Chapter 14
Genetic Aspects of Hereditary Hyperparathyroidism

Alberto Falchetti, Francesca Giusti, Loredana Cavalli, Tiziana Cavalli, and Maria Luisa Brandi

Keywords Primary hyperparathyroidism • Hereditary hyperparathyroidism • Clinical management • Mutational analysis • DNA testing • DNA polymorphisms in parathyroid diseases • Familial hypocalciuric hypercalcemia

Introduction

Primary hyperparathyroidism (PHPT) is an endocrine disorder whose onset is biochemically defined by an excessive and unregulated secretion of parathyroid hormone (PTH), from one or, more enlarged parathyroid glands and hypercalcemia. PHPT is most common in the sixth decade of life with an overall prevalence of 3/1,000 in the general population [1]. The female:male ratio has been reported to be 3:1 and women may exhibit the clinical expression of PHPT in the first menopausal decade, between 50 and 60 years [2]. PTH hypersecretion is generally caused by a solitary benign adenoma, in nearly 80% of cases, and less frequently by multiple adenomas or hyperplasia of all parathyroid glands, as observed in 15–20% of PHPT patients. Parathyroid carcinoma is a rare occurrence, representing no more than 0.5–1% of the overall PHPT cases [3].

PHPT rarely occurs in children and young adults, and when present in such subjects it is frequently within the context of a hyperparathyroid familial syndrome. Different from sporadic, nonsyndromic PHPT in which a single parathyroid adenoma constitutes the prevalent pathological finding, parathyroid hyperplasia is commonly seen in hereditary forms of PHPT: multiple endocrine neoplasia type 1 (MEN1) and type 2 (MEN2) syndromes, familial hypocalciuria hypercalcemia

A. Falchetti, MD • F. Giusti, MD • L. Cavalli, MD • T. Cavalli, MD • M.L. Brandi, MD (✉)
Department of Internal Medicine, University of Florence, Centro di Riferimento
Regionale sui Tumori Endocrini Ereditari, Azienda Ospedaliero-Universitaria Careggi,
Viale Morgagni, 85, Florence 50135, Italy
e-mail: m.brandi@dmi.unifi.it

A.A. Khan and O.H. Clark (eds.), *Handbook of Parathyroid Diseases:
A Case-Based Practical Guide*, DOI 10.1007/978-1-4614-2164-1_14,
© Springer Science+Business Media, LLC 2012

Table 14.1 Chromosomal localization and genetic defects underlying each familial form of hereditary hyperparathyroidism

Syndrome/OMIM#	Chromosomal localization	Gene/activity	Type of germline mutation
MEN1/131100	11q13	MEN1/ oncosoppressor	Inactivating
MEN2A/171400	10q11.1	RET/proto-oncogene	Activating
FIHPT/145000	11q13, 1q25-q31, 3q13.3-q21, and still unknown loci	MEN1/oncosoppres. HRPT2/oncosop- pres. CaSR/GPCR and still unknown genes	Inactivating for MEN1, HRPT2, and CaSR genes
HPT-JT/607393	1q25-q31	HRPT2/oncosoppres	Inactivating
FHH-NSHPT/ 145980-239200	3q13.3-q21	CaSR/GPCR	Inactivating
ADMH/601199	3q13.3-q21	CaSR/GPCR	Atypical inactivating

(FHH) syndrome, neonatal severe hyperparathyroidism (NSHPT) syndrome, autosomal dominant moderate hyperparathyroidism (ADMH) syndrome, hyperparathyroidism-jaw tumor (HPT-JT) syndrome, and familial isolated hyperparathyroidism (FIHPT) syndrome (Table 14.1).

In recent years, several genes have been discovered which cause parathyroid tumor(s) in hereditary forms of PHPT. Molecular tests for genetic risk assessment are now widely utilized and enable early identification of individuals at risk of developing PHPT. DNA testing has grown in its importance in the clinical management of such patients, since a large number of preventive care options have become available to patients and families with familial PHPT syndromes. This manuscript addresses general concepts on issues of genetic diagnosis, describing the role and practical usefulness of DNA-based diagnosis in patients affected by familial PHPT.

General Issues

Definition of Genetic Test

A genetic test consists of analysis of the human DNA, RNA, chromosomes, proteins, or metabolites in order to identify genetic abnormalities related to a heritable disorder. Although several different genetic strategies exist, we can briefly summarize such approaches as to direct testing, by examination of the DNA or RNA gene makeup; (a) linkage testing, by highly polymorphic DNA markers coinherited with a disease-causing gene; (b) biochemical testing, through the evaluation of specific metabolites; or (c) cytogenetic testing, by chromosome analysis.

Genetic Counseling

Genetic counseling must be performed before proceeding with any genetic testing for hereditary PTHT syndromes. It consists of an evaluation of a subject or a family to assess one or more of the following issues to (a) confirm/diagnosis or rule out a genetic condition; (b) identify medical management issues; (c) calculate and properly communicate genetic risks; and (d) provide or arrange for psychosocial support.

Genetic Consultation: For Whom?

Individuals and/or families at risk for a genetically transmitted PHPT-associated disease may benefit from genetic consultation. Information concerning the appropriateness of undergoing a genetics referral should be always given to these subjects. This approach identifies individuals who have an increased risk of having a specific genetic disorder so that treatment can be started as soon as possible.

Genetic testing may play a role in medical management (if diagnostic and/or predictive of treatment) or assist in personal decision making for education, employment, life experiences, and family planning issues.

Testing Strategy

In monogenic inherited PHPT-related syndromes, the planning for an appropriate testing strategy is mandatory.

First of all, the proband must undergo the genetic testing. When a germline disease-causing mutation, in a specific gene, has been detected in the proband, genetic counseling should be offered before testing other family members at risk (first-degree relatives). Conversely, when no germline mutation in a specific gene has been detected, the genetic testing of family members is not necessary. It has to be stressed that the disease-causing mutation must be known before testing relatives at risk. Consequently, biochemical–clinical surveillance must involve only the mutant carriers. It appears clear that the diagnosis of a genetic PHPT disorder has implications for many family members other than the affected ones.

Most of the PHPT-related genes have hundreds of disease-causing mutations (e.g., *MEN1* gene) and also benign variants, the so-called polymorphisms, which are likely to have no effect on health. Genetic tests are not usually able to detect all disease-causing mutations in a gene.

Reliability of Genetic Testing

Before ordering a mutational test, the following parameters must be considered:
(a) accuracy of the technical analysis, representing the probability of obtaining the
same result each time that the laboratory performs the test and (b) mutation detection rate, representing the probability that an individual with an inherited PHPT
disorder has an identifiable mutation (i.e., sensitivity).

DNA-Based Methods

Essentially, the following three molecular approaches can be considered: (a)
sequence analysis (nucleotide sequencing of a DNA segment); (b) mutation scanning [a segment of DNA may be screened by several methodological approaches
(e.g., SSCP, CSGE, DHPLC) to identify variant gene region(s)] that provides the
opportunity to identify variant regions to subsequently undergo sequence or
mutation analysis; and (c) targeted mutation analysis [searching for the presence
of a specific mutation, a specific type of mutation (e.g., a trinucleotide repeat
expansion, or deletions), or a set of mutations (e.g., a panel of mutations for
MEN2A), as opposed to complete gene sequencing or mutation scanning, which
detect most mutations in the tested region]. Overall, the sequence analysis has
slightly higher mutation detection rates. Mutation scanning is performed when
mutations are distributed throughout a gene, most families have different mutations, or sequence analysis would be excessively time consuming due to the size
of the gene.

Clinical Syndromes of Familial Primary Hyperparathyroidism

In general, PHPT is a sporadically occurring endocrine disorder and, as mentioned
above, can occur at any age, but it is seen most commonly in the sixth decade of life.
PHPT occurrence in children and young adults suggests the possibility of occurring
in the context of familial hyperparathyroid syndromes, such as MEN1, MEN2A,
FHH/NSHPT, ADMH, HPT/JT, and FIHPT (Table 14.1).

Most of the responsible genes for these syndromes have been identified
(Table 14.1) and their germline mutations have been demonstrated to account
for the genetic susceptibility to develop parathyroid tumors. The DNA testing has
improved diagnostic accuracy and simplified family monitoring in many cases.

The most common clinical features of familial hyperparathyroidism forms can
be briefly summarized as follows.

Table 14.2 Main clinical features of various forms of hereditary hyperparathyroidism

Syndrome	Age of onset (year)	Parathyroid glands involvement	Pathology
MEN1	20–25	Multiglandular	Hyperplasia/adenoma(s)
MEN2A	>30	Single/multiglandular	Multiple adenomas/ hyperplasia
FIHPT	Not reported	Single/multiglandular	Single, multiple adenoma(s)
HPT-JT	>30 (average age 32 year)	Single/multiglandular (generally two glands)	Single or double adenoma (cystic parathyroid adenomatosis). Parathyroid carcinoma in 10–15% of affected individuals
FHH/ NSHPT	All ages/at birth or within the first 6 months	Multiglandular	Mildly enlarged parathyroid glands/ markedly hyperplastic parathyroid glands
ADMH	44.5 ± 3.9	Single/multiglandular	Diffuse to nodular parathyroid neoplasia

Serum PTH

Higher serum PTH levels are reported in 15–100% [4] of cases according to the specific syndrome. In FIHPT and FHH, an inappropriate PTH level with respect to blood calcium levels can be found other than a clear hyperparathyroid state (Table 14.2).

Age of Onset

In general, the age of onset of familial hyperparathyroidism can be predicted in comparison to the nonsyndromic form of the disease, varying from three decades for the MEN1-PHPT to one to two decades for the other familial syndromes. Exceptions are seen in FHH, where higher/inappropriate PTH can be reported at any age, and FIHPT, in which significant data on this issue are lacking (Table 14.2).

Pathology

Hyperplastic parathyroid glands are usually seen in familial PHPT. This differs from the nonsyndromic form of PHPT in which a parathyroid adenoma is most commonly seen (Table 14.2).

Confounding Factors

Familial PHPT syndromes may not be diagnosed until later in life. This may be due to long-standing normocalcemia or the absence of symptoms of PHPT. It may also be due to limited experience of the attending physicians. Similarly a family history of renal stones or osteoporosis may not be elicited by inexperienced physicians who may not be familiar with PHPT or MEN syndromes.

Chromosomal localization and genetic defects underlying each familial form of hereditary hyperparathyroidism are described in Table 14.1. Although a molecular diagnosis can now be considered as an appropriate tool for the management of patients with familial PHPT, the real value of genetic testing is for in clinical screening and prophylactic surgery varies among these disorders.

The MEN1-Associated PHPT

MEN1-PHPT is the most common endocrinopathy associated with the syndrome, accounting for 2–4% of the overall PHPT cases. It represents the first clinical expression in approximately 90% of MEN1-affected individuals and its age of onset is typically between 20 and 25 years (Table 14.2), which is three decades earlier than sporadic, nonsyndromic, PHPT [5–7]. No evidence of sex prevalence has been described. The MEN1-PHPT penetrance reaches 100% with age and all MEN1-affected individuals are expected to exhibit hypercalcemia by age 50. However, due to the fact that MEN1-PHPT is often long-standing mild or asymptomatic, it is not surprising to diagnose it at an advanced age. In individuals affected, or at risk for MEN1 syndrome, such as asymptomatic gene mutant carriers, the biochemical evidence of hypercalcemia can be detected in the course of a periodic screening evaluation and reduced bone mass can also be observed in hyperparathyroid subjects as early as 35 years of age [8]. Finally, hypercalcemia may increase the secretion of gastrin from a gastrinoma, precipitating and/or exacerbating symptoms of Zollinger–Ellison syndrome (ZES) a clinical picture frequently associated with MEN1 syndrome [7].

MEN1 Gene Mutations and Polymorphisms

Since the cloning of the MEN1 gene in 1997 [9], more than 1,000 mutations and 20 polymorphisms have been described. More than 1,000 MEN1 families have been analyzed and gene mutations have been reported, mainly leading to truncated forms of the encoded product menin. No genotype/phenotype correlation has been found. Interestingly, the polymorphic *MEN1* gene variants could be useful for segregation analysis in informative kindreds when mutations are not detected [10, 11].

MEN1 mutations are more frequently identified in familial cases (90–94%) than in simplex cases (i.e., a single occurrence of MEN1 syndrome in a family) (6–10%) [12]. A mutation detection is most likely when one typical MEN1-associated endocrine tumor and at least one of the following conditions are present [5]: (1) a first-degree relative with a "classical" endocrine tumor; (2) an age of onset before 30 years; (3) multiple pancreatic tumors; and (4) parathyroid gland hyperplasia [10, 11, 13].

The Role of Genetic Testing in MEN1 Syndrome

It has been established that gene testing may decrease both morbidity and mortality associated with MEN1. In fact, early diagnosis of MEN1 syndrome-associated tumors and improved therapeutic strategies for management of metabolic complications have virtually eliminated ZES and complicated PHPT as causes of death [5]. Consequently, familial screening should be performed in children by the first decade of life. Although genetic testing enables the identification of a carrier status up to 20 years before the clinical manifestation of the disease, the lack of consensus on prophylactic intervention and the inability to predict the clinical pattern of future disease make this screening controversial [14]. A well-performed perspective study on *MEN1* gene mutant carriers showed that a biochemical occurrence of a neoplasm, including the MEN1-PHPT, can be identified 10 years earlier than its clinical presentation allowing early intervention [15, 16]. Moreover, it has to be considered that a negative DNA test result, in a familial member from an MEN1 family with known gene mutation, precludes the need for this subject to undergo periodic biochemical and clinical monitoring for MEN1-related disorders.

However, due to the widely reported inability of predicting tumor penetrance and malignant transformation individually, lifelong follow-up of MEN1 carriers is warranted to prevent tumor morbidity. When no mutation in the gene can be identified or genetic testing is not available, biochemical screening is a straightforward and inexpensive alternative [17].

The MEN2A-Associated PHPT

PHPT in MEN2A occurs in 15–30% of the affected subjects, less commonly than in MEN1 syndrome [5]. Although it may silently be present for several decades (asymptomatic in more than 80% of the patients), approximately 15% of MEN2A patients have nephrolithiasis [4, 5, 18]. However, its behavior is generally less aggressive than the MEN1-associated PHPT and it usually occurs after the third decade, with a median age at diagnosis of 38 years [18–20] (Table 14.2). Annual biochemical screening is recommended in case of affected individuals who have not had parathyroidectomy or parathyroid autotransplantation [21].

Since correlation between RET codon 634 mutations and MEN2A-PHPT exists, it has been suggested that patients carrying these mutations should be annually screened for PHPT by measuring serum calcium levels. Biochemical screening for PHPT in patients carrying different *RET* mutations, not localized at codon 634, and with a positive family history of PHPT should also be frequently performed [5].

RET Gene Mutations and Polymorphisms

In MEN2 syndrome, the major issue is to distinguish subjects who have MEN2-related medullary thyroid carcinoma (MTC) from those with isolated (nonsyndromic, sporadic) MTC, in particular for individuals presenting with multifocal MTC with a negative family history. The probability of a de novo *RET* mutation is 5% or less in an index case with MEN2A (50% in index case with MEN2B). However, it has been reported that 1–24% of the individuals with "sporadic" MTC have *RET* germline mutations [22–24].

Germline-activating mutations of *RET* proto-oncogene have been found in more than 90% of MEN2A and the existence of a stratification risk according to the intragenic localization of *RET* mutation has been widely accepted [5, 25]. In contrast to patients with MEN1 syndrome, here, the existence of a genotype/phenotype correlation has been clearly established. Mutations are located at exons 10, 11, 13, 14, 15, and 16 in more than 95% of MEN2 cases, indicating the existence of mutational hot spots. Several polymorphisms have been also described [26, 27], which are still of unknown clinical significance [28–34].

The Role of Genetic Testing in MEN2

Germline-activating mutations at codons 883, 918, and 922 (exons 15, 16), typical of MEN2B, have the highest risk for the development of aggressive MTC and should be operated on within the first 6 months of life; mutations at codons 611, 618, 620, and 634 (exons 10, 11), accounting for MEN2A/FMTC, have an intermediate risk and total thyroidectomy should be performed before the age of 5 years; mutations at codons 609, 768, 790, 791 804, and 891 (exons 10, 13, 14, 15), responsible for MEN2A/FMTC are generally less aggressive and, consequently, MTC should be operated on at a later stage, even if a universal consensus on this issue has not been reached. Consequently, *RET* testing can guide intervention both to prevent and treat MTC [5, 20, 21, 25, 35], providing the opportunity to significantly reduce mortality related to MTC. Similar data with *RET* genetic testing and MEN2A-PHPT are not available.

The FHH-NSHPT/NHPT Syndrome

FHH is a rare autosomal dominant disorder characterized by the occurrence of normal/increased levels of serum calcium, moderate hypophosphatemia, and normal/increased circulating PTH levels and a low calcium to creatinine clearance ratio [36]. Most of the FHH patients are asymptomatic and do not benefit from surgical resection of their mildly enlarged parathyroid glands since it cannot correct the calcium-dependent PTH secretion set-point abnormality [37, 38]. FHH-related hypercalcemia is highly penetrant at all ages [39] and, generally, these patients exhibit hypocalciuria (urinary calcium/creatinine ratio typically <0.01) in the presence of hypercalcemia and hyperparathyroidism due to inactivation of CaSR protein in renal tubules. A mild hypermagnesemia can be also found [39, 40].

FHH patients are usually asymptomatic and are identified on routine blood calcium testing.

NSHPT (Tables 14.1 and 14.2) generally represents the homozygous form of FHH, in which PHPT occurs at birth or within the first 6 months of life with poor muscle strength severe symptomatic hypercalcemia, and skeletal manifestations of PHPT. Surgery should be promptly performed to avoid a lethal outcome.

CaSR Gene Mutations and Polymorphisms

At the CaSR database (CaSR-db) (http://www.casrdb.mcgill.ca/), over 200 mutations, mostly missense, and 27 polymorphisms are reported. No definitive results have been reported on the possible role that CaSR polymorphisms may play on the development of the sporadic form of PHPT.

Role of CaSR Genetic Testing in FHH

In 150 subjects with *CaSR* mutational analysis the following was noted: (a) 52 mutant patients (15 index cases and 37 family members); (b) 16 different functional DNA variants; (c) 14 mutations were cosegregating with hypercalcemia; and (d) identification of the existence of predictive factors for *CaSR* gene mutations detection, such as (d1) the family history of hypercalcemia, the most relevant finding; (d2) the fact that 15% of the unsuccessful parathyroid operations the patients had a mutation; and (d3) the evidence that 12% of the mutant patients had elevated PTH levels [41]. Thus, a molecular genetic analysis of *CaSR* should be completed in those individuals with hypercalcemia, a positive family history or unsuccessful parathyroid surgery history.

As clinical and biochemical parameters are not always helpful in distinguishing between PHPT and FHH, DNA testing may be helpful in the diagnosis and clinical management of these conditions.

The Familial Hypercalcemia Hypercalciuria Syndrome or Autosomal Dominant Moderate Hyperparathyroidism

Carling et al. reported a large family with 20 members, from different generations, affected by this rare syndrome [42] (Table 14.2). Subjects were exhibiting hypercalcemia and hypercalciuria, with an inappropriately high serum PTH and magnesium levels and nephrolithiasis in a subset of patients.

DNA testing detected the presence of an atypical germline-inactivating mutation in the intracytoplasmic tail domain of CaSR at level in affected subjects.

Hyperparathyroidism/Jaw Tumor Syndrome

This rare autosomal dominantly inherited disorder (Tables 14.1 and 14.2) is characterized by the occurrence of fibrous-osseous tumors of the mandible and/or maxilla (ossifying fibroma), Wilms' tumor, papillary renal carcinoma, polycystic kidney disease, renal cysts, and PHPT [43]. In this syndrome, PHPT exhibits an aggressive behavior, and parathyroid carcinoma is seen in 10–15% of affected individuals, [43–47], with incomplete penetrance in HPT/JT [48, 49]. A reduced penetrance in females has also been reported [47].

Recently, the *HRPT2* gene, responsible for this syndrome, has been identified as the "tumor-suppressor gene" parafibromin, previously mapped at 1q25–q32. It appears to be also involved in the pathogenesis of sporadic forms of PHPT [50]. Fourteen germline-inactivating mutations of *HPRT2* gene have been identified in 26 kindreds [46] and approximately 60% of HPT/JT kindreds harbor a germline parafibromin mutation (Table 14.2). Mutations of *HRPT2* gene rarely occur in unselected benign parathyroid disease (<1%) and the molecular signatures of HPT/JT parathyroid "adenomas" and carcinomas are indistinguishable.

About 80% of HPT/JT patients present with PHPT [43, 47] that may develop in late adolescence or later years. When compared to MEN1-related PHPT, the HTP/JT-related PHPT seems to run a more aggressive course and the patients tend to have more severe hypercalcemia, and a hypercalcemic crisis is often the presenting feature.

The HPT/JT-associated jaw lesions have been reported to be histologically distinct from the typical bone lesions classically seen in PHPT [43, 51].

The Role of Genetic Testing of HRPT2 Gene

Most *HRPT2* mutations result in truncated parafibromin protein with loss of its expression by immunohistochemistry [52–54] (Table 14.2). Concerning the clinical management of HPT/JT patients tested for *HRPT2* mutations, we can highlight the following features: (a) the putative efficacy of early detection and treatment of HPT/JT-associated lesions; (b) *HRPT2* mutant parathyroid "adenomas" have an increased malignant potential; and (c) difficulties in managing lifelong hypoparathyroidism exist.

Somatic mutations have also been identified in the majority of sporadic, nonsyndromic parathyroid carcinomas (70%), whereas germline *HRPT2* mutations were detected in 30% of apparently sporadic parathyroid carcinomas [46]. Consequently, accurate surveillance for parathyroid, renal, and maxillary neoplasia in gene carrier is highly recommended, as well as the need to extend gene testing to other family members.

The Familial Isolated Hyperparathyroidism

FIHPT is another rare, hereditary, autosomal-dominant disorder characterized by uni- or multiglandular parathyroid lesions in the absence of other hyperfunctioning endocrine tissues (Tables 14.1 and 14.2) [55].

Due to its genetic heterogeneity, FIHPT can represent a peculiar manifestation of other familial hyperparathyroid syndromes. In fact, in FIHP cases, germline mutations have been identified in *MEN1* gene, 20–23% [56–58], in *CaSR* gene [42], 14–18% [57, 59] of families with FIHP, and, less frequently, *HRPT2* gene [50, 60, 61].

Recently, it has been reported that FIHPT can present either with symptomatic hypercalcemia, complications of primary hyperparathyroidism, such as osteoporosis and renal calculi, or remain asymptomatic, being diagnosed during investigations for an unrelated disorder.

Most of FIHPT kindreds currently have an unknown genetic background [62] (Table 14.2). To date, approximately over 100 FIHPT families have been described [59, 63].

Conclusions

The following points are noteworthy: (a) the autosomal dominant inheritance of some PHPT diseases suggests the importance of performing gene testing in family members at risk of developing a familial PHPT syndrome; (b) the identification of a gene mutation is important in life-planning decisions of affected patients; (c) the recognition of mutation has a variable weight in the clinical management of the gene mutant carriers; (d) a negative test result identifies subjects who do not require periodic screening; and (e) the great usefulness of gene testig in informing young patients about the possibility of prenatal genetic testing.

The increasing knowledge on the molecular bases of familial PHPT syndromes, together with the availability of genetic screening, greatly increases the likelihood that individuals with these syndromes will live full and normal lives, with the opportunity to develop individualized treatments in the future [64, 65]. Clinical investigations and molecular studies of the intricate molecular pathways of the involved genes are helpful to design novel therapeutic modalities.

Competing Interests The authors declared no financial or other relationship that might lead to a conflict of interest.

Acknowledgments This work was supported by grants from the Fondazione Ente Cassa di Risparmio di Firenze and F. I. R. M. O. Fondazione Raffaella Becagli to M. L. B.

References

1. Melton III LJ. Epidemiology of primary hyperparathyroidism. J Bone Miner Res. 1991;6 Suppl 2:S25–30.
2. Bilezikian JP, Silverberg SJ. Clinical spectrum of primary hyperparathyroidism. Rev Endocr Metab Disord. 2000;1(4):237–45.
3. DeLellis RA. Parathyroid carcinoma: an overview. Adv Anat Pathol. 2005;12(2):53–61.
4. Falchetti A, Brandi ML. Hereditary hyperparathyroidism. Clin Cases Miner Bone Metab. 2006;3(2):141–9.
5. Brandi ML, Gagel RF, Angeli A, et al. Guidelines for diagnosis and therapy of MEN type 1 and type 2. J Clin Endocrinol Metab. 2001;86(12):5658–71.
6. Uchino S, Noguchi S, Sato M, et al. Screening of the Men1 gene and discovery of germ-line and somatic mutations in apparently sporadic parathyroid tumors. Cancer Res. 2000;60:5553–7.
7. Marx SJ. Multiple endocrine neoplasia type 1. In: Scriver CR, Beaudet AL, Sly WS, Valle D, editors. The metabolic and molecular bases of inherited disease. 8th ed. New York: McGraw-Hill; 2001. p. 943–66.
8. Burgess JR, David R, Greenaway TM, Parameswaran V, Shepherd JJ. Osteoporosis in multiple endocrine neoplasia type 1: severity, clinical significance, relationship to primary hyperparathyroidism, and response to parathyroidectomy. Arch Surg. 1999;134:1119–23.
9. Chandrasekharappa SC, Guru SC, Manickam P, et al. Positional cloning of the gene for multiple endocrine neoplasia-type 1. Science. 1997;276(5311):404–7.
10. Tham E, Grandell U, Lindgren E, Toss G, Skogseid B, Nordenskjöld M. Clinical testing for mutations in the MEN1 gene in Sweden: a report on 200 unrelated cases. J Clin Endocrinol Metab. 2007;92(9):3389–95.
11. Lemos MC, Thakker RV. Multiple endocrine neoplasia type 1 (MEN1): analysis of 1336 mutations reported in the first decade following identification of the gene. Hum Mutat. 2008;29(1):22–32.
12. Guo SS, Sawicki MP. Molecular and genetic mechanisms of tumorigenesis in multiple endocrine neoplasia type-1. Mol Endocrinol. 2001;15(10):1653–64.
13. Schaaf L, Pickel J, Zinner K, et al. Developing effective screening strategies in multiple endocrine neoplasia type 1 (MEN 1) on the basis of clinical and sequencing data of German patients with MEN 1. Exp Clin Endocrinol Diabetes. 2007;115(8):509–17.
14. Glascock MJ, Carty SE. Multiple endocrine neoplasia type 1: fresh perspective on clinical features and penetrance. Surg Oncol. 2002;11(3):143–50.
15. Lairmore TC, Piersall LD, DeBenedetti MK, Dilley WG, Mutch MG, Whelan AJ, Zehnbauer B. Clinical genetic testing and early surgical intervention in patients with multiple endocrine neoplasia type 1 (MEN 1). Ann Surg. 2004;239(5):637–45.
16. Machens A, Schaaf L, Karges W, et al. Age-related penetrance of endocrine tumours in multiple endocrine neoplasia type 1 (MEN1): a multicentre study of 258 gene carriers. Clin Endocrinol (Oxf). 2007;67(4):613–22.
17. Herfarth KK, Wells Jr SA. Parathyroid glands and the multiple endocrine neoplasia syndromes and familial hypocalciuric hypercalcemia. Semin Surg Oncol. 1997;13(2):114–24.
18. Raue F, Kraimps JL, Dralle H, et al. Primary hyperparathyroidism in multiple endocrine neoplasia type 2A. J Intern Med. 1995;238(4):369–73.
19. Schuffenecker I, Virally-Monod M, Brohet R, et al. Risk and penetrance of primary hyperparathyroidism in multiple endocrine neoplasia type 2A families with mutations at codon 634 of the RET proto-oncogene. Groupe D'etude des Tumeurs à Calcitonine. J Clin Endocrinol Metab. 1998;83(2):487–91.
20. Frank-Raue K, Hoppner W, Frilling A, et al. Mutations of the ret proto-oncogene in German multiple endocrine neoplasia families: relation between genotype and phenotype. German Medullary Thyroid Carcinoma Study Group. J Clin Endocrinol Metab. 1996;81:1780–3.
21. Yip L, Cote GJ, Shapiro SE, et al. Multiple endocrine neoplasia type 2: evaluation of the genotype-phenotype relationship. Arch Surg. 2003;138:409–16.

22. Eng C, Mulligan LM, Smith DP, et al. Low frequency of germline mutations in the RET proto-oncogene in patients with apparently sporadic medullary thyroid carcinoma. Clin Endocrinol (Oxf). 1995;43(1):123–7.

23. Decker RA, Peacock ML, Borst MJ, Sweet JD, Thompson NW. Progress in genetic screening of multiple endocrine neoplasia type 2A: is calcitonin testing obsolete? Surgery. 1995;118(2): 257–63.

24. Kitamura Y, Goodfellow PJ, Shimizu K, et al. Novel germline RET proto-oncogene mutations associated with medullary thyroid carcinoma (MTC): mutation analysis in Japanese patients with MTC. Oncogene. 1997;14(25):3103–6.

25. Machens A, Dralle H. Multiple endocrine neoplasia type 2 and the RET protooncogene: from bedside to bench to bedside. Mol Cell Endocrinol. 2006;247(1–2):34–40.

26. Ceccherini I, Hofstra RM, Luo Y, et al. DNA polymorphisms and conditions for SSCP analysis of the 20 exons of the ret proto-oncogene. Oncogene. 1994;9(10):3025–9.

27. Sáez ME, Ruiz A, Cebrián A, Morales F, Robledo M, Antiñolo G, Borrego S. A new germline mutation, R600Q, within the coding region of RET proto-oncogene: a rare polymorphism or a MEN 2 causing mutation? Hum Mutat. 2000;15(1):122.

28. Demeester R, Parma J, Cochaux P, Vassart G, Abramowicz MJ. A rare variant, I852M, of the RET proto-oncogene in a patient with medullary thyroid carcinoma at age 20 years. Hum Mutat. 2001;17(4):354.

29. Nunes AB, Ezabella MC, Pereira AC, Krieger JE, Toledo SP. A novel Val648Ile substitution in RET protooncogene observed in a Cys634Arg multiple endocrine neoplasia type 2A kindred presenting with an adrenocorticotropin-producing pheochromocytoma. J Clin Endocrinol Metab. 2002;87(12):5658–61.

30. Gil L, Azañedo M, Pollán M, et al. Genetic analysis of RET, GFR alpha 1 and GDNF genes in Spanish families with multiple endocrine neoplasia type 2A. Int J Cancer. 2002;99(2):299–304.

31. Robledo M, Gil L, Pollán M, Cebrián A, et al. Polymorphisms G691S/S904S of RET as genetic modifiers of MEN 2A. Cancer Res. 2003;63(8):1814–7.

32. Elisei R, Cosci B, Romei C, et al. Identification of a novel point mutation in the RET gene (Ala883Thr), which is associated with medullary thyroid carcinoma phenotype only in homozygous condition. J Clin Endocrinol Metab. 2004;89(11):5823–7.

33. Ruiz A, Antiñolo G, Fernández RM, Eng C, Marcos I, Borrego S. Germline sequence variant S836S in the RET proto-oncogene is associated with low level predisposition to sporadic medullary thyroid carcinoma in the Spanish population. Clin Endocrinol (Oxf). 2001;55(3):399–402.

34. Berard I, Kraimps JL, Savagner F, et al. Germline-sequence variants S836S and L769L in the RE arranged during Transfection (RET) proto-oncogene are not associated with predisposition to sporadic medullary carcinoma in the French population. Clin Genet. 2004;65(2):150–2.

35. Schuffenecker I, Billaud M, Calender A, et al. RET proto-oncogene mutations in French MEN 2A and FMTC families. Hum Mol Genet. 1994;3(11):1939–43.

36. Marx SJ, Spiegel AM, Brown EM, Aurbach GD. Family studies in patients with primary parathyroid hyperplasia. Am J Med. 1977;62(5):698–706.

37. Thorgeirsson U, Costa J, Marx SJ. The parathyroid glands in familial hypocalciuric hypercalcemia. Hum Pathol. 1981;12(3):229–37.

38. Marx SJ, Stock JL, Attie MF, Downs Jr RW, Gardner DG, Brown EM, Spiegel AM, Doppman JL, Brennan MF. Familial hypocalciuric hypercalcemia: recognition among patients referred after unsuccessful parathyroid exploration. Ann Intern Med. 1980;92(3):351–6.

39. Marx SJ, Attie MF, Levine MA, Spiegel AM, Downs Jr RW, Lasker RD. The hypocalciuric or benign variant of familial hypercalcemia: clinical and biochemical features in fifteen kindreds. Medicine (Baltimore). 1981;60(6):397–412.

40. Kristiansen JH, Rodbro P, Christiansen C, Brochner Mortensen J, Carl J. Familial hypocalciuric hypercalcaemia. II. Intestinal calcium absorption and vitamin D metabolism. Clin Endocrinol (Oxf). 1985;23(5):511–5.

41. Nissen PH, Christensen SE, Heickendorff L, Brixen K, Mosekilde L. Molecular genetic analysis of the calcium sensing receptor gene in patients clinically suspected to have familial

hypocalciuric hypercalcemia: phenotypic variation and mutation spectrum in a Danish population. J Clin Endocrinol Metab. 2007;92(11):4373–9.

42. Carling T, Szabo E, Bai M, Ridefelt P, Westin G, Gustavsson P, Trivedi S, Hellman P, Brown EM, Dahl N, Rastad J. Familial hypercalcemia and hypercalciuria caused by a novel mutation in the cytoplasmic tail of the calcium receptor. J Clin Endocrinol Metab. 2000;85(5):2042–7.

43. Teh BT, Farnebo F, Kristoffersson U, Sundelin B, Cardinal J, Axelson R, Yap A, Epstein M, Heath III H, Cameron D, Larsson C. Autosomal dominant primary hyperparathyroidism and jaw tumor syndrome associated with renal hamartomas and cystic kidney disease: linkage to 1q21-q32 and loss of the wild type allele in renal hamartomas. J Clin Endocrinol Metab. 1996;81(12):4204–11.

44. Mallette LE, Malini S, Rappaport MP, Kirkland JL. Familial cystic parathyroid adenomatosis. Ann Intern Med. 1987;107(1):54–60.

45. Cavaco BM, Guerra L, Bradley KJ, Carvalho D, Harding B, Oliveira A, Santos MA, Sobrinho LG, Thakker RV, Leite V. Hyperparathyroidism-jaw tumor syndrome in Roma families from Portugal is due to a founder mutation of the HRPT2 gene. J Clin Endocrinol Metab. 2004;89: 1747–52.

46. Shattuck TM, Valimaki S, Obara T, Gaz RD, Clark OH, Shoback D, Wierman ME, Tojo K, Robbins CM, Carpten JD, Farnebo LO, Larsson C, Arnold A. Somatic and germ-line mutations of the HRPT2 gene in sporadic parathyroid carcinoma. N Engl J Med. 2003;349(18): 1722–9.

47. Chen JD, Morrison C, Zhang C, Kahnoski K, Carpten JD, Teh BT. Hyperparathyroidism-jaw tumour syndrome. J Intern Med. 2003;253:634–42.

48. Krebs LJ, Shattuck TM, Arnold A. HRPT2 mutational analysis of typical sporadic parathyroid adenomas. J Clin Endocrinol Metab. 2005;90(9):5015–7.

49. Kelly TG, Shattuck TM, Reyes-Mugica M, et al. Surveillance for early detection of aggressive parathyroid disease: carcinoma and atypical adenoma in familial isolated hyperparathyroidism associated with a germline HRPT2 mutation. J Bone Miner Res. 2006;21(10):1666–71.

50. Carpten JD, Robbins CM, Villablanca A, Forsberg L, Presciuttini S, Bailey-Wilson J, Simonds WF, Gillanders EM, Kennedy AM, Chen JD, Agarwal SK, Sood R, et al. HRPT2, encoding parafibromin, is mutated in hyperparathyroidism-jaw tumor syndrome. Nat Genet. 2002;32: 676–80.

51. Cavaco BM, Barros L, Pannett AA, Ruas L, Carvalheiro M, Ruas MM, Krausz T, Santos MA, Sobrinho LG, Leite V, Thakker RV. The hyperparathyroidism-jaw tumour syndrome in a Portuguese kindred. QJM. 2001;94(4):213–22.

52. Tan MH, Morrison C, Wang P, et al. Loss of parafibromin immunoreactivity is a distinguishing feature of parathyroid carcinoma. Clin Cancer Res. 2004;10(19):6629–37.

53. Gill AJ, Clarkson A, Gimm O, Keil J, Dralle H, Howell VM, Marsh DJ. Loss of nuclear expression of parafibromin distinguishes parathyroid carcinomas and hyperparathyroidism-jaw tumor (HPT-JT) syndrome-related adenomas from sporadic parathyroid adenomas and hyperplasias. Am J Surg Pathol. 2006;30(9):1140–9.

54. Cetani F, Ambrogini E, Viacava P, et al. Should parafibromin staining replace HRTP2 gene analysis as an additional tool for histologic diagnosis of parathyroid carcinoma? Eur J Endocrinol. 2007;156(5):547–54.

55. Wassif WS, Moniz CF, Friedman E, Wong S, Weber G, Nordenskjold M, Peters TJ, Larsson C. Familial isolated hyperparathyroidism: a distinct genetic entity with an increased risk of parathyroid cancer. J Clin Endocrinol Metab. 1993;77:1485–9.

56. Miedlich S, Lohmann T, Schneyer U, Lamsch P, Paschke R. Familial isolated primary hyperparathyroidism – a multiple endocrine neoplasia type 1 variant? Eur J Endocrinol. 2001; 145(2):155–60.

57. Warner J, Epstein M, Sweet A, Singh D, Burgess J, Stranks S, Hill P, Perry-Deene D, Learoyd D, Robinson B, Birdsey P, Mackenzie E, Teh BT, Prins JB, Cardinal J. Genetic testing in familial isolated hyperparathyroidism: unexpected results and their implications. J Med Genet. 2004;41:155–60.

58. Hannan FM, Nesbit MA, Christie PT, Fratter C, Dudley NE, Sadler GP, Thakker RV. Familial isolated primary hyperparathyroidism caused by mutations of the MEN1 gene. Nat Clin Pract Endocrinol Metab. 2008;4(1):53–8.

59. Simonds WF, James-Newton LA, Agarwal SK, Yang B, Skarulis MC, Hendy GN, Marx SJ. Familial isolated hyperparathyroidism: clinical and genetic characteristics of 36 kindreds. Medicine. 2002;81:1–26.
60. Teh BT, Farnebo F, Twigg S, Hoog A, Kytola S, Korpi-Hyovalti E, Wong FK, Nordenstrom J, Grimelius L, Sandelin K, Robinson B, Farnebo LO, Larsson C. Familial isolated hyperparathyroidism maps to the hyperparathyroidism-jaw tumor locus in 1q21-q32 in a subset of families. J Clin Endocrinol Metab. 1998;83:2114–20.
61. Villablanca A, Wassif WS, Smith T, Hoog A, Vierimaa O, Kassem M, Dwight T, Forsberg L, Du Q, Learoyd D, Jones K, Stranks S, Juhlin C, Teh BT, Carling T, Robinson B, Larsson C. Involvement of the MEN1 gene locus in familial isolated hyperparathyroidism. Eur J Endocrinol. 2002;147(3):313–22.
62. Carling T, Udelsman R. Parathyroid surgery in familial hyperparathyroid disorders. J Intern Med. 2005;257:27–37.
63. Huang SM, Duh QY, Shaver J, Siperstein AE, Kraimps JL, Clark OH. Familial hyperparathyroidism without multiple endocrine neoplasia. World J Surg. 1997;21:22–9.
64. Nemeth EF, Steffey ME, Hammerland LG, Hung BC, Van Wagenen BC, DelMar EG, Balandrin MF. Calcimimetics with potent and selective activity on the parathyroid calcium receptor. Proc Natl Acad Sci U S A. 1998;95(7):4040–5.
65. Falchetti A, Cilotti A, Vaggelli L, et al. A patient with MEN1-associated hyperparathyroidism, responsive to cinacalcet. Nat Clin Pract Endocrinol Metab. 2008;4(6):351–7.

Chapter 15
Hypoparathyroidism and Hypocalcemic States

Laura Masi and Maria Luisa Brandi

Keywords Hypocalcemia—acute, chronic • Differential diagnosis • Treatment • Sterol therapy • Refractoriness • Hypoparathyroidism

Clinical Case

A Caucasian 35-year-old woman 7 months pregnant was hospitalized with a spontaneous right hip fracture. She was suffering from asthenia, cramps, hypotension and tachycardia. Her height was 165 cm, weight was 60 kg. She has a history of type I diabetes diagnosed when she was 20 years old and Hashimoto's thyroiditis with hypothyroidism diagnosed when she was 30 years old. She was treated with insulin and Levo-thyroxine (L-thyroxine 125 mcg/day). In addition, vitiligo was noted before adulthood (Table 15.1).

A detailed medical history and physical examination was completed. The laboratory profile is listed below:

L. Masi, MD, (✉) • M.L. Brandi, MD
Department of Medicine, University of Florence, Centro di Riferimento Regionale sui Tumori Endocrini Ereditari, Azienda Ospedaliero-Universitaria Careggi, Florence, Italy
e-mail: m.brandi@dmi.unifi.it

A.A. Khan and O.H. Clark (eds.), *Handbook of Parathyroid Diseases:
A Case-Based Practical Guide*, DOI 10.1007/978-1-4614-2164-1_15,
© Springer Science+Business Media, LLC 2012

Table 15.1 Biochemical and hormonal characteristics of the patient

Parameters	Value	Normal value
Serum Ca	8.2*	8.2–10.7 mg/dL
Ionized calcium	4*	4.10–5.3 mg/dL
Serum P	5*	2.5–4.8 mg/dL
Urinary Ca	289	100–300 mg/24 h
Urinary P	468	400–1,000 mg/24 h
PTH	2*	1.3–7.6 pmol/L
$25(OH)D_3$	32.2	8–80 ng/mL
$1,25(OH)_2D_3$	18.2	16–65 pg/mL
Pyridinoline	7.7	2–8 µg mol/mol Cr.
Bone alkaline phosphatase	13.5	Pre-menopause: 4–14.3 µg/L
		Post-menopause: 4–22.5 µg/L
Cortisol	360	160–990 nmol/L
ACTH	18.6	9–52 ng/L
TSH	3.2	0.35–3.5 mU/L
fT3	4.3	3.5–6.4 pmol/L
fT4	14.6	10.3–19.4 pmol/L
aTPO	+	
aTG	+	
PCA	+	
AAA	−	
tTGA	−	
Ca intake	1,230	1,200–1,500 mg/day
P intake	988	800 mg/day for M; 1,000 mg/day for F

*abnormal values, + presence of serum antibodies, −absence of serum antibodies, *aTPO* thyroid preoxidase antibodies, *aTG* tyreoglobulin antibodies, *AAA* antiadrenal cortical antibodies, *PCA* parietal cells antibodies, *tTGA* transglutaminase antibodies

After delivery areal BMD (g/cm^2) was measured at the lumbar spine L1–L4 (LS-BMD) and at the left femoral neck (FN-BMD) and distal one-third radius (1/3-BMD) by dual energy X-ray absorptiometry (DXA) using the Hologic 4500 machine (Hologic, Waltham, MA, USA), with short-term *in vivo* coefficients of variation of 0.9%.

LS-BMD was low (0.840 g/cm^2). FN and 1/3-BMD were almost normal, respectively, 0.790 and 0.710 g/cm^2. Electrocardiogram (ECG) was also performed with normal layout.

The biochemical data showed low serum calcium and parathyroid hormone (PTH), mild hyperphosphatemia, normal urine Ca, inappropriately normal serum active vitamin D ($1,25(OH)_2D_3$), and normal urine P suggestive of a hypoparathyroidism.

Calcium Metabolism

Serum calcium (Ca) concentration is kept within a narrow physiological range due to complex control mechanisms involving the PTH, $1,25(OH)_2D_3$, calcitonin (CT), and calcium sensor receptors (CaSR). They act in the renal, intestinal, and bone tissues in order to maintain calcium homeostasis. Hypocalcemia occurs when homeostatic mechanisms fail or when they are not fully compensated. Dietary calcium is absorbed primarily in the small intestine with an efficiency of 30–40%. Up to half of absorbed dietary calcium is returned to the gastrointestinal (GI) tract and is excreted in the stool. Most of the remainder is excreted by the kidneys. The efficiency of absorption of dietary phosphate is greater than that of calcium (about 70%) and most is excreted by the kidneys. Approximately 99% of body calcium (the most abundant body cation) and 85% of phosphorus are found in bone, where they serve not only a structural role, but also as a reservoir for tissue and plasma calcium and phosphate. Most of the remaining phosphorus is intracellular. The majority of the 1% of calcium not found within the skeleton is located in the extracellular fluid. About half of this plasma calcium is ionized and capable of capillary diffusion into the intercellular space; the rest is bound to plasma proteins, such as albumin or other substances (citrate, sulfate, and phosphates). Ionized calcium, the physiologically active moiety, plays a vital role in many physiological processes, including bone formation, blood coagulation (prothrombin to thrombin conversion), skeletal and smooth muscle function, cardiac contractility and inotropy, nerve impulse initiation, and a host of other key physiological functions [1, 2]. Normal serum total calcium levels (generally 8.4–10.2 mg/dL or 2.12–2.55 mmol/L) and serum phosphate levels (2.5–4.5 mg/dL) are regulated to yield a calcium phosphate product of approximately 35 mg/dL. This product is important because of the potential for calcium phosphate salts to be deposited in soft tissues. Levels of the calcium phosphate product that exceed 50 are believed to place subjects at risk for ectopic soft tissue calcification.

PTH is synthesized and secreted by the parathyroid glands primarily in response to a fall in serum calcium levels. Through concerted actions on the kidney and bone, PTH is the principal regulator of plasma calcium homeostasis. In the kidney, PTH increases renal tubular reabsorption of calcium (while inversely inhibiting phosphate reabsorption) and increases the synthesis of $1,25(OH)_2D_3$ from its precursor 25-hydroxyvitamin D [$25(OH)D_3$]. Although $1,25(OH)_2D_3$ has a short in vivo half life (approximately 6 h), it directly increases intestinal calcium and phosphate absorption. In bone, PTH increases the efflux of calcium from bone, both from the rapidly exchangeable pool of calcium within bone, and by increasing the number and activity of osteoblasts and osteoclasts, thereby increasing bone turnover. As PTH also acts to inhibit the reabsorption of phosphate in the proximal nephron, it prevents an increase in plasma phosphate levels that could result from increased intestinal phosphate absorption and efflux of phosphate from bone. Calcitonin, secreted by C-cells of the thyroid gland, decreases serum calcium by inhibiting bone resorption and promoting renal tubular calcium excretion, but its effects are relatively minor in comparison to those of PTH and $1,25(OH)_2D_3$ [1, 2]. Figure 15.1 is showing an overview of the calcium homeostasis.

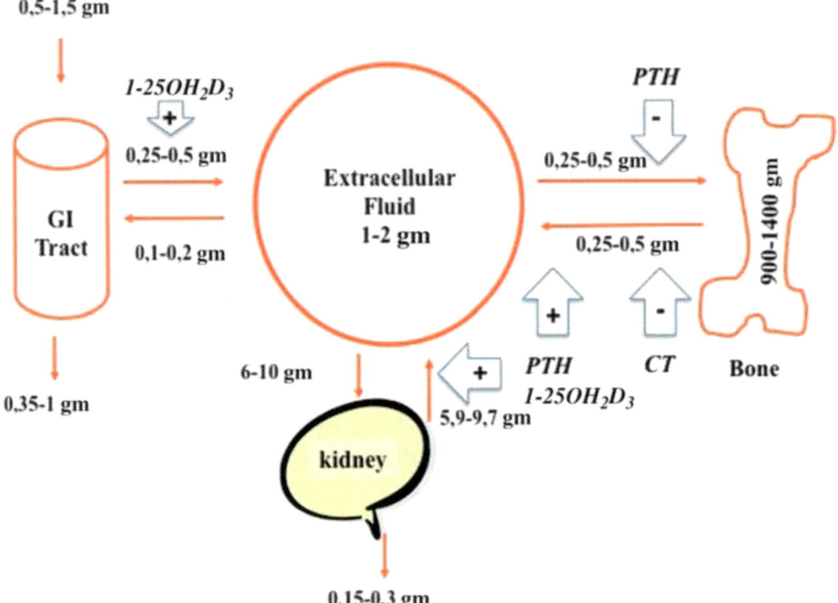

Fig. 15.1 Overview of the calcium homeostasis and the interaction between calcium and PTH, 1-25(OH)$_2$D$_3$ and calcitonin. *PTH* parathyroid hormone, *1-25(OH)$_2$D$_3$* calcitriol, *CT* calcitonin

Hypocalcemia

Hypocalcemia defined as a level of Ca that falls below the lower limit of the normal reference range. Symptoms of hypocalcemia occur when the level of ionized Ca is below 2.8 mg/dL (0.7 mmol/L), equivalent to 7.0–7.5 mg/dL (1.75–1.87 mmol/L) of total Ca [3, 4]. The severity of symptoms and clinical signs of hypocalcemia correlates with the magnitude and speed at which calcium declines, influenced by acid–base status and the presence of hypomagnesemia and/or sympathetic hyperactivity.

There are several causes for low ionized Ca. The disorder can be broadly classified as one in which there is inadequate PTH or vitamin D production, PTH or vitamin D resistance, or a miscellaneous cause. In Table 15.2, the causes of hypocalcemia are listed.

Acute Hypocalcemia

In acute and/or severe symptomatic hypocalcemia, there is a predominance of neuromuscular, neuropsychiatry, and cardiovascular abnormalities. There is an increase in neuromuscular excitability, latent or evident, with sensory and motor disruption.

Table 15.2 Etiologies for hypocalcemia

Inadequate PTH production
Genetic hypoparathyroidism
  PTH gene mutations
  X-linked hypoparathyroidism
  GCMB gene mutation with parathyroid gland agenesis
  Activating mutation of CaSR gene
Nongenetic hypoparathyroidism
  Postsurgical
  Autoimmune: isolated or polyglandular failure syndrome
  Acquired antibodies that active CaSR
  Postradiation
  Secondary to infiltrative processes (hemochromatosis; thalassemia, Wilson's disease, metastatic tumor)
  Hypo- and hypermagnesemia

Inadequate vitamin D production
Vitamin D deficiency
  Nutritional deficiency
  Lack of sunlight exposure
  Malasborption
  End-stage liver
  Chronic kidney disease

PTH resistance
  Pseudohypoparathyroidism
  Pseudo-pseudohypoparathyroidism

Vitamin D resistance
Pseudovitamin D deficiency rickets (Vitamin D-dependent rickets type 1)
Vitamin D-resistant rickets (Vitamin D-dependent rickets 2)

Others
Hungry bone syndrome: postthyroidectomy or postparathyroidectomy
Osteoblastic metastases
Rhabdomyolysis
Drugs: intravenous bisphosphonate, phenytoin, phenobarbital

Perioral or extremity paresthesia, cramps, myalgia, and muscule mild to moderate hypocalcemia can cause weakness. Smooth muscle spasms may cause biliary and intestinal cramps, dysphagia, bronchospasm, and laryngeal stridor. Severe hypocalcemia presents with spontaneous tetany, which may appear in the form of carpopedal spasm and, more rarely, laryngospasm. Neuropsychiatric manifestations include irritability, anxiety, psychosis, depression, mental confusion, and extrapyramidal abnormalities. Increased intracranial pressure, papilledema, and convulsions can also be present, and must be differentiated from severe tetany muscular spasms [5]. Hypocalcemia is well known for its effects on cardiac conduction resulting in bradycardia or ventricular arrhythmias, cardiovascular collapse, and hypotension that is non-responsive to fluids and vasopressors. In addition, a decrease in myocardial contractility occurs and prolongation of the QT-c interval is seen on the EKG.

Chronic Hypocalcemia

Patients with chronic hypocalcemia may or may not have symptoms of neuromuscular irritability, even in the presence of markedly low calcium levels. Asymptomatic cases may be detected by chance, by the presence of hypocalcemia on routine laboratory tests, during periods of greater calcium demand (i.e., gestation, lactation, menstrual cycle and states of alkalosis), or during the use of hypocalcemic drugs (i.e., bisphosphonates). Dental abnormalities suggest the time of onset of hypocalcemia. In infancy, it may lead to dental or enamel hypoplasia, the delay or absence of permanent tooth eruption, an increase in cavity occurrence, the shortening of molar roots, and, in some cases, the loss of all teeth [5].

Significant cognitive deficits, neuropsychiatric abnormalities, and extrapyramidal symptoms that resemble Parkinson's disease or chorea are associated with the calcification of basal ganglia, which occurs in all forms of chronic hypocalcemia and may be detected with greater sensitivity using computerized tomography [5]. Other findings of chronic hypocalcemia include subcapsular cataracts, an increase in bone mineral density (BMD) with unusual structural and dynamic features of bone. In particular, bone under chronic hypocalcemia due to low levels of PTH is characterized by significantly reduced osteoid width, osteoid surface, and mineral apposition. This bone alteration is associated with a low bone turnover with normal serum bone formation and bone resorption markers. The use of vitamin D to restore normal serum Ca cannot by itself restore the normal structure or dynamic properties of bone in hypoparathyroidism reflecting the unique actions of PTH on the skeleton [6].

Differential Diagnosis of Hypocalcemia

The most important biochemical parameters for diagnostic testing are determination of the serum ionized Ca, total magnesium (Mg), P, intact PTH and $25(OH)D_3$ values. Measuring intact PTH will reveal inappropriately low, low normal, or even undetectable PTH values in hypoparathyroidism. In contrast, in patients with low levels of vitamin D or with Pseudohypoparathyroidism serum calcium levels are low with high serum PTH. Phosphate levels are low in vitamin D deficiency state and high in hypoparathyroidism and pseudohypoparathyroidism. Accurate determination of 24-h urinary Ca excretion may be useful. Milder elevations are expected in hypoparathyroidism states [7].

The biochemical diagnosis of hypoparathyroidism is made in the presence of inappropriately low serum PTH with hypocalcemia and hyperphosphatemia. Primary renal failure must be excluded by evaluating creatinine clearance as this may also cause a high serum phosphate and a low $1,25(OH)_2D_3$.

DNA analysis may be of value in identifying mutations responsible for the various genetic forms of hypoparathyroidism and pseudohypoparathyroidism [8]. The

Table 15.3 Differences in the biochemical parameters in various forms of hypocalcemia

Diagnosis	Phosphate	PTH	$1\text{-}25(OH)_2D_3$
Hypoparathyroidism	↑	↓	↓
Pseudohypoparathyroidism	↑	↑↑	↓
Chronic renal failure	↑	↑	↓
Vitamin D deficiency	↓	↑	↓

goals of treatment are to alleviate symptoms and maintain acceptable ionized Ca or total serum Ca and avoid hypercalciuria in order to prevent renal dysfunction, stones, and nephrocalcinosis. In Table 15.3, the differences of biochemical parameters in the various forms of hypocalcemia are provided.

Therapy

The treatment of hypoparathyroidism is dependent on many factors including the presenting symptoms and the severity and rapidity of onset of symptoms. The aim of therapy is to maintain the serum calcium at or around the lower limit of the normal reference range (8–9 mg/dL), so that, on the one hand, hypocalcemic manifestations are limited to the mildest symptoms and, on the other hand, harmful hypercalcemia and hypercalciuria are avoided. If therapy is successful, symptoms associated with hypoparathyroidism should not affect the patient's daily life, and long-term complications should be avoided. Transient hypercalcemia should be avoided because recurrent episodes may cause irreparable kidney damage.

Management of *acute or severe* symptomatic hypocalcemia is treated with intravenous calcium. 10–30 mL of 10% calcium gluconate is given slowly over 10 min with maximum of 30 mg/min as an IV bolus (93–279 mg of elementary calcium), and repeated as many times as necessary. After the grave acute symptoms have resolved, elemental calcium levels are maintained via continuous intravenous infusion of 0.5 –1.5 mg/kg/h (maximum of 100 mg/h) of calcium for 4–6 h, using a solution with SG 5% (D5W) 900 mL + 100 mL of 10% gluconate (930 mg elementary calcium/liter).

Hyperphosphatemia, alkalosis, and hypomagnesemia, when present, must be corrected. Serum calcium levels must be measured frequently in this period, and electrocardiographic monitoring must be done, especially in those patients using digitalis as rises in serum calcium increase the risk of digitalis toxicity. Endovenous transition to oral calcium must be made as soon as possible [5].

Chronic management of hypocalcemia requires oral Ca supplements and vitamin D metabolites.

The conventional treatment for hypoparathyroidism consists of vitamin D and its analogs. These sterols, however, lack the important renal action of PTH of stimulating the distal

Table 15.4 Calciferol steroid therapy used in the therapy of hypoparathyroidism

Sterol	Average dosage (μg/kg-day)	Average T1/2 (days)	Comments
$1,25(OH)_2D_3$	0.03	1	
$1\alpha(OH)D$	0.06	2	
DHT	20	7	
25(OH)D	4	15	
D_2 and D_3	50	30	Risk of cumulative action

tubular reabsorption of calcium. A normocalcemic patient with hypoparathyroidism excretes, on average, threefold more calcium in the urine than a normal person and this increases the risk of calcium sedimentation in the kidney that may lead to nephrocalcinosis, nephrolithiasis and renal insufficiency [8–10].

Vitamin D_2 and D_3 have slow, prolonged and cumulative action because they are stored in adipose tissue. These sterols may increase the risk of severe prolonged hypercalcemia, even after years of stable maintenance of normocalcemia, and require monitoring. The biologically active metabolites of vitamin D, calcitriol, and 1α hydroxy vitamin D are the fastest and shortest acting derivates and are the best options for treatment. This therapy provides the advantage of a rapid achievement of full action (less than 1 week) allowing easy control of calcemia with a relatively short biological half-life for rapid reversal, in case of over dosage [8, 11]. Finally, dihydrotachysterol (DHT), an intermediate-acting derivate, also is an excellent drug for long-term therapy. DHT is started in a small dose and for subsequent fine adjustment the increments or the decrements in the dose should be around 10% [8]. Patients with pseudohypoparathyroidism with low urinary calcium in relation to serum calcium may achieve normal serum calcium without developing hypercalciuria. Vitamin D intoxication must be considered in patients with hypercalcemic symptoms.

The ideal long-term therapy for hypoparathyroidism includes the biologically active form of vitamin D, calcitriol given twice daily. The dose is usually 0.25 to 0.5 mcg. Calcium and sometimes magnesium supplementation is added and given in small increments three to four times daily. Hypoparathyroidism also requires a calcium supplement of approximately 1 g/day, divided into three or four doses, given orally. The usual doses of vitamin D analogs are listed in Table 15.4.

Thiazide diuretics may offer a complementary strategy to limit the risk of nephrocalcinosis in cases of persistently severe hypocalcemia and hypercalciuria. The product of calcium x phosphate must be kept below 55. These patients must have their kidneys radiologically evaluated regularly in order to rule out nephrocalcinosis [12]. The administration of thiazide diuretics in the usual antihypertensive doses and sodium restriction in patients with hypoparathyroidism lowers urinary calcium excretion. Hypercalciuric Hypocalcemia due to a CaSR mutation when treated with hydrochlorothiazide and vitamin D_3 can successfully reduce the patient's urinary calcium excretion [13]. This hypocalciuric effect allows the calcium and vitamin D supplements to be reduced. The treatment also may protect against the development of kidney stones. Although this approach is beneficial in some patients, the use of diuretics may be problematic in patients with concurrent adrenal insufficiency (due to polyglandular disease) or impaired renal function.

Some forms of hypoparathyroidism require special attention and monitoring. For example, in cases of hypocalcemia due to an activating mutation of the Ca receptor (CaSR) there is a tendency to excessive hypercalciuria even at low or below normal serum calcium levels. The aim of vitamin D administration is to correct or prevent the occurrence of clinical symptoms of severe hypocalcemia and to concurrently avoid hypercalciuria. All severely symptomatic patients should be treated. The decision to initiate treatment, however, should be carefully evaluated on a case-by-case basis in mildly symptomatic patients. Based on a retrospective analysis of patients with CaSR mutations, treatment recommendations have been published [14, 18].

Refractoriness to Sterol Therapy

Some patients become refractory to oral steroid therapy. This is most common in patients with hypoparathyroidism associated with autoimmune polyglandular syndrome [8]. In these patients, one contributing factor to their chronic hypocalcemia and refractoriness to vitamin D therapy is fat malabsorption. Dietary and supplemental calcium is poorly absorbed. In addition, these patients are prone to vitamin D deficiency which further exacerbates their tendency to hypocalcemia. Magnesium deficiency is also common which can be managed with $MgCl_2$ supplementation in daily doses of 2 mmol/kg divided into four doses.

PTH1-34 treatment has the advantage of normalizing calcemia without increasing calciuria, reducing the risk of nephrocalcinosis and renal insufficiency, and, theoretically, the antagonists of the CaSR may be utilized in the treatment to promote the inactivation of the receptor and, consequently, increase PTH secretion, but there still have not been sufficient studies [15].

Clinical Case Conclusion

Diagnosis

1. Patient showed biochemical findings suggestive of hypoparathyroidism.
2. The association of hypoparathyroidism with diabetes type I, Hashimoto's thyroiditis and vitiligo is consistent with a diagnosis of autoimmune polyglandular syndrome [16]. Autoimmune celiac disease or Addison's disease were not present.
3. The clinical status was complicated by osteoporosis at the lumbar spine with normal value for cortical bone mass. We thought that the sudden hip fracture which occurred in the patient could be the result of multiple factors:

(a) The possibility that the low levels of PTH could be the cause of:
a low bone modeling during childhood followed by achievement of low peak bone mass, an anomalous remodeling characterized by markedly unusual structural and dynamic properties of bone [6].

(b) The loss of bone mass during pregnancy

4. Remember: Type I diabetes may be associated with [16]:

(a) Celiac disease: tTGA antibodies (8–12% in the type I diabetes vs. 0.5–1% in general population) were negative in this case.

Addison's disease: AAA antibodies (0.7–3% in type I diabetes vs. 0.005% in general population) were negative in this patient.

Pernicious anemia: not present in this patient.

Autoimmune Gastritis: PCA antibodies (15–20% in type I diabetes vs. 0.15–1% in general population) were positive in this patient.

Therapy

The absence of severe signs of hypocalcemia was due to a chronic hypocalcemic state. In addition, during pregnancy hypoparathyroid women may have fewer hypocalcemic symptoms and require less supplemental calcium. This is consistent with a limited role for PTH in the pregnant women where a PTH independent increase of $1\text{-}25(OH)_2D$ is present. This is due to the fact that the renal 1-alpha hydroxylase is up-regulated in response to factors such as the increasing levels of PTH-related peptide (PTH-rP) and estradiol in maternal circulation [17].

The therapy of choice in this patient is oral administration of calcium and vitamin D.

Recommendation

Patient with Hypocalcemia

A detailed family history (which may suggest a genetic cause) and relevant medical history (particularly regarding neck surgery and autoimmune disease) are required.

↓

Measurements of serum total and ionized calcium, albumin, phosphorus, magnesium, and intact PTH levels.

↓

Severe symptoms: Therapy with intravenous calcium should be initiated immediately

Absence of symptoms: Outpatient treatment with calcium carbonate three times daily and calcitriol once or twice daily would be appropriate, with adjustment as needed to maintain a target level of albumin-corrected serum calcium at the lower end of the normal range [approximately 8.0–8.5 mg/dL (2.00–2.12 mmol/L)], a 24-h urinary calcium level well below 300 mg, and a calcium–phosphate product below 55.

References

1. Leibrandt T, editor. Diagnostics. Nurse's Reference Library, Nursing Books; 1983; pp. 1–1089.
2. Shoback D. Hypoparathyroidism. N Engl J Med. 2008;359:391–403.
3. Broadus AE. Mineral balance and homeostasis. In: Favus MJ, editor. Primer on the metabolic bone diseases and disorders of mineral metabolism. 5th ed. Washington DC: American Society for Bone and Mineral Research; 2003. p. 105–11.
4. Bushinsky DA, Monk RD. Electrolyte quintet: calcium. Lancet. 1998;352:306–11.
5. Maeda SS, Fortes EM, Oliveira MU, Borba VCZ, Lazaretti-Castro M. Hypoparathyroidism and pseudohypoparathyroidism. Arq Bras Endocrinol Metab. 2006;50–4:664–73.
6. Rubin MR, Dempster DW, Zhou H, Shane E, Nickolas T, Sliney Jr J, Silverberg SJ, Bilezikian JP. Dynamic and structural properties of the skeleton in hypoparathyroidism. J Bone Miner Res. 2008;23:2018–24.
7. Shoback D. Hypocalcemia: definition, etiology, pathogenesis, diagnosis and management. In: Rosen CJ, Compston JE, Lian JB, editors. Primer on the metabolic bone diseases and disorders of mineral metabolism, chapter 68. 7th ed. Washington DC: ASBMR; 2008. p. 313–7.
8. Masi L, Winer KK, Potts JP, Brandi ML. Management of hypoparathyroidism. Clin Cases Miner Bone Metab. 2004;2:127–8.
9. Litvak J, Moldawer MP, Forbes AP, Henneman PH. Hypocalcemic hypercalciuria during vitamin D and dihydrotachysterol therapy of hypoparathyroidism. J Clin Endocrinol Metab. 1958;18:246–71.
10. Weber G, Cazzuffi MA, Frisone F, et al. Nephrocalcinosis in children and adolescents: sonographic evaluation during long-term treatment with 1,25-dihydrocholecalciferol. Child Nephrol Urol. 1988;89:273, 2762–2763.
11. Bouillon R, Okamura WH, Norman AW. Structure-function relationship in the vitamin D endocrine system. Endocr Rev. 1995;36:200–57.
12. Levine M. Hypoparathyroidism and pseudohypoparathyroidism. In: DeGroot LJ, Jameson JL, editors. Endocrinology. 4th ed. Philadelphia: WB Saunders; 2001. p. 1133–53.
13. Sato K, Hasegawa Y, Nake J, Nanao K, Takahashi I, Tajima T, Shinohara N, Fujieda K. Hyrochlorothiazide effectively reduces urinary calcium excretion in two Japanese patients with gain-of-function mutations of the calcium-sensing receptor gene. J Clin Endocrinol Metab. 2002;87:3068–73.

14. Lienhardt A, Bai M, Lagarde JP, Rigaud M, Zhang Z, Jiang Y, Kottler ML, Brown EM, Garabedian M. Activating mutations of the calcium-sensing receptor: management of hypocalcemia. J Clin Endocrinol Metab. 2001;86:5313–23.
15. Winer KK, Ko CW, Reynolds JC, Dowdy K, Keil M, Peterson D, et al. Long-term treatment of hypoparathyroidism: a randomized controlled study comparing parathyroid hormone-(1–34) versus calcitriol and calcium. J Clin Endocrinol Metab. 2003;88:4214–20.
16. Van Den Driessche A, Eenkoorn V, Van Gall L, De Block C. Type 1 diabetes and autoimmune polyglandular syndrome: a clinical review. Neth J Med. 2009;67:376–87.
17. Kovacs CS, Kronenberg HM. Pregnancy and lactation. In: Rosen CJ, editor. Primer on the metabolic bone diseases and disorders of mineral metabolism, chapter 18. 7th ed. Washington DC: ASBMR; 2008. p. 90–5.
18. Bilezikian J, Khan A, Potts J, Brandi ML, Clarke B, Shoback D, et al. Hypoparathyroidism in the adult: epidemiology, diagnosis, pathophysiology target-organ involvement, treatment and challenges for future research. JBMR. 2011;26:2317–37.

Chapter 16
Molecular Pathogenesis of Primary Hyperparathyroidism

Kelly Lauter and Andrew Arnold

Keywords Hyperparathyroidism • Cyclin D1 • MEN1 • CDKN1B • CTNNB1 • p27 • B-Catenin • RET • CASR • HRPT2 • Parathyroid carcinoma • Parathyroid adenoma • Multiple endocrine neoplasia • Calcium sensing receptor • Hyperparathyroidism jaw tumor syndrome • Familial isolated hyperparathyroidism • Parafibromin • Ectopic PTH secretion • FHH • Neonatal severe hyperparathyroidism

Molecular Oncologic Principles and the Parathyroids

The molecular pathogenesis of primary hyperparathyroidism has recently been elucidated to a great extent, but many questions remain. While the molecular genetics of parathyroid disease have notable specific features, the general principles of parathyroid tumorigenesis are shared with those of tumor formation in other neoplastic diseases.

Parathyroid adenomas and carcinomas are monoclonal neoplasms, and many examples of "parathyroid hyperplasia" have also been shown to contain clonal outgrowths [1, 2]. This clonality indicates that the growth originated from a single cell, which acquired a selective growth advantage. Such a selective advantage is typically conferred by changes in the genome, potentially from external stimuli like ionizing

K. Lauter, MD
Center for Molecular Medicine, University of Connecticut, School of Medicine,
Farmington, CT, USA

A. Arnold, MD (✉)
Center for Molecular Medicine, University of Connecticut, School of Medicine,
263 Farmington Avenue, Farmington, CT 06030-3101, USA
e-mail: molecularmedicine@uchc.edu

A.A. Khan and O.H. Clark (eds.), *Handbook of Parathyroid Diseases:
A Case-Based Practical Guide*, DOI 10.1007/978-1-4614-2164-1_16,
© Springer Science+Business Media, LLC 2012

irradiation or chemical carcinogens, or from intrinsic errors in DNA/chromosomal replication [3]. Additionally, epigenetic changes such as methylation or acetylation of a gene, may play a role in tumor formation.

Clonal growth of a tumor can result from DNA alterations in two main categories of growth controlling genes, tumor suppressor genes and protooncogenes. Tumor suppressor genes contribute to tumorigenesis through their inactivation. Typically, the inactivation occurs by a genetic mutation or deletion which renders the gene product either absent from the cell or nonfunctional [4, 5]. Conversion from a protooncogene to an oncogene can result from a variety of genetic lesions, such as amplification (increased gene copy number), gain-of-function point mutation, or gene rearrangement that creates a novel gene fusion or increases expression of the structurally normal gene product [6].

In practical terms, exploring the changes in chromosome/gene copy number can uncover the location tumor suppressors and protooncogenes that may contribute to tumorigenesis, providing important initial clues to their eventual identification. For classical tumor suppressor genes following Knudson's two-hit formulation [7], independent events that inactivate both alleles in the tumor progenitor cell are needed to impart a selective growth advantage. Loss of heterozygosity (LOH), in which an individual's normal genome contains two distinguishable alleles for a particular gene, and the tumor cell only possesses one allele, can result from various genetic mechanisms, including allelic deletion that commonly serve to somatically inactivate tumor suppressors. The recurrent presence of LOH in a chromosomal region carries the strong suggestion that a tumor suppressor gene may be present in the region, but often such regions are large and consequently it is difficult to identify the true tumor suppressor gene among scores of innocent bystander genes in the region of LOH. Tumor suppressor validation in these instances generally requires identification of an intragenic inactivating mutation of the remaining allele since bystander genes would not be expected to have suffered a second hit. Microarray technology has enabled the genome-wide survey of large numbers of single nucleotide polymorphisms (SNPs) which can reveal genomic deletions and amplifications that are present within a tumor. Newer technologies using massively parallel DNA sequencing can also yield such information as well as identify intragenic mutations on a genome-wide basis.

Molecular Genetic Drivers of Parathyroid Tumorigenesis

The discovery that parathyroid adenomas were monoclonal indicated that, while these growths are benign, they would have specific acquired genetic alterations which contribute to the tumor cells' selective advantage. Additionally, linkage analysis and testing of candidate genes in familial diseases have revealed the genetic basis of many of these heritable predispositions. In the following pages, we describe the genes which have been directly implicated in the molecular pathogenesis of primary parathyroid disease (Table 16.1).

Table 16.1 Germ line and somatic genetics of primary hyperparathyroidism

Parathyroid disease	Gene(s) involved
Sporadic parathyroid adenoma	*CCND1 (PRAD1), MEN1, CDKN1B* pending confirmation: *CTNNB1*
Sporadic parathyroid carcinoma	*HRPT2*
MEN1	*MEN1*
"MEN4" and related states	*CDKN1B*, other CDK inhibitor genes
MEN2A	*RET*
HPT-JT	*HRPT2*
Familial hypocalciuric hypercalcemia (FHH) Neonatal severe hyperparathyroidism	*CASR*
Familial isolated hyperparathyroidism (FIHP)	*MEN1, HRPT2, CASR*, others

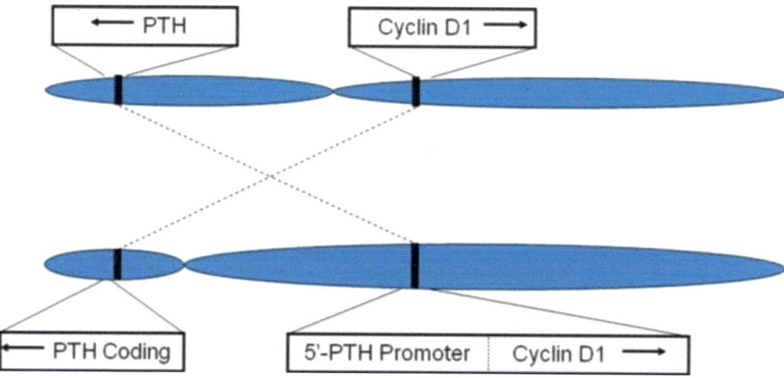

Fig. 16.1 Schematic diagram of the DNA rearrangement on chromosome 11 which induces tumor formation in a subset of parathyroid adenomas. This pericentromeric inversion places the *PTH* gene upstream regulatory region adjacent to the *Cyclin D1* oncogene

Cyclin D1

DNA rearrangements, such as translocations, can activate oncogenes, and these events have been well-characterized in many different neoplastic diseases. For example, the translocation t(14;18) in follicular lymphoma places the *BCL-2* protooncogene in close proximity to the strong regulatory sequences of the immunoglobulin heavy-chain gene, activating BCL2 expression in B lymphoid cells. *Cyclin D1 (PRAD1, CCND1)* is an oncogene that is activated by a similar mechanism in a subset of parathyroid adenomas, and is also involved in many types of human cancers [8].

The type of rearrangement that activates *cyclin D1* in parathyroid adenomas is diagrammed in Fig. 16.1. Its juxtaposition near the strong PTH gene control sequences leads to overexpression of cyclin D1 mRNA and protein, which in turn drives excessive parathyroid cell proliferation. Cyclin D1 acts by binding to the cyclin-dependent

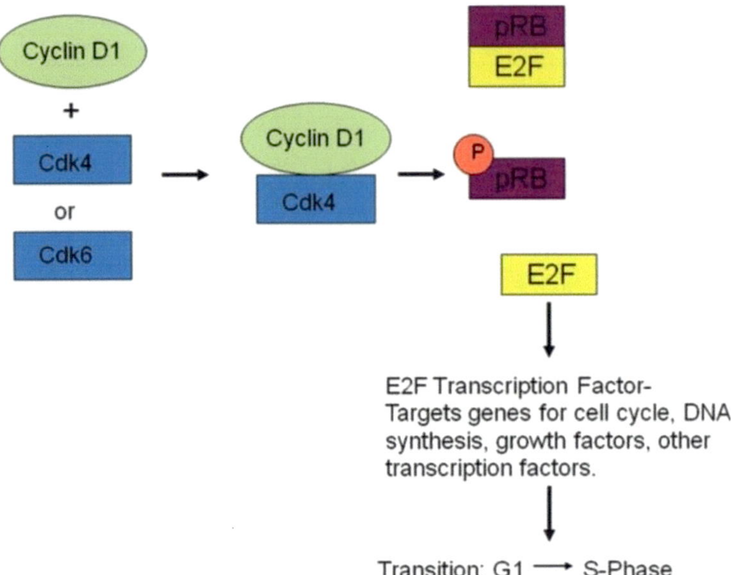

Fig. 16.2 Schematic diagram of cyclin D1 function binding to CDK4/6 to promote the transition from G1 to the S-phase of the cell cycle

kinase (CDK) proteins, specifically CDK4 and CDK6. This complex can then phosphorylate pRB, a tumor suppressor, which normally binds to the E2F transcription factor, acting as a repressor (Fig. 16.2). An inhibitory protein, such as p27 or p21, can bind the Cyclin-CDK complex, making it unable to phosphorylate pRB. Upon phosphorylation, pRB releases E2F, which can then bind DNA in the nucleus, targeting many genes involved in cell cycle progression, including CDK2 and 4 as well as the cyclins A, D1, and E [9]. Additionally, cyclin D1/CDK4 complexes can sequester p27, making it unable to interact with CDK2, resulting in increased cellular proliferation despite adequate quantities of p27 [10], or p27 can bind to a cyclin-CDK complex to inhibit its kinase activity and repress progression of the cell cycle.

Southern blotting has detected *CCND1-PTH* rearrangements in about 5–8% of adenomas; however, because of insensitivity of the detection method used, such rearrangements may be more common [11–13]. Even if rearrangements are somewhat more frequent, overexpression of *CCND1* has been found in as many as 20–40% of parathyroid adenomas, strongly suggesting that mechanisms other than rearrangement also participate in tumorigenic cyclin D1 activation. Of importance, parathyroid-targeted overexpression of cyclin D1 is sufficient to drive parathyroid tumorigenesis in transgenic mice.

Future work will include additional analyses of translocations in parathyroid tumors to determine if a different promoter could participate in *CCND1* upregulation, if the *PTH* promoter could upregulate expression of a different oncogene, or if there are entirely different translocations which participate in parathyroid tumorigenesis.

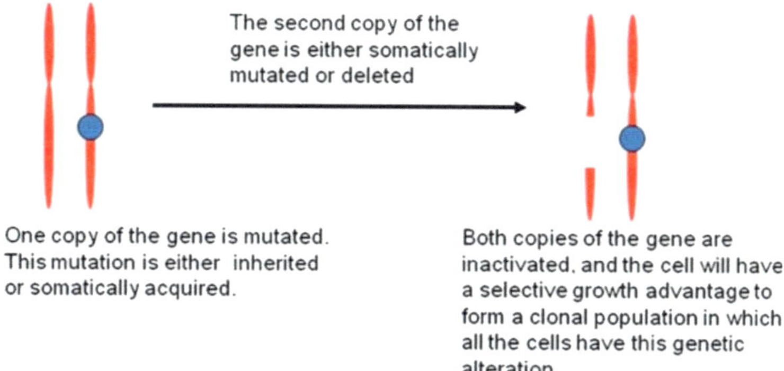

Fig. 16.3 Schematic diagram of Knudson's 2-hit mechanism illustrating inactivation of a tumor suppressor gene

MEN1

The *MEN1* tumor suppressor gene was originally found in the search for the genetic basis of the familial syndrome Multiple Endocrine Neoplasia Type 1 (MEN1). Linkage analysis of families harboring this autosomal dominant predisposition pointed to a location on chromosome 11q13 [14, 15]. Although *CCND1* is located on the same cytogenetic band, *MEN1* was mapped to an area several million base pairs upstream. One candidate gene in this region was determined to be *MEN1* based on the detection of inactivating germ line mutations within the gene in multiple families with MEN1. Tumors from patients with MEN1 had acquired LOH at markers in the 11q region, and the allele which was lost originated from the unaffected parent [15]. Thus, *MEN1* inactivation generally follows Knudson's two-hit model characteristic of a classic tumor suppressor gene, in which the patient inherits a mutant allele from one parent, and subsequently acquires an alteration in the remaining allele, rendering the gene nonfunctional (Fig. 16.3).

Subsequently, *MEN1* was investigated in sporadic parathyroid adenoma, and about 12–20% of tumors were found to have an acquired *MEN1* mutation, clearly demonstrating that somatic mutation of the gene in the parathyroid gland contributes to sporadic parathyroid adenoma development [16–18].

MEN1 has also been implicated in familial isolated hyperparathyroidism (FIHP) [19]. FIHP accounts for about 1% of primary hyperparathyroidism, and is due to either incomplete expression of a syndrome, such as MEN1 or HPT-JT, or (apparently in most instances) a genetically distinct syndrome. Like *MEN1*, other genes, such as *HRPT2* and *CASR* that are involved in specific familial hyperparathyroid syndromes have been occasionally associated with FIHP. These genes are discussed in further detail below.

Sequencing of *MEN1* in familial MEN1 cases has revealed over 300 distinct germ line mutations [20] which are dispersed throughout the gene. While some minor clustering has been reported [20], generally speaking the large spectrum of mutations reflects the multiple ways in which a gene can be inactivated and is consistent with a classical tumor suppressor mechanism.

MEN1 contains 10 exons, 9 of which are coding, that span 7.2 kb of DNA. It encodes menin, a 610 amino acid protein (68 kDa) which is not highly homologous to other proteins. Despite its specificity for the development of a narrow spectrum of endocrine and nonendocrine tumors when mutated, menin is normally expressed in a large variety of tissue types [21]. A mouse model with selective homozygous loss of menin in the liver, illustrated that despite a 97% reduction in the Men1 transcript in hepatocytes, liver abnormalities did not develop [22]. Therefore, menin may have a more crucial or nonredundant function in certain tissues, or regulate/complex with specific proteins that are only functional in those tissues with a tendency to develop MEN1-related tumors [22].

While studies have revealed many binding partners for menin, the function of this protein is still under investigation. At least two nuclear localization signals (NLSs) have been identified in the C-terminal portion of menin [23]. It has been suggested by immunohistochemical analysis that menin, while typically localized in the nucleus, is translocated to the cytoplasm during the M phase of the cell cycle [24]. A similar study approached this question with western blotting, and found no difference in menin localization throughout the cell cycle [21].

Menin has been associated with regulation of many different cellular functions, including gene transcription, cell proliferation, and apoptosis [25]. It has been shown to interact with many proteins, such as JunD, where it aids in repressing transcriptional activation [26]. Menin interacts with activator of S-phase kinase (ASK) [27] and the NF-κB proteins p50, p52, and p65 [28] to repress cell proliferation; menin also effects TGF-β-induced growth inhibition [29], specifically through interaction with Smad3 and the resultant blockage of Smad3-DNA binding [30]. Additionally, menin can bind directly to several secondary DNA structures, an interaction which is mediated by the carboxy-terminus of the protein [31]. Overexpression of menin leads to Bax/Bak-induced apoptosis, and deletion of menin reduces UV and TNF-α-induced apoptosis [32]. Menin also can bind to the loci of genes such as p27, p18, and Hoxc8, and a reduction of menin reduces their expression, a relationship which would be expected between these tumor suppressor genes [25]. While menin represses these genes, it increases expression of IGFBP-2, which regulates cell growth. Importantly, menin has been shown to bind the mixed-lineage leukemia (MLL) proteins, which form a complex that functions as the histone methyltransferase (HMT) necessary for *CDKN1B* and *CDKN2C* (p27 and p18) expression [25]. This interaction illustrates the role of menin as a scaffold protein, regulating transcription of target genes through chromatin modification [25, 33]. Thus, while menin seems to participate in many cellular pathways, its exact function in normal physiology and in tumorigenesis remains under investigation.

RET

Multiple Endocrine Neoplasia Type 2A (MEN2A) manifests parathyroid tumors in about 20% of patients. MEN2A is mainly associated with medullary thyroid carcinoma, and pheochromocytomas, both with higher penetrance than the parathyroid disease; parathyroid tumors very rarely occur in MEN type 2B, which features MTC, pheochromocytoma, and mucosal neuromas. MEN2A is due to an activating mutation, typically in the cysteine-rich domain, of the *RET* protooncogene, which encodes a receptor tyrosine kinase [34]. It has also been suggested that a specific mutation may be associated with the parathyroid disease phenotype [35]. *RET* has been examined as a candidate gene for somatic mutation in sporadic parathyroid adenomas, and despite its role in MEN2A-related parathyroid disease, such mutations rarely if ever contribute to sporadic parathyroid adenoma formation [36].

CDKN1B

The findings that up to 30% of patients who develop classical familial MEN1-like disease, and up to 89% of patients who develop a variant disease with sporadic parathyroid and pituitary tumors, are negative for *MEN1* mutation [37–40], suggest that there are additional gene(s) which contribute to this type of endocrine disease. Recently, a syndrome in rats termed MENX, consisting of a combination of the human MEN1 and MEN2 characteristics, namely parathyroid hyperplasia, bilateral pheochromocytomas, multifocal thyroid C cell hyperplasia, paragangliomas, and pituitary adenoma [41], was found to result from a mutation of the *CDKN1B* gene [42]. *CDKN1B* encodes the $p27^{Kip1}$, or p27, protein, which is a CDK inhibitor. By binding to and inhibiting cyclin/CDK complexes, p27 can inhibit cell cycle progression from G1 to the S phase, thus having the potential to act as a tumor suppressor gene [43, 44]. Additionally, p27 expression is significantly decreased in human parathyroid adenomas as compared to normal parathyroid glands [45, 46].

Thus, the potential for *CDKN1B* mutation to cause MEN1-like disease in patients who lacked *MEN1* mutation was explored, and *CDKN1B* mutation was found in a 48-year-old female with a pituitary adenoma and primary hyperparathyroidism [42]. The mutation was also present in an older sister who was diagnosed with renal angiomyolipoma, and their father suffered from acromegaly; a brother died at age 39 from hypertension, suggesting the possibility (unproven) of pheochromocytoma [42]. *CDKN1B* was also examined in a population of 37 patients with MEN1-like disease who were negative for MEN1 mutation and 19 familial and 50 sporadic acromegaly/pituitary adenoma patients, and one of the 37 MEN1-like patients (2.8%) possessed a duplication in *CDKN1B* which led to a truncated p27 protein [47]. Subsequently, *CDKN1B* was examined in 27 individuals with multiple endocrine tumors and the absence of identifiable *MEN1* mutations, but no *CDKN1B* mutations were uncovered [40]. Thus, germ line *CDKN1B* mutations appear to be important in a small minority of individuals or families with MEN1-like phenotypes who have no detectable *MEN1* mutation. Furthermore, alterations of p27 or one of three other genes encoding cdk inhibitors p15, p18, and p21, were implicated in a few percent of *MEN1* mutation-negative patients with MEN1-like features [48]. Finally, evidence for a role of p27 DNA alterations in common, sporadically presenting parathyroid adenomas was recently reported [49].

CTNNB1

The contribution of clonally selected mutations in *CTNNB1*, which encodes β-catenin and, more generally, the potential role of the Wnt signaling pathway, in parathyroid adenoma tumorigenesis, is currently uncertain and continues to be investigated. β-catenin is a primarily cytoplasmic protein that is targeted for degradation via phosphorylation in the absence of growth signals. If β-catenin is not phosphorylated, it can accumulate in the cytoplasm and be translocated into the nucleus, where it binds other proteins and acts as a transcription factor for numerous genes, including *c-myc*, *cyclin D1*, *E-cadherin*, and *RET*.

One group used immunohistochemistry to find accumulated β-catenin in all 37 parathyroid adenomas analyzed [50], whereas another group failed to detect these abnormalities [51]. In the former study, a single homozygous protein-stabilizing somatic mutation in the phosphorylation site, located in exon 3, was found in 3 of 20 parathyroid adenomas (15%) [50]. A follow-up study from this group identified additional cases of the identical somatic mutation S37A, although at a lower frequency of 5.8%, with the combined results from both studies revealing 7.3% of parathyroid adenomas with this alteration [52], and uniformly increased β-catenin expression in typical adenomas. However, neither S37A nor any other exon 3 mutation was found in series of adenomas from the USA and Japan [51, 53, 54]. The explanation for this discrepancy remains unclear, and further investigations are necessary to clarify this situation.

CASR

The calcium sensing receptor (CaSR), encoded by the *CASR* gene, is a seven-membrane-spanning G-protein coupled receptor which can sense extracellular calcium levels and control PTH secretion [55]. Mutation of *CASR* thus leads to an altered "set point," which is defined as the calcium concentration at which PTH secretion is half of its maximal value. An increase in this setpoint, in this case due to decreased function of CaSR, would thus result in hypercalcemia. Germ line mutation of *CASR* has been implicated as the major cause of familial hypocalciuric hypercalcemia (FHH) and neonatal severe hyperparathyroidism (NSHPT) [56]. FHH is an autosomal-dominant condition involving lifelong elevated serum calcium levels, lower than expected fractional urinary excretion of calcium, and elevated or inappropriately normal PTH levels. NSHPT is the homozygous form of

FHH, which leads to dangerously elevated serum calcium and PTH, and "floppy," slow to develop, children. NSHPT is typically lethal if total parathyroidectomy is not performed early in life. Numerous inactivating *CASR* mutations have been documented, and there is not one specific "hot spot" which can be preferentially tested for mutations [57]. *CASR* mutations also account for a small number of FIHP cases [58]. Due to its major role in FHH and NSHPT, *CASR* has been examined for somatic mutations in sporadic parathyroid adenomas, carcinomas, and secondary/tertiary hyperplasias, and the dearth of detectable mutations implies that such mutations, if acquired in an otherwise normal parathyroid cell in adult life, do not confer a significant selective advantage upon the cell [59]. This is in contrast to the dramatic proliferative outcome of homozygous *CASR* mutation when present in all cells throughout embryonic development (in NSHPT). That said, decreased expression of the CaSR could well contribute to the altered setpoint found in sporadic parathyroid adenomas.

HRPT2

Primary hyperparathyroidism is also present in the hyperparathyroidism-jaw tumor syndrome (HPT-JT), an autosomal dominant condition in which patients may also develop ossifying fibromas of the jaw, bilateral renal cysts, renal hamartomas, or Wilms tumors. The *HRPT2* gene, which encodes a 531 amino acid protein termed parafibromin, was linked to chromosome 1q25-q32 and subsequently identified through positional cloning in families with HPT-JT [60]. Germ line mutation in *HRPT2* is also responsible for a small subset of kindreds with FIHP [61].

Parathyroid tumors in HPT-JT are primarily benign adenomas, which may develop asynchronously, but parathyroid carcinomas also occur with increased frequency (about 15–20%) in HPT-JT. Accordingly, the possible role of acquired mutation of the *HRPT2* gene in sporadic parathyroid carcinoma was studied, and inactivating *HRPT2* mutations have been detected in over 75% of these tumors [62–64]. Because noncoding mutations would have escaped detection, it is likely that virtually all parathyroid carcinomas are driven by inactivation of *HRPT2*. In contrast, such mutations are exceedingly rare in typical sporadic parathyroid adenomas [65]. Furthermore, a subset of patients with apparently sporadic parathyroid carcinoma bears a germ line mutation of *HRPT2*, and may transmit the increased risk of parathyroid malignancy to offspring [62]. This finding warrants consideration of *HRPT2* DNA testing in such individuals.

Parafibromin has homology to the cdc73 protein in yeast, which is important in regulation of gene expression as part of the Paf1 complex. For example, parafibromin interacts with the proteins Paf1, Leo1, and Ctr9, and RNA polymerase II to play a role in transcription elongation and 3′ end processing [66], and its downregulation promotes entry into the S phase of the cell cycle [67, 68]. Parafibromin has an NLS at amino acids 136–139, which is required for proper localization and function of the protein [69, 70]. Immunohistochemistry has identified proper nuclear localization in parathyroid adenomas, while carcinomas, which typically contain *HRPT2* mutations, frequently have decreased or absent nuclear parafibromin staining. The possible utility of immunohistochemical testing for parafibromin expression in clinical diagnosis is being examined.

Other Candidate Genes in Sporadic Adenoma

A number of candidate genes have been investigated for a primary role, evidenced by intragenic somatic mutation, in adenoma formation, including *RAS*; *p53*; *the vitamin D receptor* (*VDR*); *CASR*; *RET*; *RAD51; and RAD54* [71], with no mutations being detected. Nonetheless, the existence of various clonal chromosomal and genetic alterations in parathyroid tumors suggests that a number of additional contributing oncogenes and tumor suppressors do participate and await discovery [72, 73].

Ectopic PTH Secretion

The ectopic secretion of PTH by nonparathyroid tumors is a very rare cause of biochemical primary hyperparathyroidism. Ectopic PTH may occur with or without accompanying PTHrP production. Ectopic PTH secretion has been reported in a variety of tumor types, including small cell lung cancer, thymoma, neuroectodermal/neuroendocrine cancers, ovarian and papillary thyroid carcinomas. Although the molecular basis for ectopic PTH expression was not identified in most instances, rearrangement and amplification of the *PTH* gene was responsible in an ovarian clear cell carcinoma [74], and transcriptional transactivation of PTH was found in a pancreatic neuroendocrine carcinoma [75].

Summary

While the genetics of primary hyperparathyroidism have recently advanced, there is still much to learn. Alterations in genes, such as *Cyclin D1*, *MEN1*, and *HRPT2*, have been implicated as drivers of parathyroid tumorigenesis. *Cyclin D1* alterations have also been implicated in the cause of many other human tumors. Multiple additional genetic contributors to parathyroid neoplasia must exist but are yet unknown. Much of the genetics of familial syndromes, such as MEN1, MEN2, FHH, and HPT-JT, have been elucidated. Future research will investigate how these genes and their pathways might converge, and knowledge of the exact functions of proteins such as menin, could provide important information regarding the mechanisms of neoplastic transformation. These future advances should lead to new diagnostic, prognostic, and treatment strategies for patients with all forms of primary hyperparathyroidism.

References

1. Arnold A, Staunton CE, Kim HG, Gaz RD, Kronenberg HM. Monoclonality and abnormal parathyroid hormone genes in parathyroid adenomas. N Engl J Med. 1988;318(11):658–62.
2. Arnold A, Brown MF, Urena P, Gaz RD, Sarfati E, Drueke TB. Monoclonality of parathyroid tumors in chronic renal failure and in primary parathyroid hyperplasia. J Clin Invest. 1995;95(5):2047–53.
3. Lengauer C, Kinzler KW, Vogelstein B. Genetic instabilities in human cancers. Nature. 1998;396(6712):643–9.
4. Marshall CJ. Tumor suppressor genes. Cell. 1991;64(2):313–26.
5. Haber D, Harlow E. Tumour-suppressor genes: evolving definitions in the genomic age. Nat Genet. 1997;16(4):320–2.
6. Koss LG. The mystery of chromosomal translocations in cancer. Cytogenet Genome Res. 2007;118(2–4):247–51.
7. Knudson Jr AG. Mutation and cancer: statistical study of retinoblastoma. Proc Natl Acad Sci USA. 1971;68(4):820–3.
8. Motokura T, Bloom T, Kim HG, et al. A novel cyclin encoded by a bcl1-linked candidate oncogene. Nature. 1991;350(6318):512–5.
9. Tashiro E, Tsuchiya A, Imoto M. Functions of cyclin D1 as an oncogene and regulation of cyclin D1 expression. Cancer Sci. 2007;98(5):629–35.
10. Matsuda Y. Molecular mechanism underlying the functional loss of cyclin-dependent kinase inhibitors p16 and p27 in hepatocellular carcinoma. World J Gastroenterol. 2008;14(11): 1734–40.
11. Williams ME, Swerdlow SH, Rosenberg CL, Arnold A. Chromosome 11 translocation breakpoints at the PRAD1/cyclin D1 gene locus in centrocytic lymphoma. Leukemia. 1993;7(2): 241–5.
12. Williams ME, Swerdlow SH, Rosenberg CL, Arnold A. Characterization of chromosome 11 translocation breakpoints at the bcl-1 and PRAD1 loci in centrocytic lymphoma. Cancer Res. 1992;52(19 Suppl):5541s–4s.
13. Rosenberg CL, Kim HG, Shows TB, Kronenberg HM, Arnold A. Rearrangement and overexpression of D11S287E, a candidate oncogene on chromosome 11q13 in benign parathyroid tumors. Oncogene. 1991;6(3):449–53.
14. Larsson C, Skogseid B, Oberg K, Nakamura Y, Nordenskjold M. Multiple endocrine neoplasia type 1 gene maps to chromosome 11 and is lost in insulinoma. Nature. 1988;332(6159): 85–7.
15. Bystrom C, Larsson C, Blomberg C, et al. Localization of the MEN1 gene to a small region within chromosome 11q13 by deletion mapping in tumors. Proc Natl Acad Sci USA. 1990;87(5):1968–72.
16. Heppner C, Kester MB, Agarwal SK, et al. Somatic mutation of the MEN1 gene in parathyroid tumours. Nat Genet. 1997;16(4):375–8.
17. Farnebo F, Teh BT, Kytola S, et al. Alterations of the MEN1 gene in sporadic parathyroid tumors. J Clin Endocrinol Metab. 1998;83(8):2627–30.
18. Carling T, Correa P, Hessman O, et al. Parathyroid MEN1 gene mutations in relation to clinical characteristics of nonfamilial primary hyperparathyroidism. J Clin Endocrinol Metab. 1998;83:2960–3.
19. Hannan FM, Nesbit MA, Christie PT, et al. Familial isolated primary hyperparathyroidism caused by mutations of the MEN1 gene. Nat Clin Pract Endocrinol Metab. 2008;4(1):53–8.
20. Lemos MC, Thakker RV. Multiple endocrine neoplasia type 1 (MEN1): analysis of 1336 mutations reported in the first decade following identification of the gene. Hum Mutat. 2008;29(1):22–32.
21. Wautot V, Khodaei S, Frappart L, et al. Expression analysis of endogenous menin, the product of the multiple endocrine neoplasia type 1 gene, in cell lines and human tissues. Int J Cancer. 2000;85(6):877–81.

22. Scacheri PC, Crabtree JS, Kennedy AL, et al. Homozygous loss of menin is well tolerated in liver, a tissue not affected in MEN1. Mamm Genome. 2004;15(11):872–7.
23. Guru SC, Goldsmith PK, Burns AL, et al. Menin, the product of the MEN1 gene, is a nuclear protein. Proc Natl Acad Sci USA. 1998;95(4):1630–4.
24. Huang SC, Zhuang Z, Weil RJ, et al. Nuclear/cytoplasmic localization of the multiple endocrine neoplasia type 1 gene product, menin. Lab Invest. 1999;79(3):301–10.
25. Yang Y, Hua X. In search of tumor suppressing functions of menin. Mol Cell Endocrinol. 2007;265–266:34–41.
26. Agarwal SK, Guru SC, Heppner C, et al. Menin interacts with the AP1 transcription factor JunD and represses JunD-activated transcription. Cell. 1999;96(1):143–52.
27. Schnepp RW, Hou Z, Wang H, et al. Functional interaction between tumor suppressor menin and activator of S-phase kinase. Cancer Res. 2004;64(18):6791–6.
28. Heppner C, Bilimoria KY, Agarwal SK, et al. The tumor suppressor protein menin interacts with NF-kappaB proteins and inhibits NF-kappaB-mediated transactivation. Oncogene. 2001;20(36):4917–25.
29. Sowa H, Kaji H, Kitazawa R, et al. Menin inactivation leads to loss of transforming growth factor beta inhibition of parathyroid cell proliferation and parathyroid hormone secretion. Cancer Res. 2004;64(6):2222–8.
30. Kaji H, Canaff L, Lebrun JJ, Goltzman D, Hendy GN. Inactivation of menin, a Smad3-interacting protein, blocks transforming growth factor type beta signaling. Proc Natl Acad Sci USA. 2001;98(7):3837–42.
31. La P, Silva AC, Hou Z, et al. Direct binding of DNA by tumor suppressor menin. J Biol Chem. 2004;279(47):49045–54.
32. Schnepp RW, Mao H, Sykes SM, et al. Menin induces apoptosis in murine embryonic fibroblasts. J Biol Chem. 2004;279(11):10685–91.
33. Yokoyama A, Cleary ML. Menin critically links MLL proteins with LEDGF on cancer-associated target genes. Cancer Cell. 2008;14(1):36–46.
34. Thakker RV. Multiple endocrine neoplasia. Horm Res. 2001;56 Suppl 1:67–72.
35. Mulligan LM, Eng C, Healey CS, et al. Specific mutations of the RET proto-oncogene are related to disease phenotype in MEN 2A and FMTC. Nat Genet. 1994;6(1):70–4.
36. Pausova Z, Soliman E, Amizuka N, et al. Role of the RET proto-oncogene in sporadic hyperparathyroidism and in hyperparathyroidism of multiple endocrine neoplasia type 2. J Clin Endocrinol Metab. 1996;81(7):2711–8.
37. Sakurai A, Katai M, Yumita W, Minemura K, Hashizume K. Clinical and genetic features of patients with multiple endocrine tumors who have neither family history nor MEN1 germline mutations. Endocrine. 2004;23(1):45–9.
38. Namihira H, Sato M, Matsubara S, et al. No evidence of germline mutation or somatic deletion of the MEN1 gene in a case of familial multiple endocrine neoplasia type 1 (MEN1). Endocr J. 1999;46(6):811–6.
39. Hai N, Aoki N, Shimatsu A, Mori T, Kosugi S. Clinical features of multiple endocrine neoplasia type 1 (MEN1) phenocopy without germline MEN1 gene mutations: analysis of 20 Japanese sporadic cases with MEN1. Clin Endocrinol (Oxf). 2000;52(4):509–18.
40. Ozawa A, Agarwal SK, Mateo CM, et al. The parathyroid/pituitary variant of MEN1 usually has causes other than p27Kip1 mutations. J Clin Endocrinol Metab. 2007;92:1948–51.
41. Fritz A, Walch A, Piotrowska K, et al. Recessive transmission of a multiple endocrine neoplasia syndrome in the rat. Cancer Res. 2002;62(11):3048–51.
42. Pellegata NS, Quintanilla-Martinez L, Siggelkow H, et al. Germ-line mutations in p27Kip1 cause a multiple endocrine neoplasia syndrome in rats and humans. Proc Natl Acad Sci USA. 2006;103(42):15558–63.
43. Sgambato A, Cittadini A, Faraglia B, Weinstein IB. Multiple functions of p27(Kip1) and its alterations in tumor cells: a review. J Cell Physiol. 2000;183(1):18–27.
44. Toyoshima H, Hunter T. p27, a novel inhibitor of G1 cyclin-Cdk protein kinase activity, is related to p21. Cell. 1994;78(1):67–74.

45. Buchwald PC, Akerstrom G, Westin G. Reduced p18INK4c, p21CIP1/WAF1 and p27KIP1 mRNA levels in tumours of primary and secondary hyperparathyroidism. Clin Endocrinol (Oxf). 2004;60(3):389–93.
46. Erickson LA, Jin L, Wollan P, Thompson GB, van Heerden JA, Lloyd RV. Parathyroid hyperplasia, adenomas, and carcinomas: differential expression of p27Kip1 protein. Am J Surg Pathol. 1999;23(3):288–95.
47. Georgitsi M, Raitila A, Karhu A, et al. Germline CDKN1B/p27Kip1 mutation in multiple endocrine neoplasia. J Clin Endocrinol Metab. 2007;92(8):3321–5.
48. Agarwal SK, Mateo CM, Marx SJ. Rare germline mutations in cyclin-dependent kinase inhibitor genes in multiple endocrine neoplasia type 1 and related states. J Clin Endocrinol Metab. 2009;94:1826–34.
49. Costa-Guda J, Marinoni I, Molatore S, Pellegata NS, Arnold A. Somatic mutation and germline sequence abnormalities of *CDKN1B*, encoding p27^{Kip1}, in sporadic parathyroid adenomas. J Clin Endocrinol Metab. 2011;96:E701–6.
50. Bjorklund P, Akerstrom G, Westin G. Accumulation of nonphosphorylated beta-catenin and c-myc in primary and uremic secondary hyperparathyroid tumors. J Clin Endocrinol Metab. 2007;92(1):338–44.
51. Ikeda S, Ishizaki Y, Shimizu Y, et al. Immunohistochemistry of cyclin D1 and beta-catenin, and mutational analysis of exon 3 of beta-catenin gene in parathyroid adenomas. Int J Oncol. 2002;20(3):463–6.
52. Bjorklund P, Lindberg D, Akerstrom G, Westin G. Stabilizing mutation of CTNNB1/beta-catenin and protein accumulation analyzed in a large series of parathyroid tumors of Swedish patients. Mol Cancer. 2008;7:53.
53. Costa-Guda J, Arnold A. Absence of stabilizing mutations of beta-catenin encoded by CTNNB1 exon 3 in a large series of sporadic parathyroid adenomas. J Clin Endocrinol Metab. 2007;92(4):1564–6.
54. Semba S, Kusumi R, Moriya T, Sasano H. Nuclear accumulation of B-Catenin in human endocrine tumors: association with Ki-67 (MIB-1) proliferative activity. Endocr Pathol. 2000;11(3):243–50.
55. Brown EM, Gamba G, Riccardi D, et al. Cloning and characterization of an extracellular Ca(2+)-sensing receptor from bovine parathyroid. Nature. 1993;366(6455):575–80.
56. Pollak MR, Brown EM, Chou YH, et al. Mutations in the human Ca(2+)-sensing receptor gene cause familial hypocalciuric hypercalcemia and neonatal severe hyperparathyroidism. Cell. 1993;75(7):1297–303.
57. Pearce SH, Trump D, Wooding C, et al. Calcium-sensing receptor mutations in familial benign hypercalcemia and neonatal hyperparathyroidism. J Clin Invest. 1995;96(6):2683–92.
58. Warner J, Epstein M, Sweet A, et al. Genetic testing in familial isolated hyperparathyroidism: unexpected results and their implications. J Med Genet. 2004;41(3):155–60.
59. Hosokawa Y, Pollak MR, Brown EM, Arnold A. Mutational analysis of the extracellular Ca(2+)-sensing receptor gene in human parathyroid tumors. J Clin Endocrinol Metab. 1995;80(11):3107–10.
60. Carpten JD, Robbins CM, Villablanca A, et al. HRPT2, encoding parafibromin, is mutated in hyperparathyroidism-jaw tumor syndrome. Nat Genet. 2002;32(4):676–80.
61. Simonds WF, Robbins CM, Agarwal SK, Hendy GN, Carpten JD, Marx SJ. Familial isolated hyperparathyroidism is rarely caused by germline mutation in HRPT2, the gene for the hyperparathyroidism-jaw tumor syndrome. J Clin Endocrinol Metab. 2004;89(1):96–102.
62. Shattuck TM, Valimaki S, Obara T, et al. Somatic and germ-line mutations of the HRPT2 gene in sporadic parathyroid carcinoma. N Engl J Med. 2003;349(18):1722–9.
63. Cetani F, Pardi E, Borsari S, et al. Genetic analyses of the HRPT2 gene in primary hyperparathyroidism: germline and somatic mutations in familial and sporadic parathyroid tumors. J Clin Endocrinol Metab. 2004;89(11):5583–91.
64. Howell VM, Haven CJ, Kahnoski K, et al. HRPT2 mutations are associated with malignancy in sporadic parathyroid tumours. J Med Genet. 2003;40(9):657–63.

65. Krebs LJ, Shattuck TM, Arnold A. HRPT2 mutational analysis of typical sporadic parathyroid adenomas. J Clin Endocrinol Metab. 2005;90(9):5015–7.
66. Rozenblatt-Rosen O, Hughes CM, Nannepaga SJ, et al. The parafibromin tumor suppressor protein is part of a human Paf1 complex. Mol Cell Biol. 2005;25(2):612–20.
67. Yart A, Gstaiger M, Wirbelauer C, et al. The HRPT2 tumor suppressor gene product parafibromin associates with human PAF1 and RNA polymerase II. Mol Cell Biol. 2005;25(12):5052–60.
68. Zhang C, Kong D, Tan MH, et al. Parafibromin inhibits cancer cell growth and causes G1 phase arrest. Biochem Biophys Res Commun. 2006;350(1):17–24.
69. Bradley KJ, Bowl MR, Williams SE, et al. Parafibromin is a nuclear protein with a functional monopartite nuclear localization signal. Oncogene. 2007;26(8):1213–21.
70. Hahn MA, Marsh DJ. Identification of a functional bipartite nuclear localization signal in the tumor suppressor parafibromin. Oncogene. 2005;24(41):6241–8.
71. Arnold A. Molecular basis of primary hyperparathyroidism. In: Bilezikian JP, Marcus R, Levine MA, editors. The parathyroids. 2nd ed. San Diego, CA: Academic; 2001. p. 331–47.
72. Palanisamy N, Imanishi Y, Rao PH, Tahara H, Chaganti RS, Arnold A. Novel chromosomal abnormalities identified by comparative genomic hybridization in parathyroid adenomas. J Clin Endocrinol Metab. 1998;83(5):1766–70.
73. Tahara H, Smith AP, Gas RD, Cryns VL, Arnold A. Genomic localization of novel candidate tumor suppressor gene loci in human parathyroid adenomas. Cancer Res. 1996;56(3):599–605.
74. Nussbaum SR, Gaz RD, Arnold A. Hypercalcemia and ectopic secretion of parathyroid hormone by an ovarian carcinoma with rearrangement of the gene for parathyroid hormone. N Engl J Med. 1990;323(19):1324–8.
75. VanHouten JN, Yu N, Rimm D, et al. Hypercalcemia of malignancy due to ectopic transactivation of the parathyroid hormone gene. J Clin Endocrinol Metab. 2006;91(2):580–3.

Chapter 17
Cost-Effectiveness of Parathyroidectomy for Primary Hyperparathyroidism

Kyle Zanocco and Cord Sturgeon

Keywords Cost-effectiveness in primary hyperparathyroidism • Surgery vs. medical follow-up decision analysis • Treatment modality and quality of life outcome • Age variability and cost-effectiveness in treatment strategies

What is Cost-Effectiveness Analysis?

Cost-effectiveness analysis (CEA) is a method to assess the outcomes of various treatment options when the costs incurred and the subsequent changes in the quality of life (QOL) are known. Guidelines for formal CEA were outlined by the Panel on Cost-Effectiveness in Health and Medicine in 1996 [1]. Many studies in the literature claim to evaluate cost-effectiveness, but often they fail to conform to these guidelines and are therefore not considered formal analyses. Formal CEA looks at a problem not by the charges incurred, but by the actual costs. CEA can be performed from any of several perspectives: for example, the hospital, the patient, the society, or the third-party payer. CEA can be used to compare the effects of two or more competing strategies to determine which one is less costly and/or more effective. CEA asks the question, "How much does it cost to save 1 year of healthy life?" Comparisons between two or more interventions are expressed as incremental cost-effectiveness ratios (ICERs) and the units are dollars per quality-adjusted life year (QALY). Sensitivity analysis is performed to determine the level of uncertainty of the results. Each variable can be changed either individually or simultaneously to determine the cumulative impact of errors on the final conclusion. CEA is not a substitute for head-to-head analyses of competing treatment regimens in prospective trials, nor is it designed to make treatment decisions for individual patients.

K. Zanocco, MD • C. Sturgeon, MD (✉)
Section of Endocrine Surgery, Department of Surgery, Northwestern University Feinberg
School of Medicine, 676 North Saint Clair Street, Suite 650, Chicago, IL 60611, USA
e-mail: csturgeo@nmh.org

A.A. Khan and O.H. Clark (eds.), *Handbook of Parathyroid Diseases:*
A Case-Based Practical Guide, DOI 10.1007/978-1-4614-2164-1_17,
© Springer Science+Business Media, LLC 2012

Literature Review Methods

The PubMed and Embase databases were queried with the keywords "primary hyperparathyroidism" and "cost effectiveness." The search was limited to publications between January 1996 and November 2008. Thirty nine articles were retrieved from the Pubmed database and 44 from Embase. Results were cross referenced and 59 unique articles were identified. Abstracts were reviewed for relevance. Pertinent articles are reviewed herein.

CEA in Asymptomatic Primary Hyperparathyroidism

There are very few formal CEA on asymptomatic primary hyperparathyroidism published in the English language literature. Only three formal studies are available to date that compare surgical vs. nonsurgical treatments and meet the methodological standards to be considered formal analyses (Table 17.1):

- Sejean et al. Surgery vs. medical follow-up in patients with asymptomatic primary hyperparathyroidism: a decision analysis [2].
- Zanocco et al. Cost-effectiveness analysis of parathyroidectomy for asymptomatic primary hyperparathyroidism [3].
- Zanocco et al. How should age at diagnosis impact treatment strategy in asymptomatic primary hyperparathyroidism? A cost-effectiveness analysis [4].

The competing strategies evaluated in these three studies were observation, parathyroidectomy, and pharmacologic therapy for hypercalcemia. In each study, the strategy of medical monitoring was found to be less effective than surgery. Surgery was found to be less costly and more effective than pharmacologic therapy. Minimally invasive surgery was more cost-effective than traditional surgical approaches.

Sejean et al. compared bilateral neck exploration, unilateral neck exploration, video-assisted parathyroidectomy, and monitoring. The base case scenario was a 55-year-old woman with asymptomatic sporadic primary hyperparathyroidism and the time horizon was the remaining life expectancy. Crossover from monitoring to surgery for progression of disease was modeled. Complications from surgery considered in the model included hematoma, vocal cord paralysis, death, persistent hyperparathyroidism, postoperative hypocalcemia, and sternotomy. Costs were calculated from the perspective of the healthcare delivery system. Included in the analysis were costs incurred from imaging, specialist consultation, surgery, and labwork. The costs of pharmacologic therapy for hypercalcemia were not included in this study. All surgical patients underwent yearly lifelong medical follow-up. Quality of life (QOL) indices were calculated through a survey of healthy volunteers using the time trade-off method. QOL outcomes were adjusted based on probability of complications and cure of hyperparathyroidism. The authors found that monitoring was less costly, but less effective than surgery. Both minimally invasive strategies were more effective than bilateral neck exploration or monitoring, although slightly more

Table 17.1 Cost-effectiveness of different treatment strategies for asymptomatic primary hyperparathyroidism

Strategy	Patient Age	Cost	Effectiveness	Incr C/E (ICER[a])	References
Observation	60	$4,209[b]	15.766[c]	–	Zanocco et al. [3]
Parathyroidectomy	60	$4,986[b]	15.929[c]	4,778[d]	Zanocco et al. [3]
Pharmacologic treatment (cinacalcet)	60	$181,083[b]	15.937[c]	20,995,772[d]	Zanocco et al. [3]
Medical followup and bilateral neck exploration for disease progression	55	€2,538[e]	15.7469[c]	–	Sejean et al. [2]
Medical followup and unilateral neck exploration for disease progression	55	€2,563[e]	15.7543[c]	3,378[f]	Sejean et al. [2]
Bilateral neck exploration	55	€3,537[e]	17.0329[c]	762[f]	Sejean et al. [2]
Unilateral neck exploration	55	€3,766[e]	17.118[c]	2,688[f]	Sejean et al. [2]
Video-assisted parathyroidectomy	55	€3,835[e]	17.1221[c]	17,250[f]	Sejean et al. [2]

[a]Incremental cost-effectiveness ratio
[b]2005 US dollars
[c]Quality-adjusted life years
[d]Dollars per quality-adjusted life years
[e]2002 Euros
[f]Euros per quality-adjusted life years

costly due to the cost of localization studies. The ICERs for surgical therapy were all considered within the cost-effective range. Sensitivity analysis found that surgery remained more effective than monitoring when the age used in the base-case scenario was varied between 40 and 80 years old.

Zanocco et al. compared monitoring, pharmacologic therapy (i.e., calcimimetics, bisphosphonates, calcitonin, etc.), and parathyroidectomy for sporadic asymptomatic primary hyperparathyroidism. The model's reference case scenario was a 60-year-old patient with no prior neck surgery who did not meet the 2002 criteria [5] for parathyroidectomy and had no contraindication to surgery. The time horizon for the analysis was the patient's remaining life expectancy. Crossover between monitoring, surgery, and pharmacologic therapy was modeled, as well as multiple operations. Complications considered in the model included persistent hyperparathyroidism, unilateral permanent recurrent laryngeal nerve (RLN) damage and permanent hypoparathyroidism. Extremely low frequency events, such as death, sternotomy, and bilateral RLN damage, were not modeled. The long-term effects of transient complications, such as hematoma, infection, temporary dysphonia, and temporary hypocalcemia were not modeled. Treatment outcomes, their probabilities, and costs were identified based on literature and cost database review. Costs were estimated from the third-party payer perspective. Cost included sestamibi scintigraphy and ultrasonography for all patients. The costs incurred by additional operations for persistent hyperparathyroidism, procedures to medialize a paralyzed vocal cord, and lifelong calcium and calcitriol for permanent hypoparathyroidism were also included in the model. Outcomes were weighted using published QOL utility factors from surveys conducted on patients with asymptomatic primary hyperparathyroidism. Sensitivity analysis was used to examine the uncertainty of costs and utility estimates in the model. The authors found that monitoring was the least expensive but least effective option. Both inpatient and outpatient parathyroidectomy were cost-effective. Pharmacologic therapy was not cost-effective unless the annual cost was less than $221 (2005 US dollars). The ICER for cinacalcet, a calcimimetic, was greater than $20 million per QALY.

In a follow-up study, Zanocco et al. examined how age at diagnosis impacts treatment decisions in sporadic asymptomatic primary hyperparathyroidism. Once again, they compared monitoring, pharmacologic therapy, and parathyroidectomy for sporadic asymptomatic primary hyperparathyroidism. In the base-case scenario the age at diagnosis was varied. Treatment outcomes, their probabilities, and costs were the same as in the earlier study. Threshold analysis identified the optimal treatment strategy for patients with remaining life expectancies ranging from 6 months to 75 years. Multivariate sensitivity analysis was performed with Monte Carlo simulation. The authors found that parathyroidectomy was cost-effective for patients with a predicted life-expectancy of 5 years (outpatient parathyroidectomy) or 6.5 years (inpatient parathyroidectomy). For patients with a shorter life expectancy, observation was the most cost-effective strategy. Pharmacologic therapy was not found to be cost-effective at any age modeled.

In the above studies, the cost-effectiveness of the different treatment strategies was affected by the time horizon evaluated by the study. When a treatment strategy is evaluated over a short time horizon, such as a few months or years, interventions with a lower daily cost (such as pharmacologic therapy) will appear to be less costly than curative interventions with a large up-front cost (such as surgical therapy). When costs are examined and outcomes compared over a patient's lifetime, however, chronic (i.e., pharmacologic) therapy will almost always be more costly.

In summary, monitoring is the least costly, but least effective option. Surgery was more costly, but more effective than observation, and was considered to be cost-effective, even for patients with a relatively short life expectancy. Pharmacologic therapy had an unacceptably high ICER (i.e., >$50,000/QALY) when compared to surgery, and was not found to be cost-effective.

CEA in Symptomatic Primary Hyperparathyroidism

There is no debate in the medical or surgical community that parathyroidectomy is the preferred treatment for patients with symptomatic primary hyperparathyroidism. For those patients who are unwilling or unable to undergo surgery, monitoring or targeted medical therapies are appropriate. Numerous studies have explored the cost-effectiveness of various surgical approaches, intraoperative or preoperative localization studies, and other surgical adjuncts. The authors are not aware of any formal cost-effectiveness analyses specifically comparing surgery with observation or medical therapy for patients with symptomatic primary hyperparathyroidism.

Conclusions

Only three formal cost-effectiveness analyses were identified in the PubMed and Embase databases that compare surgery with observation or pharmacologic therapy for asymptomatic primary hyperparathyroidism. No studies were identified comparing these three treatment options for patients with symptomatic primary hyperparathyroidism. By modeling asymptomatic disease over a variety of age ranges, surgery was found to be the most costly but most effective treatment option with an ICER that was well within the acceptable range to declare cost-effectiveness. These data cannot be directly extrapolated to symptomatic disease, but a surgical strategy should demonstrate an even higher utility in patients with overt symptomatology affecting their quality of life.

References

1. Gold MR. Cost-effectiveness in health and medicine. New York: Oxford University Press; 1996.
2. Sejean K, Calmus S, Durand-Zaleski I, et al. Surgery versus medical follow-up in patients with asymptomatic primary hyperparathyroidism: a decision analysis. Eur J Endocrinol. 2005; 153(6):915–27.

3. Zanocco K, Angelos P, Sturgeon C. Cost-effectiveness analysis of parathyroidectomy for asymptomatic primary hyperparathyroidism. Surgery. 2006;140(6):874–81. discussion 881–2.
4. Zanocco K, Sturgeon C. How should age at diagnosis impact treatment strategy in asymptomatic primary hyperparathyroidism? A cost-effectiveness analysis. Surgery. 2008;144(2):290–8.
5. Bilezikian JP, Potts Jr JT, Fuleihan Gel H, et al. Summary statement from a workshop on asymptomatic primary hyperparathyroidism: a perspective for the 21st century. J Clin Endocrinol Metab. 2002;87(12):5353–61.

Index

A.A. Khan and O.H. Clark (eds.), *Handbook of Parathyroid Diseases:*
A Case-Based Practical Guide, DOI 10.1007/978-1-4614-2164-1,
© Springer Science+Business Media, LLC 2012

Made in the USA
Monee, IL
07 July 2026

56551496R00178